Microbial Diseases

Notes, Reports, Summaries, Trends

Microbial Diseases
Notes, Reports, Summaries, Trends

Compiled by Carl W. May
Editor
The Biology Bookist

WILLIAM KAUFMANN, INC.
Los Altos, California

Preface

In any dynamic scientific field communication gaps exist between primary research workers and teachers, between current journal papers and reference tomes, and between research news reports and textbook examples. Thus it is no surprise that this situation also exists in the general realm of pathogenic microbiology and infectious disease. Here, as elsewhere, the time required for the synthesis, writing, production, and eventual revision of standard texts and references usually adds up to a period of several years before the latest information about new or variant pathogens, diagnoses, and methods of treatment and prevention makes its way into the standard books.

This premier edition of *Microbial Diseases*—the first of a new series—is designed to help plug the information gap; it will do double duty as an inexpensive ancillary text for courses on medical microbiology and infectious disease and as a new shelf reference for office, library, or laboratory.

The material in *Microbial Diseases* is reproduced directly from *The Morbidity and Mortality Weekly Report*—better known as *MMWR*—which emanates from the Center for Disease Control, a branch of the U.S. Public Health Service in Atlanta, Georgia. Each issue of that unique publication contains tables of data on the incidence of specific notifiable diseases (most of which are organized by state and region in the United States) and on mortality in major U.S. cities. The data are the best available as of the week prior to the publication of *MMWR*. Surrounding the tables are articles that report outbreaks of various kinds of disease or summarize the status of one disease or another over a recent period. Every autumn an *MMWR Annual Summary* reviews data for the previous year and graphs trends over recent years for various notifiable and non-notifiable diseases. *Microbial Diseases* includes both selected articles from the weekly reports and items from the annual summary for 1978, and it is divided into major parts by type of pathogen and then subdivided into chapters on diseases.

Most articles in *MMWR* are, in their own succinct way, remarkable. An initial report on the outbreak of a disease typically presents case reports (including symptoms, diagnostic procedures, and treatment employed), epidemiological investigations, and public health measures; editorial notes place the outbreak in context and remind the reader of important information. All of this is done in a few pages of text and within a few weeks after the first events. Other types of articles include follow-ups on previous reports, current recommendations on vaccination, new developments and recommendations for diagnosis and treatment, international situations of potential significance to the U.S., and updated summaries and trends for various diseases based on recent data. All of these forms are well represented in *Microbial Diseases*.

A long-time editor of textbooks on microbiology, I find that my favorite pieces of writing from *MMWR* are the brief editorial notes that close most articles; in a few sentences these often say as much as entire pages of educational texts, and they serve to tie basic knowledge and terminology to the article at hand. (Some instructors may wish to have students read these notes first rather than last, as introductions to the specifics to follow.) Perhaps health practitioners will focus on the portions of the articles most relevant to their individual interests. Students, on the other hand, may appreciate most the current, real-world cases, which provide more stimulating examples than the less immediate ones in most texts.

A feature of *MMWR* that is not apparent in individual weekly issues and perhaps is best displayed in a compilation such as *Microbial Diseases* is the continuity among articles about a specific disease. These articles may have appeared weeks or months apart. For example, reasonably complete stories about a cholera outbreak in Louisiana, polio in an unimmunized Amish population, and laboratory-associated smallpox in England are achieved in Chapters 11, 22, and 31, respectively, offering a dimension of value to readers of *Microbial Diseases* beyond that obtained from individual articles. A few years ago this book would have covered the recognition of Legionnaire's disease; now, however, the proper function of Chapter 1 is to present ongoing development contributing to the increasing body of knowledge about this disease. New editions of *Microbial Diseases* will appear every two years, and it should be interesting to witness trains of information provided by *MMWR* over the longer run.

Material for *Microbial Diseases* was not chosen at random. Initial decisions were made to cover infectious diseases as broadly and with as much balance as possible. Articles superseded by more recent articles, case reports with nothing new or different to say, and other types of redundant information were instant candidates for culling. Emphasis was placed on the more recent information, so almost all articles are taken from volumes 27 and 28 of *MMWR*, extending coverage through January 4, 1980. Where insufficient information precluded separate chapters for one disease or another, diseases were collected in more general chapters. (See Chapter 20 on "Various Nosocomial Infections" or Chapter 28 on "Hemorrhagic Fevers" as examples.) An attempt was made to correct as many errata as possible (there are remarkably few, considering the rapid publication schedule of *MMWR*), but no other rearrangement, abbreviation, or editing of articles was allowed. Because an occasional article covers more than one disease entity, information on a few diseases occurs outside its normal position. A case in point is the inclusion of malaria in the piece on "Health Status of Indochinese Refugees" in Chapter 2. Reference to the index should allow all information on various diseases and etiological agents to be easily located.

Initial selections were subjected to review by experienced professors in the health sciences. Though these critics sometimes disagreed, the process resulted in a substantial tightening of concept and organization. No clear-cut consensus was reached on the question of whether or not to include articles on vaccination, but a final decision was made to provide articles on new vaccines, procedures that have been changed in recent years, or vaccination against particularly widespread diseases. Following the wishes of several reviewers, most chapters progress from specific information on cases or outbreaks to articles and graphs of a more general and summary nature.

As compiler and editor, I am, of course, responsible for this work in its present form. *Microbial Diseases* is an experimental effort—the first of its kind among publications in microbiology and the health sciences, to the best of my knowledge. But I must pay homage here to the editors and contributing authors of *MMWR*. That consistently worthy publication is certainly one of the best uses of our tax dollars. I also want to thank Tyler Buchenau, formerly College Editor of W.B. Saunders Company, for my editorial training in scientific publishing and to express my gratitude to Dr. Arthur C. Giese of Stanford University for his selfless friendship and his encouragement of my various academic endeavors over the years. I thank the entire staff of William Kaufmann, Inc., well known for innovative publishing efforts, for its unfailing support and help.

Readers' comments and suggestions are invited and may be sent to me in care of the publisher. All comments received will be given careful consideration in the preparation of the next volume in this series.

Carl W. May

Acknowledgements

All material in this book was taken directly from *The Morbidity and Mortality Weekly Report*, which is published weekly by the U.S. Public Health Service's Center for Disease Control in Atlanta, Georgia. Over the entire period of more than two years that is represented here, the editor of *MMWR* was Michael B. Gregg, M.D., and the managing editor was Anne D. Mather, M.A.

Tentative selections for the volume were reviewed by several experienced practitioners and instructors representing a variety of perspectives on infectious disease. Although the final list of articles is entirely the responsibility of the editor, the reviewers had a profound, constructive effect on the organization and balance of selections. They were:

Thomas W. Huber
Houston Health Department Laboratory and
The University of Texas School of Public Health

Russell C. Johnson
Department of Microbiology
University of Minnesota Medical School

Lee Anne McGonagle
Department of Laboratory Medicine
University of Washington School of Medicine

Wesley A. Volk
Department of Microbiology
University of Virginia School of Medicine

Contents

Part I

Diseases Caused by Prokaryotes

CHAPTER 1

Legionnaire's Disease

MMWR 27:293 (8/11/78)

Identification of a New Serogroup of Legionnaires' Disease Bacterium

A new serogroup of Legionnaires' disease bacterium (LDB) has been identified by the Bureau of Laboratories, CDC.

A patient in Togus Veterans Administration Center, Maine, contracted atypical pneumonia on April 2, 1978, and died April 5. Twenty-two days following the onset of illness of this patient, a case of atypical pneumonia occurred in a second patient in the hospital. There was no known contact between the 2 patients. Acute and convalescent phase serum specimens (Togus acute and Togus convalescent) were obtained from the second patient. An LDB (Togus strain) isolated at CDC from a postmortem lung specimen of the first patient was found to be negative in direct fluorescent antibody (FA) staining tests with fluorescein isothiocyante (FITC) conjugates of antibodies prepared in rabbits against 16 other strains of LDB. Conversely, FITC conjugates of antibodies produced in rabbits against cells of the Togus strain stained Togus cells brightly and were negative with cells of the other 16 strains of LDB.

IFA staining titers were performed with the Togus acute and convalescent phase serum specimens using cells of the Philadelphia 1, Detroit, and Togus strains, LDB, as antigens. The convalescent serum specimen obtained from the Detroit-strain case served as the positive control serum. The greater than 4-fold rise in titer (1:32 to 1:256) to Philadelphia 1 antigen of the Togus serum from acute to convalescent phase was indicative of a recent infection with LDB. However, the rise in titer from 1:32 to 1:8,192 when the serum specimens were tested with the Togus antigen indicated that this patient had probably been infected with LDB of the Togus serogroup. Serogroup difference was also shown by the titer (1:128) of the Detroit control serum when it was tested with the Togus antigen; by contrast, the titer was 1:262,144 when tested with either Philadelphia 1 or Detroit antigen.

Reported by HE Lind, PhD, Public Health Laboratory, Maine State Dept of Human Services; Bacteriology Div, Pathology Div, and Virology Div, Bur of Laboratories, Bacterial Diseases Div, Bur of Epidemiology, CDC.

Editorial Note: Adequate screening or diagnostic direct FA staining of the currently recognized LDB groups requires the use of conjugates prepared against strains such as Philadelphia 1 and Togus group. The Togus strain of LDB should be considered in diagnostic procedures for LD based on immunologic reactions. Attempts are underway to identify other LDB strains with serologic characteristics of the Togus group.

MMWR 27:352 (9/15/78)

Legionnaires' Disease — New York, Tennessee

New York: Six confirmed and 118 suspected cases of Legionnaires' disease have recently been reported in workers in the garment district in New York City—an area from W. 34th Street to W. 39th Street between 5th and 9th Avenues.

Cases are defined as follows: *confirmed:* a 4-fold rise in reciprocal antibody titer to ⩾128 or positive direct fluorescent antibody test on lung tissue; and *suspected:* fever of 38.8 C (102 F) or pneumonia since August 1 in a person who works or lives in the garment district.

Two of the confirmed cases and 1 of the suspected cases were fatal. Dates of onset for confirmed cases range from August 11 to August 24, and for suspected cases from August 1 to September 9.

In an effort to evaluate whether this represents an outbreak, and if so, where it is localized, 4 populations are being surveyed for illness that meets the definition of a suspected case and for seroreactivity to the Legionnaires' disease bacterium. These include: 1) all 27 workers at Establishment A, where 1 of the patients with confirmed disease and 4 of those with suspected Legionnaires' disease were employed; 2) all workers in selected establishments throughout the garment district (approximately 500 workers); 3) a control group of approximately 300 garment workers outside the garment district; and 4) a control group of approximately 300 non-garment workers outside the garment district.

Preliminary results from the first population show that 4 out of 4 persons with illness meeting the case definition and 4 out of 13 completely well individuals at Establishment A had reciprocal titers ⩾256. This suggests that acute illness in that building is statistically associated with antibody titers to Legionnaires' disease (p=.03, Fisher's exact test). However, no association between antibody titer and illness that matches the definition of a suspected case has yet been found in the survey of other areas of the garment district. The overall prevalence of elevated titers (29% ⩾128) appears high in comparison to other populations which have been studied. The remaining survey results are pending.

Establishment A, where illness in workers is associated with elevated titers to Legionnaires' disease, occupies 2 stories within a much larger structure situated on the northern side of 35th Street. There is no evidence of increased illness or seroreactivity in other workers at the larger building. The ventilation systems are apparently separate; further environmental investigation of the site is underway.

Hospitals in New York City are being surveyed to determine if there has also been an increased number of cases of Legionnaires' disease outside the garment district.

Tennessee: Five confirmed cases of Legionnaires' disease, 1 of them fatal, have been diagnosed by the laboratory at Baptist Hospital, Memphis. Two occurred in hospital employees and 3 in patients with previous contact with the hospital. The dates of onset of cases were between August 14 and August 25. Inspection of infection-control surveillance records suggests an increased number of pneumonia cases from August 12 through September 7.

A flood occurred in portions of Memphis, including the hospital, on August 8; it inactivated several portions of the hospital's air-conditioning system for several weeks. Testing of environmental samples for the Legionnaires' disease bacterium is in progress. Investigations are currently underway by the hospital, local and state health departments, and CDC to evaluate cases of pneumonia at Baptist Hospital and at other hospitals in the Memphis area to define the situation.

Reported by Health and Hospitals Corporation of New York; JS Marr, MD, New York City Epidemi-

ologist, New York City Dept of Health; RP Kelly, MD, R Rendtorff, MD, Baptist Memorial Hospital, Memphis; J Levy, MD, G Lovejoy, MD, Memphis-Shelby County Health Dept; RH Hutcheson Jr, MD, State Epidemiologist, Tennessee Dept of Public Health; Field Services Div, Epidemic Investigations Laboratory Br, Hospital Infections Br, Special Pathogens Br, Bacterial Diseases Div, Bur of Epidemiology, CDC.

MMWR 27:365 (9/22/78)

Follow-up on Legionnaires' Disease — New York, Tennessee

To date, 8 confirmed and 136 suspected cases of Legionnaires' disease have been identified in workers in the New York City garment district since August 1, 1978. Data from survey control groups are under analysis.

In Tennessee, 7 confirmed and 3 presumptive cases of Legionnaires' disease have been identified to date by the laboratory of Baptist Memorial Hospital in Memphis and the Tennessee State Public Health Laboratory. Intensive surveillance efforts have revealed no new suspected cases with onset after September 12.

Reported by Health and Hospitals Corporation of New York; JS Marr, MD, New York City Epidemiologist, New York City Dept of Health; R Rendtorff, MD, Baptist Memorial Hospital, Memphis; J Levy, MD, G Lovejoy, MD, Memphis-Shelby County Health Dept; RH Hutcheson Jr, MD, State Epidemiologist, Tennessee Dept of Public Health; Field Services Div, Epidemiologic Investigations Laboratory Br, Hospital Infections Br, Special Pathogens Br, Bacterial Diseases Div, But of Epidemiology, CDC.

MMWR 27:368 (9/29/78)

Isolation of Organisms Resembling Legionnaires' Disease Bacterium — Tennessee

Organisms closely resembling the Legionnaires' disease bacterium (LDB) have been isolated from water from an auxiliary air conditioning cooling tower at Baptist Memorial Hospital in Memphis, Tennessee. Nine confirmed and 6 presumptive* cases of Legionnaires' disease (LD) with dates of onset from August 12 through September 1, 1978, have been identified either by the laboratory of that hospital or by the state public health laboratory. Prior to the isolation of the organism, a case-control study had found a significant association between cases and working or being a patient at the hospital during the 2 weeks before onset of illness.

The auxiliary air conditioning system was employed from August 8 to September 7 because a flood had inactivated the hospital's main air conditioning unit. The auxiliary cooling tower was sealed off with polyethylene sheeting on September 15, and its fan disconnected. Water in the tower has been sufficiently chlorinated to maintain free residual levels of greater than or equal to 3 parts per million.

The isolate, made by the Bacteriology Laboratory at the hospital, is pathogenic on passage to guinea pigs and embryonated eggs; grows on charcoal-yeast extract agar but not on conventional media; stains faintly gram-negative; resembles LDB in smears stained by the Gimenez method; and stains strongly in direct immunofluorescence testing using

---

*presumptive: X-ray evidence of pneumonia and indirect fluorescent antibody titer $\geq 1:256$

conjugated antiserum from rabbits immunized with LDB. A subculture submitted to CDC showed a pattern of cellular fatty acids on gas-liquid chromatography typical of the LDB. Further taxonomic studies at CDC are in progress.

Despite intensive surveillance, no case of suspected LD has been identified in the Memphis area with onset after September 16.

Reported by RT Kelly, MD, R Rendtorff, MD, WA Rightsel, PhD, Baptist Memorial Hospital, Memphis; J Levy, MD, G Lovejoy, MD, Memphis-Shelby County Health Dept; RH Hutcheson Jr, MD, State Epidemiologist, Tennessee Dept of Public Health; Bacteriology Div, Bur of Laboratories, Field Services Div, Epidemiologic Investigations Laboratory Br, Hospital Infections Br, Special Pathogens Br, Bacterial Diseases Div, Bur of Epidemiology, CDC.

Editorial Note: This represents the third isolation of organisms resembling the LDB from water from an air conditioning cooling tower at the site of an outbreak (1,2). In Pontiac and Memphis, there was a temporal correlation between the interval of cooling tower use and the occurrence of cases of LD. Possible explanations of this association may be that the cooling towers and cases were both exposed to airborne organisms from other sources; that LDB in the cooling tower water was a coincidental finding unrelated to these outbreaks; or that the organisms from the cooling towers were in fact responsible for some or all of the cases in the outbreaks. Although the temporal association in Memphis with the use of the auxiliary air conditioning system makes the third hypothesis appear the most plausible, outbreaks apparently spread by the airborne route have occurred in Washington, D.C. and Spain (3,4) that were not associated with cooling towers or air conditioning systems. Studies are in progress with cooling tower water from sites not associated with an outbreak to test the second hypothesis.

The ability of chlorine concentrations of 3 ppm to eliminate LDB from in-use cooling tower water, which is exposed to ultraviolet light, organic material, and aeration, has not been documented. Studies are in progress to define the need for decontaminating cooling towers and the best means for decontamination if it is indicated.

MMWR 27:415 (10/27/78)

Isolation of Organisms Resembling Legionnaires' Disease Bacterium — Georgia

Organisms resembling the Legionnaires' disease bacterium (LDB) have been isolated from water obtained from the evaporative condensor at a country club in Atlanta, Georgia, by intraperitoneal inoculation of guinea pigs. The organism shows typical appearance on F-G agar, is positive by direct immunofluorescence, and has a characteristic cellular fatty acid profile on gas chromatographic analysis. DNA relatedness studies are pending. From July 2-7, 1978, a cluster of 3 confirmed and 5 presumptive cases of Legionnaires' disease occurred among member golfers (1). The water sample was obtained on August 23. The output vent of the evaporative condensor faces the tenth tee of the golf course, approximately 150 feet away. Decontamination of the evaporative condensor has been attempted, and post-decontamination water samples are presently being tested for the bacterium.

Reported by WR Elsea, MD, Fulton County Dept of Health; J McCroan, PhD, State Epidemiologist, Georgia Dept of Human Resources; Bacteriology Div and Pathology Div, Bur of Laboratories, Bacterial Diseases Div, Bur of Epidemiology, CDC.

Editorial Note: This is the fourth isolation of an organism resembling LDB from a cooling tower or evaporative condensor at the site of an outbreak (2-4). Epidemiologic analysis indicates that the golfers may have been exposed to airborne LDB coming from the evaporative condensor. Laboratory evaluation of chemical agents that might be effective in decontamination or preventive maintenance of evaporative condensors and cooling towers has been initiated by CDC, in consultation with the Environmental Protection Agency and the American Society of Heating, Refrigeration and Air Conditioning Engineers.

References
1. MMWR 27:293, 1978
2. MMWR 27:283, 1978
3. MMWR 27:268, 1978
4. Glick TH, Gregg MB, Berman B, et al: Pontiac fever: An epidemic of unknown etiology in a health department: I. Clinical and epidemiologic aspects. Am J Epidemiol 107:149-160, 1978

MMWR 27:523 (1/5/79)

Legionnaires' Disease — Australia

Australia has reported its first confirmed case of Legionnaires' Disease (LD). The patient and a presumptive case were identified through a retrospective serologic survey conducted on 32 patients admitted with atypical pneumonia to Fairfield Hospital in Melbourne, Australia, in 1976 and 1977 and tested at CDC.

The confirmed case, documented by sequential reciprocal indirect immunofluorescent (IF) titers of 64 and 256 in specimens collected 14 days apart, was in a 46-year-old Australian man who died. The patient with presumptive LD, documented by a single reciprocal IF titer of 256, was a 56-year-old Spanish man who moved to Australia 13 years before the onset of illness. He had visited Spain 3 years before onset, but denied severe respiratory illness relating to that visit. He recovered after prolonged treatment for severe pneumonia. Neither patient responded to penicillin or chloramphenicol.

Reported by P Cavanagh, Fairfield Hospital, Melbourne, Australia; The World Health Organization in the Weekly Epidemiological Report, October 27, 1978; Bacteriology Div, Bur of Laboratories, Special Pathogens Br, Bacterial Diseases Div, Bur of Epidemiology, CDC.

Editorial Note: In addition to Australia, LD has now been reported from Canada, England, Israel, the Netherlands, Scotland, Sweden, and Denmark. A presumptive case of LD also has been identified in a 29-year-old man hospitalized in New South Wales, Australia, who had onset of illness in early April 1978. Investigation of suspected LD among Scottish travelers to Benidorm has suggested that *Legionella pneumophila,* the proposed name for the LD bacterium, may be acquired in Spain (1). The patient with presumptive LD reported here may well have been previously exposed to *L. pneumophila* in Spain or elsewhere prior to onset of pneumonia.

Reference
1. MMWR 26:344, 1977

MMWR 28:286 (6/22/79)

Preliminary Studies on Environmental Decontamination of *Legionella pneumophila*

Nine months ago, CDC, after consultation with the American Society of Heating, Refrigerating and Air-Conditioning Engineers (ASHRAE) and the Environmental Protection Agency (EPA), initiated studies to test the ability of chemicals in commercially available, EPA-registered biocides to inhibit growth of *Legionella pneumophila* in tap water. Such studies were indicated because of the isolation of *L. pneumophila* from water taken from cooling towers and evaporative condensers at the sites of outbreaks of legionellosis (Legionnaires' disease; Pontiac fever) and the implication of such air-conditioning units in the dissemination of the organism (1-3).

Preliminary data from the testing of 6 compounds—including a chlorinated phenol, a quaternary ammonium; an isothiazolin; a dithiocarbamate; 2, 2-dibromo-3-nitrilopropionamide; and calcium hypochlorite—are now available. Fixed concentrations of L. pneumophila were exposed in hypochlorite-free, sterile tap water to several concentrations of each compound; aliquots of the tap water were then inoculated at various time periods on artificial media and in yolk sacs of embryonated eggs for growth of L. pneumophila. A compound with 50% didecyl dimethyl ammonium chloride (a quaternary ammonium compound), 20% isopropanol, and 30% inert ingredients was effective at concentrations of 70, 140, and 630 ppm in preventing recovery of L. pneumophila from aliquots of water taken 3, 6, 24, and 168 hours after initial exposure. Calcium hypochlorite and 2, 2-dibromo-3-nitrilopropionamide also appeared effective, but testing is not complete. The other 3 compounds appeared to be less rapidly effective in inhibiting recovery of L. pneumophila in laboratory testing.

Reported by Epidemiologic Investigations Laboratory Br and Special Pathogens Br, Bacterial Diseases Div, Bur of Epidemiology, CDC.

Editorial Note: These studies identify certain commercially available water disinfectants that might be tested for their ability to decontaminate evaporative condensers and cooling towers implicated in the transmission of L. pneumophila. However, the efficacy of any such decontamination procedures in actually inhibiting growth of L. pneumophila in cooling tower or evaporative condenser water and preventing transmission of the organism remains to be demonstrated. Protocols are being designed to test the use of chemical disinfectants in decontaminating evaporative condensers and cooling towers implicated in dissemination of L. pneumophila in outbreaks.

These findings also do not address the problem of long-term preventive maintenance of evaporative condensers and cooling towers. Although CDC and ASHRAE advise that routine preventive maintenance measures may be effective in controlling slime, scale, algae, and bacterial growth in such air-conditioning units, they have no information about the utility of such procedures in preventing legionellosis.

References
1. MMWR 27:283, 1978
2. MMWR 27:368, 1978
3. Glick TH, Gregg MB, Berman B, Mallison G, Rhodes WW, Kassanoff I: Pontiac fever: An epidemic of unknown etiology in a health department. I. Clinical and epidemiologic aspects. Am J Epidemiol 107:149-160, 1978

MMWR 27:439 (11/10/78)

Legionnaires' Disease — United States

As of October 31, 1978, 453 sporadic cases of infection with the Legionnaires' disease bacterium (LDB) have been confirmed in the United States* by ≥4-fold rise in antibody titer to a reciprocal titer of ≥128, as measured by indirect immunofluorescence, demonstration of the organism in tissue by direct immunofluorescence, or culture of the organism. The earliest case had onset in May 1973.

_____

*As of November 7, 43 more sporadic cases have been reported that are not included in these analyses—2 from Oregon, and 41 from Michigan. Dates of onset in most cases are since January 1, 1978.

FIGURE 1. Sporadic cases of Legionnaires' disease,† by state, United States, May 1973 through October 1978

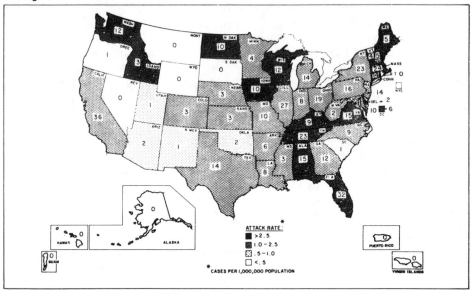

†Numbers within states indicate total reported cases per state.

These 453 cases, which are in addition to the confirmed outbreak-associated cases in Ohio, Vermont, Tennessee, California, Georgia, New York, Michigan, Indiana, Texas, Pennsylvania, and the District of Columbia, have occurred in 43 states and the District of Columbia. Outbreaks associated with apparent common exposure in Indiana and Texas each predominantly affected travelers from several states. The majority of sporadic cases have been in eastern and midwestern states (Figure 1). The geographic distribution of the 13 known outbreaks is similar.

The number of sporadic cases by month of onset of symptoms peaked in September 1977 and has averaged approximately 20 cases per month over the past year (Figure 2). The rising number of cases with onset from August 1976 to September 1977 is partly due to increased numbers of specimens being submitted in late 1977, when LD testing became widely available. The progressive decrease from September 1977 to a low in February 1978, and the progressive increase since then may indicate a true seasonality paralleling that demonstrated by outbreak cases (Figure 3).

Where the sex of the patient was known, the sporadic cases included 309 men and 128 women. The youngest patient was a 2-year-old boy; the oldest patient was an 84-year-old man. The median age for males is 54 years, for females 56 years. Death directly attributable to Legionnaires' disease (LD) has occurred in 86 (19%) of the sporadic cases in which the outcome was known. Among 244 cases in which race was known, 210 occurred in whites and 34 occurred in blacks.

Among 558 cases of LD associated with 10 outbreaks,* 412 were male and 146 were female. There were 70 deaths among these 558 cases, representing 14% of cases present-

---

*excluding 95 cases among 100 office workers in Pontiac, Michigan, and excluding outbreaks in Memphis, Tennessee; Texas; and California because data collection is ongoing.

FIGURE 2. Confirmed sporadic cases* of Legionnaires' disease, by month of onset, United States, August 1976 through October 1978

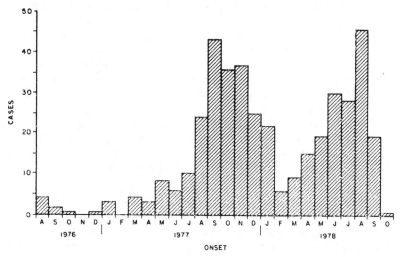

*453 cases, as of October 31, 1978; excludes 51 cases in which the month of onset is not known

FIGURE 3. Seasonal distribution of Legionnaires' disease outbreaks, by location, 1965 through 1978

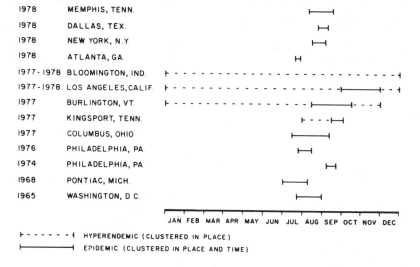

ing with pneumonia. The relatively large number of sporadic cases confirmed by direct immunofluorescence (a test that generally has been performed on autopsy material) may partly explain the higher case-fatality rate associated with sporadic cases.

Among sporadic cases in which death was directly attributable to LD, the median age was 56 years; among cases in which the sex was known, 59 were males and 19 were females. The case-fatality rate for men was 19%, for women 15%. There was no significant change in the case-fatality rate with increasing age.

As a result of investigations of outbreaks in Bloomington, Ind., Memphis, Tenn., and Atlanta, Ga., LDB has been isolated from water from 2 cooling towers, 2 evaporative condensers, and a creek.

Three hundred seventy-four cases have been confirmed by serology alone, 59 by direct immunofluorescence alone, 4 by culture alone, 8 by serology and direct immunofluorescence, 4 by culture and direct immunofluorescence, 1 by serology and culture, and 1 by all 3 methods. In 2 cases the method of diagnosis is unknown. Among 59 cases confirmed by direct immunofluorescence in which the sources of the specimens are known, 52 have been confirmed from lung specimens obtained by biopsy or autopsy alone, 2 from lung aspirates, 1 from a bronchoscopy specimen, 1 from pleural fluid alone, 1 from a transtracheal aspirate, 1 from sputum, and 1 from lung and pleural fluid specimens. Among 3 culture-confirmed cases in which the sources of the specimens are known, 1 has been confirmed from pleural fluid, 1 from lung, and 1 from pleural fluid and lung.

Reported by State Epidemiologists from 43 states and the District of Columbia; Virology Div, Bacteriology Div, Bur of Laboratories, and Bacterial Diseases Div, Bur of Epidemiology, CDC.

Editorial Note: In April 1978, the Conference of State and Territorial Epidemiologists agreed to make LD a reportable disease for 3 years. As specific testing is more widely used, LD is being diagnosed with increasing frequency. Serum specimens for diagnosis should include an acute-phase specimen drawn in the first week of illness and a convalescent-phase specimen drawn at least 22 days after onset of illness; another specimen drawn up to 6 weeks after onset may permit recognition of late seroconversion. Lung tissue specimens providing greatest yield in establishing the diagnosis of LD include the combination of fresh refrigerated or frozen tissue for culture and wet formalin-fixed tissue for direct immunofluorescence testing.

While the CDC has no new or specific recommendations on routine maintenance of cooling towers in relation to the presence of LDB, adherence to standard procedures for the control of algae and bacteria that may interfere with satisfactory mechanical operation is advised. Laboratory work to determine procedures for decontamination of air-conditioning systems is underway.

CHAPTER 2

Tuberculosis

MMWR 27:108 (3/31/78)

Bovine Tuberculosis — Maryland

Two cases of tuberculosis caused by *Mycobacterium bovis* were reported in Maryland in 1976.

The first case was a 29-year-old woman from India who was admitted to a hospital in June 1976 because of fever, cough, chest pain, and general malaise. A chest X-ray examination showed an infiltrate in the right upper lung area with possible cavitation. When sputum smears were reported positive for acid-fast bacilli, she was started on isoniazid (INH), ethambutol, and streptomycin. Subsequent culture results showed the infective organism to be *M. bovis.* She responded well to treatment, and the lesion seen on her chest X ray completely resolved. She had left India in 1971, worked in England for about 4 years, and arrived in the United States in 1975. Her chest X ray at the time of arrival in the United States was negative.

The second patient was a 41-year-old female who participated in a routine tuberculin skin-test screening program. She had a positive reaction (12 mm), and a follow-up chest X ray in September 1976 demonstrated soft infiltrates with cavitation in the right upper lung. Sputum smears were positive for acid-fast bacilli, and cultures were subsequently positive for *M. bovis.* The patient was asymptomatic. She responded well to therapy with rifampin and ethambutol. Born in Lebanon to native-born American parents, the patient had received BCG vaccination as a child. She had traveled throughout the world and had spent extensive time in India and Bangladesh. On 2 occasions after her diagnosis her husband and 2 children had negative tuberculin skin tests.

Reported by H Passes, MD, Montgomery County Health Dept; D Glasser, MD, Baltimore City Health Dept; Division of Laboratories, J Flynn, MD, MPH, KH Acree, MDCM, State Epidemiologist, Maryland Dept of Health and Mental Hygiene; Bacteriology Div, Bur of Laboratories, Tuberculosis Control Div, Bur of State Services, CDC.

Editorial Note: *M. bovis* is an infrequent cause of tuberculosis in the United States. Pasteurization of milk products and systematic testing and destruction of tuberculin-positive cattle have contributed to the virtual disappearance of this type of tuberculosis in this country. The cultures from these 2 patients, confirmed by CDC, were the only such isolations from Maryland received at CDC in the past 5 years. Including these 2 cases, the CDC laboratory has identified *M. bovis* organisms in cultures from only 28 patients residing in 13 different states from July 1, 1972 to December 31, 1977.

M. bovis can be transmitted between animals, between animals and humans, and between humans. Tuberculosis caused by *M. bovis* is treated the same way as that caused by *M. tuberculosis*. Contact examination for cases of bovine tuberculosis should include both human and animal contacts. When indicated, INH can be used for preventive therapy in human contacts.

Because the disease in cattle has not been controlled in many other parts of the world, it is noteworthy that both of these patients were born outside of the United States and spent a considerable amount of time abroad. In addition to such cases of foreign acquisition, cases may occur in older people in the United States who may have been infected in this country many years ago.

MMWR 27:355 (9/22/78)

Follow-up on Drug-Resistant Tuberculosis — Mississippi

On December 23, 1977, an outbreak of drug-resistant tuberculosis was described in a rural northern Mississippi county (1). Since then 5 more cases of tuberculosis due to organisms with confirmed primary resistance to isoniazid, para-aminosalicylic acid, and streptomycin (INH-PAS-SM) have been reported. This brings the total of such cases in the county to 19 since 1964.

Three of 5 new cases are known to be epidemiologically linked to cases previously reported with INH-PAS-SM resistance in the county. All 19 patients known to have this drug-resistant disease have been placed on alternative drug regimens, and all but one have had a good response. One patient was started on therapy but relapsed because of poor compliance. She is currently hospitalized in Illinois. Her 2-year-old son has been clinically diagnosed as having tuberculosis with negative bacteriology.

Two of the 5 newly confirmed cases due to drug-resistant organisms occurred in 1 household. The first was in a 17-year-old woman who was a sophomore in the same high school as were some of the other patients previously reported (1). She did not receive a tuberculin test during the attempts to complete the school screening in 1976 because she had dropped out of school. However, her private physician has reported that she had a normal chest X ray in September 1976. This patient was admitted to a local hospital in late March 1978 with cavitary tuberculosis, bacteriologically confirmed, due to organisms resistant to INH-PAS-SM. The second such case in this household was in this patient's 10-month-old daughter.

During the evaluation of the 17-year-old's 21 other close contacts, 4 more cases were discovered. Since organisms were not recovered, a drug-resistance pattern could not be determined. However, all the patients were placed on INH, ethambutol, and rifampin. These 4 cases were the mother of the 17-year-old, age 42, who had been tuberculin-negative in October 1977 but had an 18-mm reaction to tuberculin, PPD, with an abnormal X ray on April 10, 1978; a 4- year-old sister, who converted (11 mm) and had an abnormal X ray; a 22-month-old nephew, who had an 18-mm reaction with an abnormal X ray; and a 33-year-old uncle, who had a 6-mm reaction with an abnormal X ray. Of the 17 remaining contacts, 11 were tuberculin-positive (9 of these were placed on INH preventive therapy), and 6 were tuberculin-negative (one was placed on INH preventive therapy).

Of the 19 cases of drug-resistant tuberculosis reported in this county, 4 occurred since 1976 in individuals who had received INH as preventive therapy. Records show that 3 of the 4 persons took INH irregularly; the fourth patient had taken 10 months of INH medication over a 12-month period. However, it is possible that this person had not been infected with *Mycobacterium tuberculosis* at the time he received INH, since his tuberculin test results were questionable (5-mm reaction to tuberculin, PPD).

Reported by DL Blakey, MD, State Epidemiologist, Mississippi Board of Health; IE Imm, State Epidemiologist, Wisconsin Dept of Health and Social Services; EA Piszczek, MD, MPH, Suburban Cook County Tuberculosis Sanitorium District; BJ Francis, MD, MPH, State Epidemiologist, AB Grant, Illinois Dept of Public Health; Tuberculosis Control Div, Bur of State Services, Field Services Div, Bur of Epidemiology, CDC.

Editorial Note: Although transmission of drug-resistant tuberculosis in families and households has been previously documented (2), this outbreak of tuberculosis is unusual because it is the first documented community outbreak of drug-resistant tuberculosis. Also unusual is the fact that this strain exhibits considerable catalase activity. The catalase activity of INH-resistant strains is usually absent or weak, and such strains demonstrate diminished virulence in laboratory animals. The fact that these organisms have retained their catalase activity may explain their apparent virulence. Officials from the Mississippi State Board of Health and CDC are conducting ongoing surveillance and containment activities for this outbreak. Special long-term follow-up activities are being initiated for cases and contacts thought to be infected with this drug-resistant strain. Additional screening activities are being planned in September for schools in the outbreak area. These will be followed by selected community screening activities designed to assess transmission and to uncover any possible remaining foci of drug-resistant disease.

Patients from Mississippi with disease due to organisms resistant to INH-PAS-SM have traveled to Tennessee, Wisconsin, and Illinois. Epidemiologic investigations in these states have not uncovered any additional cases of bacteriologically confirmed disease related to the Mississippi outbreak. Because of the possibility of interstate transmission, it is recommended that health departments carefully assess any case of tuberculosis due to organisms resistant to INH-PAS-SM to determine if any link to the Mississippi outbreak can be established (especially in persons never previously treated with INH-PAS-SM).

On July 31 and August 1, experts in the fields of tuberculosis, infectious disease, public health, and medical ethics reviewed the management of the Mississippi outbreak. They agreed that, since there is no known effective preventive treatment under these circumstances, prolonged careful follow-up of infected contacts is indicated regardless of what preventive measures might be taken. Recognizing that there were several options from which to choose, including INH preventive treatment (the option which had been chosen in Mississippi), they generally concurred that the CDC plan of action be continued in Mississippi, but that other options be considered in similar future episodes. CDC is now in the process of preparing a summary of the expert opinions and will issue recommendations on the management of contacts to INH-resistant tuberculosis.

References
1. MMWR 26:417-418, 1977
2. Steiner M, Chaves AD, Lyons HA, Steiner P, Portugaleza C: Primary drug-resistant tuberculosis: Report of an outbreak. N Engl J Med 283:1353-1358, 1970

MMWR 28:241 (6/1/79)

BCG Vaccines

INTRODUCTION

Tuberculosis cases and deaths in the United States have declined steadily since reporting began in the 19th century. In 1977 there were approximately 30,000 reported cases and 3,000 deaths, for rates of 13.9 (cases) and 1.4 (deaths) per 100,000 population. These rates are 40% and 60% lower than the corresponding rates for 1967. The rate of infection, judged by the prevalence of positive tuberculin skin tests, has also declined, particularly for susceptible groups, such as young children. The prevalence of positive reactors among children entering school is now estimated to be 0.2%, and among adolescents, 0.7%. The current annual infection rate is estimated to be 0.03%, based on the prevalence among 6-year-olds.

The incidence of tuberculosis cases varies broadly among different segments of the population and in different localities. Cases occur twice as frequently in males as in females. Rates increase sharply with age in both sexes and all races. More than 80% of reported cases are in persons over 25 years of age, most of whom were infected several years previously. Reported cases are generally typical post-primary pulmonary disease. The risk of infection is greatest for those who have repeated exposure to persons with unrecognized or untreated sputum-positive pulmonary tuberculosis. Chemotherapy rapidly reduces the infectivity of cases.

Efforts to control tuberculosis in the United States are directed toward the early identification and treatment of cases and preventive therapy with isoniazid for infected persons at high risk of developing disease. In this country, vaccine prepared from the Bacillus of Calmette and Guérin (BCG) has been used mainly for selected groups of uninfected persons who live or work where they have an unavoidable risk of exposure to tuberculosis.

BCG VACCINES

BCG was derived from a strain of *Mycobacterium bovis* attenuated through years of serial passage in culture by Calmette and Guérin at the Pasteur Institute, Lille, France. It was first administered to humans in 1921.

There are many BCG vaccines* available in the world today; all are derived from the original strain, but they vary in immunogenicity, efficacy, and reactogenicity. Variation probably has been the result of genetic changes in the bacterial strains; differences in

---

*Official name: BCG Vaccine.

techniques of production; methods and routes of vaccine administration; and characteristics of the populations and environments in which vaccine has been studied. Controlled trials—all conducted prior to 1955—of liquid vaccines prepared from different BCG strains showed protection ranging from 0 to 80%.

The vaccines now available in the United States differ from products used in the field trials in that additional culture passages have since taken place, and there have been various modifications in methods of preparation and preservation. The efficacy of these current vaccines has not been demonstrated directly and can only be inferred.

Production standards for BCG vaccines (Bureau of Biologics, Food and Drug Administration) specify that they be freeze-dried products containing live bacteria from a documented strain of the Bacillus of Calmette and Guérin. The strain must demonstrate various specified characteristics of safety and potency and be capable of inducing tuberculin sensitivity in guinea pigs and humans. (The assumed relationship between sensitivity and immunity has not been proven.)

Freeze-dried vaccine should be reconstituted, protected from exposure to light, and used within 8 hours.

VACCINE USAGE

General Recommendations

Modern methods of case detection, chemotherapy, and preventive treatment can be highly successful in controlling tuberculosis. Nevertheless, an effective BCG vaccine may be useful under certain circumstances. In particular, BCG may benefit uninfected persons with repeated exposure to infective cases who cannot or will not obtain or accept treatment.

Recommended Vaccine Recipients

1. BCG vaccination should be seriously considered for individuals, such as infants in a household, who are tuberculin skin-test negative (1) but who have repeated exposure to persistently untreated or ineffectively treated patients with sputum-positive pulmonary tuberculosis.

2. BCG vaccination should be considered for groups in which an excessive rate of new infections can be demonstrated and the usual surveillance and treatment programs have failed or are not feasible. Such groups might exist among those without a regular source of health care.

Adequate surveillance and control measures should be possible to protect groups such as health workers (2). However, some health workers may be at increased risk of repeated exposure, especially those working in institutions serving major urban population centers in which the endemic prevalence of tuberculosis is relatively high. BCG vaccine should be considered when the frequency of skin-test conversion representing new infections (3) exceeds 1% annually.

Schedule

BCG should be reserved for persons who are skin-test negative to 5 TU* of tuberculin, PPD.† Those who receive BCG should have a tuberculin skin test 2-3 months later. If that skin test is negative and the indications for BCG remain, a second dose of vaccine should be given. Dosage is indicated by the manufacturer in the package labeling; one-half of the usual dose should be given to persons under 28 days old. If the indications

---

*Tuberculin unit.
†Purified protein derivative of tuberculin.

for immunization persist, these children should receive a full dose after attaining 1 year of age.

Administration Technique

The World Health Organization recommends that BCG be given by the intradermal route in order to provide a uniform and reliable dose. In the United States, however, vaccines for intradermal and for percutaneous administration are licensed, and vaccination should be only by the route indicated in the package labeling.

RISKS AND SIDE EFFECTS

BCG vaccine has been associated with adverse reactions including severe or prolonged ulceration at the vaccination site, lymphadenitis, and—very rarely—osteomyelitis, lupoid reactions, disseminated BCG infection, and death. Available data on adverse reactions do not necessarily pertain to the vaccines currently licensed in the United States, and the reported frequency of complications has varied greatly, depending in part on the extent of the surveillance effort. For example, the frequency of ulceration and lymphadenitis has been reported to range from 1% to 10%, depending on the vaccine, the dosage, and the age of vaccinees. Osteomyelitis has been reported to occur in 1 per 1,000,000 vaccinees, although limited information indicates that with newborns it may be higher. Disseminated BCG infection and death are very rare (1-10 per 10,000,000 vaccinees) and occur almost exclusively in children with impaired immune responses.

PRECAUTIONS AND CONTRAINDICATIONS

Altered Immune States

BCG for prevention of tuberculosis should not be given to persons with impaired immune responses such as occur with congenital immunodeficiency, leukemia, lymphoma, or generalized malignancy, and when immunologic responses have been suppressed with steroids, alkylating agents, antimetabolites, or radiation.

Pregnancy

Although no harmful effects of BCG on the fetus have been observed, it is prudent to avoid vaccination during pregnancy unless there is an immediate excessive risk of unavoidable exposure to infective tuberculosis.

Interpretation of Tuberculin Test

After BCG vaccination, it is usually not possible to distinguish between a tuberculin reaction caused by virulent supra-infection and one resulting from persistent postvaccination sensitivity. Therefore, caution is advised in attributing a positive skin test to BCG (except in the immediate postvaccination period), especially if the vaccinee has recently been exposed to infective tuberculosis.

Tuberculosis in Vaccinated Persons

Since full, lasting protection from BCG vaccination cannot be assured, tuberculosis should be included in the differential diagnosis of any tuberculosis-like illness in a BCG vaccinee.

SURVEILLANCE

All suspected adverse reactions to BCG should be carefully investigated and reported to health authorities. These reactions occasionally occur as long as a year or more after vaccination.

References
1. American Lung Association: Diagnostic standards and classification of tuberculosis and other mycobacterial diseases. New York, American Lung Association, 1974
2. CDC: Guidelines for Prevention of TB Transmission in Hospitals (HEW Pub. No. [CDC] 79-8371). Atlanta, CDC, Jan 1979
3. Thompson N, Glassroth JL, Snider D, Farer LS: The booster phenomenon in serial tuberculin testing. Am Rev Respir Dis 119:587-597, 1979

SELECTED BIBLIOGRAPHY

CDC: Tuberculosis in the United States 1977 (HEW Pub. No. [CDC] 79-8322). Atlanta, CDC, Mar 1979

Eickhoff TC: The current status of BCG immunization against tuberculosis. Annu Rev Med 28:411-423, 1977

National Institutes of Health: Status of Immunization in Tuberculosis in 1971: Report of a Conference on Progress to Date, Future Trends, and Research Needs (HEW Pub. No. [NIH] 72-68). Washington, Government Printing Office, 1972

Rouillon A, Waaler H: BCG vaccination and epidemiological situation: A decision making approach to the use of BCG. Adv Tuberc Res 19:64-126, 1976

World Health Organization: Ninth Report of the Expert Committee on Tuberculosis (WHO Tech Rep No. 552). Geneva, WHO, 1974

MMWR 28:313 (7/13/79)

Tuberculosis — United States, 1978

In 1978, 28,521 cases of tuberculosis were reported to CDC, for a case rate of 13.1 per 100,000. This represents a decrease, since 1977, of 5.4% in the number of cases reported and of 5.8% in the case rate (Table 1). Case rates for the 50 states in 1978 ranged from 32.3 per 100,000 in Hawaii to 1.9 per 100,000 in Nebraska. Case rates decreased in 34 states and the District of Columbia. The percent decrease ranged from 2.3% in Idaho to 50.5% in Hawaii. However, case rates increased in 15 states. The percent increase ranged from 1.5% in Florida to 43.6% in Wisconsin.

Tuberculosis case rates continued to be higher in areas with large Black, Asian, American Indian, and Hispanic populations (Figure 1) and in urban areas. The case rate of persons living in cities of 250,000 or more was 22.5 per 100,000—1.7 times the national case rate. Urban rates ranged from 50.4 per 100,000 in San Francisco, California, to 2.4 per 100,000 in Douglas County (Omaha), Nebraska. In 1978, the case rate increased in 21 (38%) of the country's 56 largest cities.

Reported by Tuberculosis Control Div, Bur of State Services, CDC.

Editorial Note: The observed decreases in cases and in the case rate in 1978 are more consistent with the progressive decline in the incidence of tuberculosis over the last 25 years than the earlier predictions for 1978 based on preliminary figures (1). However, 36.5% of the decrease in cases is attributable to Hawaii and New York City, both of which established more stringent criteria for case reporting in 1978. The marked increase in Wisconsin is thought to have been caused, in part, by improved surveillance.

Tuberculosis remains an important public health problem in spite of an impressive decline in national incidence during this century. Pockets with persistently high case rates remain in areas with large numbers of socioeconomically deprived persons or immigrants from high-prevalence areas such as Asia, Africa, and Latin America. Groups of these persons often congregate in urban areas, accounting in large part for the high rates observed in major cities.

Reference
1. MMWR 28:57, 1979

TABLE 1. Tuberculosis cases and case rates, by state, 1978 and 1977

State	Tuberculosis cases		Case rate		Rank according to rate	
	1978	1977	1978	1977	1978	1977
United States	28,521	30,145	13.1	13.9	–	–
Alabama	672	704	18.0	19.1	10	9
Alaska	94	92	23.3	22.5	2	2
Arizona	406	358	17.2	15.6	11	17
Arkansas	417	392	19.1	18.3	7	11
California	3,351	3,465	15.0	15.8	16	15
Colorado	143	149	5.4	5.7	41	41
Connecticut	186	247	6.0	7.9	39	35
Delaware	58	67	9.9	11.5	30	24
District of Columbia*	314	342	46.6	49.6	–	–
Florida	1,724	1,674	20.1	19.8	4	7
Georgia	876	916	17.2	18.1	12	12
Hawaii	290	584	32.3	65.3	1	1
Idaho	38	38	4.3	4.4	45	45
Illinois	1,645	1,727	14.6	15.4	17	18
Indiana	544	560	10.1	10.5	28	28
Iowa	103	99	3.6	3.4	46	47
Kansas	116	153	4.9	6.6	43	40
Kentucky	649	719	18.6	20.8	8	4
Louisiana	648	615	16.3	15.7	15	16
Maine	70	82	6.4	7.6	38	38
Maryland	755	827	18.2	20.0	9	6
Massachusetts	580	647	10.0	11.2	29	25
Michigan	1,260	1,290	13.7	14.1	19	20
Minnesota	175	211	4.4	5.3	44	42
Mississippi	549	460	22.8	19.3	3	8
Missouri	456	497	9.4	10.4	31	30
Montana	58	68	7.4	8.9	37	32
Nebraska	30	42	1.9	2.7	50	49
Nevada	73	58	11.1	9.2	25	31
New Hampshire	21	22	2.4	2.6	49	50
New Jersey	1,003	1,162	13.7	15.9	20	14
New Mexico	149	152	12.3	12.8	21	23
New York	2,060	2,434	11.6	13.6	24	21
North Carolina	943	1,042	16.9	18.9	13	10
North Dakota	33	32	5.1	4.9	42	44
Ohio	890	845	8.3	7.9	34	36
Oklahoma	346	305	12.0	10.9	22	27
Oregon	204	171	8.3	7.2	33	39
Pennsylvania	1,278	1,282	10.9	10.9	27	26
Rhode Island	72	78	7.7	8.3	36	34
South Carolina	563	643	19.3	22.4	6	3
South Dakota	76	58	11.0	8.4	26	33
Tennessee	842	864	19.3	20.1	5	5
Texas	2,160	2,326	16.6	18.1	14	13
Utah	42	43	3.2	3.4	48	48
Vermont	41	37	8.4	7.7	32	37
Virginia	722	742	14.0	14.4	18	19
Washington	305	384	8.1	10.5	35	29
West Virginia	216	239	11.6	12.9	23	22
Wisconsin	260	181	5.6	3.9	40	46
Wyoming	15	20	3.5	4.9	47	43
American Samoa†	7	8	22.6	26.1	–	–
Guam†	67	67	58.8	67.0	–	–
Puerto Rico†	375	NA	11.4	NA	–	–
Trust Territory Pacific Is.†	59	77	45.3	60.3	–	–
U.S. Virgin Is.†	NA	7	NA	7.1	–	–

*District of Columbia is not ranked with the states but is included in totals.
†Not included in totals.
(–)=Not ranked.
NA=Not available.

FIGURE 1. Tuberculosis case rates, by state, 1978

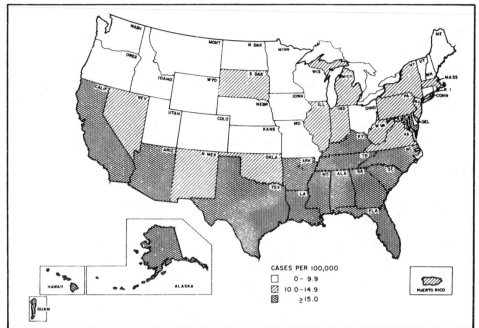

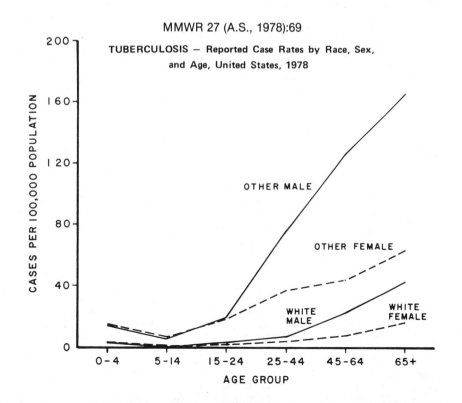

MMWR 28:385 (8/24/79)

Health Status of Indochinese Refugees

INTRODUCTION

Last month the President announced that by September 1979, 14,000 Indochinese refugees would be accepted monthly for resettlement in the United States. Within the Public Health Service (PHS), CDC shares federal responsibility for the health of refugees with the Health Services Administration (HSA). CDC is responsible for the medical screening of refugees while they are still abroad and for the inspection of refugees upon arrival at U.S. ports of entry. By law, health screening of refugees in Asia includes examination for tuberculosis, leprosy, venereal disease, and mental defects and disorders.* The HSA provides—or helps private, local, or state sources provide—immediate medical services, as well as a more comprehensive medical assessment of refugees after their arrival in the United States. State and local health departments are being notified of the arrival of each refugee to their communities. Both CDC and HSA are seeking to insure that adequate documentation on refugees with special health problems is acquired and distributed to state and local health authorities.

PHS teams have recently visited areas in California, Oregon, Washington, and Hawaii that have already received large numbers of refugees, as well as refugee camps and embarkation areas in Southeast Asian countries. From these visits, as well as from limited surveillance data and the experience gained in the resettlement of over 150,000 Vietnamese refugees in the United States since May 1975, the following may be expected:

1. The majority of refugees will be free of major contagious diseases;
2. Where an illness is present, it will likely represent a personal rather than a public health problem, and;
3. The main health problems, perhaps exceeded only by the stress of resettlement itself, will include tuberculosis and parasitic diseases.

This report represents a summary of recommendations that have been prepared by CDC as a guide to practitioners and state and local health departments concerning some of the more significant infectious disease problems that may be encountered. As surveillance information becomes available, these data will appear in the *MMWR.*

TUBERCULOSIS

Tuberculosis is the most serious potential public health problem of Indochinese refugees. Data from San Francisco, Los Angeles, and the state of Washington, indicate that 1%-2% of refugees who have arrived during 1979 and have been examined have been found to have "active" tuberculosis. This estimate may be high because refugees in whom tuberculosis was identified overseas are more likely to have been examined upon arrival in the United States than other refugees. In San Francisco, 41% (136 of 333) of refugees

---

*Conditions for which a person would be excluded entry into the United States are designated as Class A by the Immigration and Naturalization Service. These are as follows: 1) syphilis, gonorrhea, chancroid, granuloma inguinale, and lymphogranuloma venereum. These conditions are not excludable if they are adequately treated. 2) active tuberculosis. 3) infectious leprosy. 4) mental retardation, insanity (past, present), and severe personality disorders, including chronic alcoholism and drug addiction. Mental retardation and previous attacks of insanity are waiverable under certain circumstances, as established in the Immigration and Nationality Act.

less than 18 years of age had a skin test that was positive for tuberculosis. In Los Angeles and Washington state, about half of the refugees—of all age groups—had a positive skin test. The proportion who had received BCG vaccination is not known.

Screening and Notification Procedures

At present, refugees 2 years and older are screened in the refugee camps in Southeast Asia with a chest X ray.* "Active" or suspected "active" (Immigration Class A†) tuberculosis is an excludable condition. Refugees so classified must remain in Asia under treatment until their disease is no longer "active," unless excludability is waived. Persons with Class A tuberculosis who are eligible for a waiver of excludability can travel immediately if their disease is non-contagious. If their disease is contagious they must remain under treatment in Asia until their disease is judged non-contagious. Refugees classified as having "active" or suspected "active" (Class A) tuberculosis or tuberculosis "not considered active" (Class B), are referred for medical evaluation upon arrival. In either case, local and state health departments in the United States are notified of the arrival of the person to facilitate initiation or continuation of treatment.

A Class A refugee who is eligible to enter the United States must have at least 2 sputum smears, taken at least 1 day apart, that are negative for acid-fast organisms, before he or she is considered noninfectious and permitted to travel. Any form of extrapulmonary tuberculosis, as well as pulmonary tuberculosis designated Class B, is considered noninfectious for travel purposes. The medical examination form (OF-157, formerly FS-398) must specify if the individual has Class A or Class B tuberculosis, give the results of bacteriologic studies, describe X-ray findings, and detail the treatment. A copy of the OF-157 and the chest X rays remain with the refugee. A copy of the OF-157 should be forwarded to the local health department along with a copy of either the "Report of Alien with Tuberculosis Waiver" (CDC 4.451)—for Class A cases—or the "Report of Alien with Tuberculosis Not Considered Active" (CDC 4.447)—for Class B cases. A copy of the CDC 4.451 or the CDC 4.447 also should be sent to the state health department at the refugee's destination and a copy given to the refugee. Appropriate follow-up procedures then become the responsibility of the refugee and the health department.

CDC has recommended that Class A tuberculosis cases with positive bacteriology and/or cavitary lesions on chest X ray be started on treatment consisting of isoniazid (INH), rifampin, and ethambutol. Ethambutol has been included because, based on drug-resistance studies done in the United States, it is estimated that approximately 10% of the refugees with tuberculosis may be infected with an organism resistant to INH. Children too young to be assessed for alterations of visual acuity should receive INH, rifampin, and streptomycin. The doses of drugs for adults are INH, 300 mg daily; rifampin, 600 mg daily (450 mg daily for persons weighing less than 50 kg); ethambutol, 15-20 mg per kg body weight daily (the dose can be rounded off, e.g., 800 mg, 1000 mg, 1200 mg). For children the doses are INH, 10 mg per kg of body weight daily up to a maximum of 300 mg; rifampin, 10 to 20 mg per kg of body weight daily; ethambutol, 15 to 20 mg per kg of body weight daily; streptomycin, 20 mg per kg of body weight up to the maximum of 1 g daily. Class A tuberculosis cases other than those with positive bacteriology and/or cavitary lesions on chest X ray may be started on treatment at the discretion of the examining physician, or treatment may be deferred until arrival in the United States.

---

*The 2 exceptions are Indonesia and Singapore, where only refugees 15 years of age or older are screened for tuberculosis.
†For a description of the Class A designations, see footnote on page 385.

Follow-up and Treatment after Arrival in the United States

If treatment has not been started abroad on a refugee with Class A tuberculosis, specimens should be obtained for bacteriologic examination (smear and culture) and for drug-susceptibility tests. Depending on the examining physician's clinical judgment, treatment may be started after specimens have been obtained or deferred until the results of the tests are available. Treatment started in the United States should follow the regimens outlined above. When drug-susceptibility results are available, treatment can be adjusted accordingly. However, it is important that the regimen always contain at least 2 drugs to which the organisms are known to be, or thought to be, susceptible. If cultures are negative, precluding drug-susceptibility testing, then INH, rifampin, and ethambutol should all be continued for the duration of therapy. Treatment should continue for a period of 12 months after sputum specimens are negative. For patients with negative bacteriology, the total period of treatment should be 12 months.

If treatment has been started abroad on a refugee with Class A tuberculosis, the refugee would have negative sputum smears before being permitted to travel. Upon arrival, treatment should be continued, but specimens should be obtained for attempted culture and drug-susceptibility tests. If the culture results are positive, proceed as above and adjust regimen, if necessary, according to the drug-susceptibility test results. If the cultures are negative, precluding drug-susceptibility testing, it is necessary to continue a regimen of INH, rifampin, and ethambutol for a period of 12 months after sputum specimens are negative.

Class B tuberculosis patients are a high-risk group and should be re-evaluated upon arrival in the United States. If "active" disease is found, indicating either incorrect classification or development of progressive disease after the initial medical examination, consider the person as a case of tuberculosis and treat as described above. If the Class B designation is correct, these refugees are candidates for preventive therapy with INH. Even though as many as 10% of Class B patients may be infected with an INH-resistant organism, it is not possible to identify these individuals. Therefore, it is recommended that INH be used for preventive therapy; if tuberculosis caused by INH-resistant organisms should develop later in any of these persons, it can be treated appropriately with other drugs at that time.

Preventive therapy is recommended for contacts of tuberculosis patients and other infected persons who may be identified. Since a positive reaction from BCG vaccination cannot be distinguished from natural infection, the tuberculin test should be interpreted without regard to BCG vaccination. INH is recommended unless the person is known to have been exposed to a source case with INH-resistant tubercle bacilli. In that situation, 1 of the following 3 alternative approaches may be selected: 1) treat with INH; 2) treat with rifampin (alone or in combination with INH or another drug); or 3) use no drugs for preventive treatment but assure close clinical follow-up and provide treatment with appropriate drugs if tuberculosis develops.

Depending upon the number of refugees in the community and the resources available, health departments will have varying degrees of difficulty in accommodating the increased case load presented by Indochinese refugees. The recommended priorities for tuberculosis control in Indochinese refugees are as follows: 1) evaluation, management, and contact investigation of Class A cases; 2) evaluation, management, and contact investigation (if indicated) of Class B cases; 3) tuberculin screening and preventive therapy programs for children, e.g., testing of all refugee children entering the community's school system; 4) evaluation and follow-up of the family and other close associates of children found to be infected; and 5) tuberculin screening and preventive therapy programs for adult refugees under 35 years of age. Screening programs are not recommended for older refugees because the vast majority would not be candidates for preventive therapy. (The exception would be those with abnormal chest X rays who have already been identified as Class B patients at the time of their arrival in the United States).

Although there is some risk of transmission of tuberculosis from refugees to the U.S. population, the current methods of detection and the use of appropriate containment procedures make the risks minimal. Efforts are being made to improve the medical evaluation of refugees overseas, including the interpretation of X rays and performance of laboratory bacteriologic procedures, and to assure that health departments are properly notified of the arrival of refugees who have tuberculosis.

MALARIA

Diagnosis

Malaria can be definitively diagnosed only through the careful microscopic examination of blood films. Both thick and thin blood films should be made from each patient's blood. Thick films provide the best opportunity to detect the lowest number of parasites but require some training and experience to read. Thin films are used for species identification. Blood films should be prepared from specimens from all refugees who have a fever. The films should be promptly stained (Giemsa stain preferred) and examined for parasites, and the species and approximate density of parasites (i.e., number per 100 white blood cells on thick films) should be noted, if possible.

Signs and symptoms other than fever that suggest the possibility of malaria also dictate a blood film examination. These would include anemia, splenomegaly, chills, headache, backache, and malaise. Negative blood films on at least 2 consecutive days aid in ruling out malaria infection. Although detectable parasitemia almost always accompanies a clinical attack of malaria, parasitemia may occur in the absence of significant symptoms.

Treatment

Presumptive Therapy: Identification of the species of *Plasmodium* should be done as soon as possible. However, presumptive therapy should be instituted to prevent serious complications and death before the diagnosis can be confirmed parasitologically. Since many refugees will be coming from areas of Southeast Asia where chloroquine-resistant *P. falciparum* malaria is endemic, presumptive antimalarial therapy for such refugees must be undertaken with the possibility of chloroquine-resistant *P. falciparum* malaria in mind. For patients who are seriously ill with the presumptive diagnosis of *P. falciparum* malaria, parenteral or oral quinine is indicated. Parenteral quinine should be used with extreme caution and is chiefly indicated for patients who cannot take oral medication. For clinically stable patients chloroquine may be started as an alternative to quinine in initial presumptive therapy, but the patient should be kept under careful observation.

Therapy of Laboratory-Confirmed Cases: When the species has been identified, specific therapy should be instituted along the following guidelines:*

---

*All chloroquine and primaquine doses are expressed in terms of the base. Dosages of all drugs are given as the adult dose. Proportional reduction in dosage would be necessary for children.
†Use of trade names does not imply endorsement by the PHS or the U.S. Department of Health, Education, and Welfare.

1. *P. falciparum*: Because of the high proportion of chloroquine-resistant *P. falciparum* in Southeast Asia, all *falciparum* infections seen in refugees should be assumed resistant, and one of the following regimens should be used:

    a. Quinine sulfate, 650 mg, t.i.d. x 3 days
       plus pyrimethamine, 25 mg, b.i.d. x 3 days
         plus sulfadiazine, 500 mg, q.i.d. x 5 days; these 3 drugs must be administered concurrently (*1*).

    b. Quinine sulfate, 650 mg, t.i.d x 3 days
       plus Bactrim Double Strength† (160 mg trimethoprim and 800 mg sulfamethoxazole), 2 tablets, b.i.d. x 5 days, administered concurrently.

    c. Quinine sulfate, 650 mg, t.i.d. x 3 days
       plus tetracycline, 250 mg, q.i.d. x 10 days, administered concurrently (*2*).

Several points about the above therapy should be noted.

Sulfonamides are used in combination with a folic acid antagonist (e.g., pyrimethamine or trimethoprim) because they are synergistic. The type of sulfonamide used is not critical, provided that a sufficient blood level is maintained for at least 5 days. While combinations of sulfonamide, a folic acid antagonist, and a tetracycline are effective schizonticides, their rate of action is slow. Thus, at least 3 days of quinine therapy is important to rapidly reduce the parasite density to safe levels. Treatment of *P. falciparum* malaria is effective in up to 95% of cases; however, such patients should be carefully followed up for at least 90 days to detect recurring symptoms or parasitemia. Recurrences are usually within the first 30 days, but may occur later. Retreatment may be with the same or another drug combination.

2. *P. vivax*: The recommended treatment for *P. vivax* infections is a total dose of 1.5 g of chloroquine (base) over a 3-day period (600 mg initial dose, followed by 300 mg at 6, 24, and 48 hours). There have been no reports of resistance of this species to chloroquine, and this regimen should eliminate the parasitemia and symptoms within 24 to 72 hours. Relapses may occur after chloroquine treatment unless radical curative therapy is administered to eliminate the exoerythrocytic schizonts in the liver. The 2 accepted regimens for radical curative therapy are as follows:

    a. Primaquine, 15 mg (base) daily for 14 days. The initial dose should be in association with chloroquine, either with the normal therapeutic course, or, if administered later, with a single dose 600 mg (base) of chloroquine.

    b. Primaquine, 45 mg (base) weekly for 8 weeks.

For a closely supervised patient, the 14-day regimen may be preferable because regular drug-taking would be assured and the likelihood of missing doses during the longer 8-week course of treatment would be avoided.

The administration of primaquine or chloroquine-primaquine mixtures may cause gastrointestinal symptoms in some patients. Patients with glucose-6-phosphate dehydrogenase (G6PD) deficiency may experience mild to severe hemolysis during primaquine therapy. Because an estimated 10%-12% of nationals from Southeast Asia may have at least some level of deficiency of this enzyme, it is recommended that all patients be screened for G6PD deficiency before primaquine treatment is begun and that periodic determinations of hematocrit be done during therapy. Those with a G6PD deficiency should be placed on the once-weekly dosage schedule rather than the daily regimen. The hemolysis is reversible upon cessation of the drug, and a significant and persistent fall in hematocrit should dictate cessation of treatment.

3. *P. malariae*: Most authorities believe that *P. malariae* is not a relapsing species of malaria. There are no reports of *P. malariae* resistance to chloroquine. Therefore, this

species may be treated with chloroquine in the doses outlined above for *P. vivax*; no primaquine therapy is indicated.

PARASITIC INFECTIONS OTHER THAN MALARIA

Parasitic infections are common in the Indochinese refugees who are now entering the United States. For example, a survey of 165 Laotian refugees examined in Illinois in February 1979 found hookworm to be the most common intestinal parasite in this group (64%), followed by *Giardia* (18%), *Trichuris* (12%), and *Ascaris* (9%) (*3*). Many of these are infections with which most American physicians have had little or no experience.

Refugees infected with intestinal helminths (worms) do not pose a significant public health hazard since adequate sewage disposal interrupts transmission of the helminths, which require several days of incubation in the soil before becoming infective. Adequate hygienic practices will also minimize the risk posed by intestinal protozoa. Although CDC does not consider it necessary to screen routinely all Indochinese refugees for intestinal parasites, testing for such parasites is indicated as part of a complete examination of individual refugees requiring medical care.

Physicians who want consultation on the diagnosis or therapy of parasitic infections, including malaria, should call the Parasitic Diseases Division, Bureau of Epidemiology, CDC, (404) 329-3676.

SEXUALLY TRANSMITTED DISEASES

Adult refugees receive a medical examination and a syphilis serologic test as part of routine medical screening for obtaining a visa. Patients with obvious genital infections or reactive serologic tests are referred to local health-care facilities for further evaluation and treatment before departure for the United States. Preliminary results of special studies that screened refugee groups for the presence of sexually transmitted diseases indicate that the prevalence of these diseases is very low. Upon arrival in the United States, refugees are invited to attend any PHS hospital or state or local health-care facility for full evaluation of new or pre-existing conditions.

Recommended treatment regimens for syphilis and gonorrhea have been published (*4,5*) and should be followed when treating refugees who develop a sexually transmitted disease after arrival in the United States. Although isolates of *Neisseria gonorrhoeae* from Southeast Asia may be relatively resistant to a variety of antibiotics, initial therapy should consist of procaine penicillin G, ampicillin, amoxicillin, or tetracycline in adequate doses, as recommended by CDC. Follow-up cultures 3-5 days after therapy are important to detect treatment failures caused by resistant organisms. Positive follow-up cultures should be tested for the presence of penicillinase (B-lactamase)-producing *N. gonorrhoeae*.

CHILDHOOD IMMUNIZATIONS

Refugee children who have been immunized in the camps should carry a record of such immunizations with them. Current indications are, however, that most refugee children are not receiving routine immunizations before leaving Southeast Asia. CDC is seeking to improve the immunization status of refugees before they enter the United States, but prudence dictates that all children be evaluated carefully to determine their immunization status upon arrival in the United States.

The purpose of these recommendations is to protect immigrants and persons already residing in the United States from vaccine-preventable diseases. The objective is to ensure that all immigrants receive, when appropriate, vaccines recommended for routine use in the U.S. population. These recommendations are adapted from those of the PHS Advisory Committee on Immunization Practices (ACIP).

Because of immunization requirements for U.S. public schools, all refugee children 2 months through 18 years (up to the 19th birthday) should be up to date on diphtheria, tetanus, and pertussis (DTP) vaccine or tetanus-diphtheria toxoid, adult type (Td); oral polio vaccine (OPV); and measles, mumps, and rubella (MMR) vaccinations. Girls 14 through 19 years old may be immunized with MMR vaccine if they are not pregnant and understand that they should avoid pregnancy for 3 months after the vaccine is given. Use of a standard vaccination record facilitates the recording and transfer of immunization records.

Certain vaccines can be given simultaneously without increasing the rate of adverse reactions or interfering with the immune response. Two acceptable combinations are DTP with OPV, and OPV with MMR. While the effectiveness of the combined administration of DTP and MMR is not certain, it is reasonable to give OPV, DTP, and MMR simultaneously under certain circumstances: if the individual is thought to have had no previous immunizations, if further follow-up is questionable, or if the time available to immunize the person is limited.

None of the live-virus vaccines discussed here has been associated with allergic reactions. Allergy to eggs is not a contraindication to their use. However, these vaccines should not be given to persons known to have compromised immune systems from disease or medical therapy. MMR vaccines should not be given to women known to be pregnant, and women receiving them should avoid pregnancy for 3 months after vaccination.

Previous serious reactions with DTP or Td are a contraindication to the subsequent administration of these vaccines.

Diphtheria-Tetanus-Pertussis

Children 6 weeks through 6 years of age should receive a primary series of DTP vaccine consisting of 4 doses, 3 given at 4- to 8-week intervals and a fourth given 1 year after the third. Immunization should begin at 2 to 3 months of age, if possible. A booster dose of DTP is recommended when the child is 4 to 7 years of age, usually just before entering school.

Persons 7 years of age or older who have not previously received a primary series of DTP vaccine should receive a primary series consisting of 3 doses of Td, with 2 doses 4 to 8 weeks apart and the third dose 6 to 12 months later. A routine booster of Td is recommended only every 10 years.

Persons who have received a partial series of DTP or Td vaccine can simply complete the series and be considered up to date. DTP and Td vaccine received in Southeast Asia should be considered of adequate immunogenicity for purposes of these recommendations. Unnecessary additional doses of these vaccines should not be given, since adverse reactions may occur more frequently when larger numbers of doses have been administered.

Poliomyelitis

Only persons under 19 years of age need to be vaccinated against polio. Most adults from Southeast Asia will be naturally immune if they have not already been vaccinated.

Vaccination may be completed with OPV or inactivated polio vaccine (IPV).

A primary series of OPV consists of 3 doses, 2 given 6 to 8 weeks apart and the third given 8 to 12 months later. Ideally, polio vaccination is initiated during infancy. A booster of OPV is recommended before school entry; other booster doses should not be necessary for persons immigrating to the United States.

A primary series with IPV consists of 4 doses, 3 given at 4- to 8-week intervals and the fourth given 6 to 12 months later. Booster doses of IPV are recommended every 5 years. IPV is the vaccine of choice for persons with compromised immune systems since OPV is contraindicated in this situation.

Measles-Mumps-Rubella

Refugees aged 15 months to 20 years should receive a single dose of combined MMR vaccine.

LEPROSY

Leprosy has been a relatively uncommon problem among refugees from Southeast Asia. Currently, persons diagnosed as having infectious leprosy are excluded from admission to the United States. However, persons with leprosy under appropriate treatment can be admitted and present a minimal health risk to the U.S. population. Such persons will be reported to the state and local health department in the jurisdiction to which they are destined for follow-up. Guidance on medical management can be obtained from U.S. PHS hospitals in Carville (Louisiana), San Francisco, and Staten Island, and from Leahi Hospital in Honolulu.

References
1. Hall AP, Doberstyn EB, Mettaprakong V, Sonkom P: *Falciparum* malaria cured by quinine followed by sulfadoxine-pyrimethamine. Br Med J 2:15-17, April 1975
2. Colwell EJ, Hickman RL, Intraprasert R, Tirabutana C: Minocycline and tetracycline treatment of acute *falciparum* malaria in Thailand. Am J Trop Med Hyg 21:144-149, 1972
3. MMWR 28:346-347, 1979
4. MMWR 25:101-102, 107, 1976
5. MMWR 28: 13-16, 21, 1979

CHAPTER 3

Diphtheria

MMWR 28:451 (9/28/79)

Diphtheria — California

On May 10, 1979, a 68-year-old man with no history of diphtheria immunization was seen at a Los Angeles County Health Department clinic with a sore throat. When a pharyngeal membrane was noted, a throat culture was taken, and the patient was referred to a hospital with a diagnosis of diphtheria. A physician in the ear, nose, and throat clinic of the hospital stripped the membrane and sent it for culture, made a diagnosis of pharyngitis, and sent the patient home on oral penicillin. The next day, the county health department again referred the patient to the hospital because of the suspicion of diphtheria, but he was sent home with no change in the diagnosis or treatment.

Corynebacterium diphtheriae was cultured from the throat membrane fragments, and guinea pigs were inoculated to test for toxigenicity. When the test was found to be positive on June 1, the county health department was informed of the culture results.

The patient, whose throat had healed, was hospitalized on June 4. An electrocardiogram showed a right bundle branch block which had not changed from the pattern a year earlier. The patient was discharged without parenteral penicillin or antitoxin treatment. Two throat cultures taken during admission were reported as negative on June 12 and 13. On June 25, the patient returned to the hospital with trouble swallowing and a nasal quality to his voice. He was admitted with a diagnosis of diphtheritic bulbar neuropathy and was put on tube feeding for the dysphagia. At present, he has a neurologic deficit involving the muscles of the soft palate.

On June 4, the county health department cultured the throats of 20 family members, all of whom had been well. The culture of a 9-year-old granddaughter, who had been previously immunized, was positive for *C. diphtheriae*; that culture was also toxigenic. The granddaughter received 10 days of oral penicillin, and a booster dose of tetanus-diphtheria toxoid was given. The immunizations of all family members have been brought up to date, and all remain well. Because the index patient had made a trip to Albuquerque, New Mexico, 4 weeks before the onset of illness, the New Mexico State Health and Environment Department was notified about the case. All family members in New Mexico who were visited by the patient were followed up for immunizations; all have remained well.

Reported by S Fannin, MD, Los Angeles County Health Dept; J Chin, MD, State Epidemiologist, California Dept of Health Services; RE Hoffman, MD, Acting State Epidemiologist, New Mexico State Health and Environment Dept; Immunization Div, Bur of State Services, Field Services Div, Bacterial Diseases Div, Bur of Epidemiology, CDC.

Editorial Note: The number of reported diphtheria cases has declined since 1975, with fewer than 100 cases reported annually in 1977 and 1978. The mortality rate from diphtheria has also declined since 1970. However, the case-fatality ratio for noncutaneous diphtheria has remained unchanged at 5%-10% since 1920 (1). Diphtheria is likely to be more severe or fatal in individuals with no or unknown histories of immunization. Though the incidence rate of noncutaneous diphtheria decreases with age, adults and children under 5 are less likely to be adequately immunized. This case illustrates the importance of keeping adults up to date with recommended immunizations and of considering the diagnosis of "childhood" diseases in unimmunized adults.

Persons with suspected or proven diphtheria should receive both parenteral penicillin and diphtheria antitoxin after their skin has been tested for hypersensitivity (2). In addition, asymptomatic, unimmunized household contacts should be managed by (1) either benzathine penicillin or a 7-day course of oral erythromycin, with cultures before and after treatment; (2) vaccination with diphtheria toxoid; and (3) daily surveillance for 7 days for evidence of diphtheria. Where close surveillance is impossible or unreliable, diphtheria antitoxin should be given (3).

References
1. CDC: Diphtheria Surveillance Report No. 12, Issued July 1978, p 2
2. American Academy of Pediatrics: Report of the Committee on Infectious Diseases. 18th ed. Evanston, Illinois, AAP, 1977, p 62
3. Public Health Service Advisory Committee on Immunization Practices: Diphtheria and tetanus toxoids and pertussis vaccine. MMWR 26:401-402, 407, 1977

MMWR 28:509 (11/2/79)

Diphtheria in Indochinese Refugees from Thailand

At the Lumphini refugee transit center in Bangkok, Thailand, a 2-year-old girl developed clinical evidence of diphtheria and was hospitalized on October 20. She had arrived by bus the night before from Leoi Camp in northern Thailand, where in the preceding month a child had died with pharyngitis and fever of unknown cause. On October 22, the flow of refugees into Lumphini Center was stopped, and active surveillance for diphtheria was initiated at both the camp and the center and among refugees arriving into the United States from Lumphini.

Among 96 refugees who arrived in Los Angeles on October 26, 7 were found to have pyrexia and pharyngitis without pharyngeal exudate or pseudomembrane and were cultured for *Corynebacterium diphtheriae*. One was culture positive: a 32-year-old man, with no known prior diphtheria immunization, who along with 5 well family members traveled to Denver to join his sponsor family before the culture results were available. Biotyping and toxigenicity testing of his isolate are not complete. Among 29 refugees who arrived in Honolulu on October 29, one, a 1-year-old Cambodian boy, had possible signs of diphtheria. The boy was transferred to Tripler Air Force Medical Center for evaluation. Cultures of the boy and 3 family contacts are pending. Culture or clinical evidence of diphtheria was not identified in refugees from 5 other flights arriving in the United States through October 29.

Reported by S Fannin, MD, Los Angeles County Health Dept; J Chin, MD, State Epidemiologist, California Dept of Health Services; RS Hopkins, MD State Epidemiologist, Colorado State Dept of Health; K Wells, MD, USPHS Outpatient Clinic, Honolulu; NH Wiebenga, MD, State Epidemiologist, Hawaii State Dept of Health; Quarantine Div, Field Services Div, and Special Pathogens Br, Bacterial Diseases Div, Bur of Epidemiology, CDC.

Editorial Note: Evidence of diphtheria in refugees at Lumphini Center and possibly at Leoi Camp has prompted several control measures. Attempts have been increased to initiate diphtheria immunization of all persons at the Lumphini Center and other transit camps. The goal is to immunize all refugees at least twice, including once on arrival at a camp and once 3 weeks later. A waiting period of at least 1 week is planned between the second toxoid immunization and departure from Thailand. Until the immunization program is fully implemented and shown to be effective, refugees scheduled to leave Bangkok will be screened within 24 hours of departure for clinical evidence of diphtheria. Those with pyrexia and pharyngitis, exudative pharyngitis, or pseudomembranes will be detained, cultured, and, if indicated, treated for diphtheria. Upon arrival in the United States, refugees will again be screened for evidence of diphtheria. Any persons suspected to have the disease will be cultured and isolated pending results of culture.

MMWR 27 (A.S., 1978): 23

DIPHTHERIA – Reported Case and Death Rates by Year, United States, 1920–1978

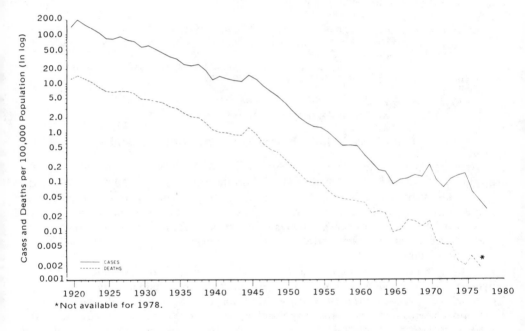

*Not available for 1978.

CHAPTER 4

Pneumonia

MMWR 27:25 (1/27/78)

Pneumococcal Polysaccharide Vaccine

INTRODUCTION

Polyvalent polysaccharide vaccine against disease caused by *Streptococcus pneumoniae* (pneumococcus) has recently been licensed in the United States. This statement summarizes current knowledge about this vaccine and provides initial guidance for its use in this country in reducing the incidence of pneumococcal disease.

PNEUMOCOCCAL DISEASE

Pneumococcal pneumonia, meningitis, otitis media, and bacteremia occur throughout the United States. Before 1950, significant epidemics of pneumococcal disease were described in closed populations such as military recruits. Since then epidemics have been rare, perhaps because of the use of effective antibiotics. Of the 83 capsular types of pneumococci, 14 cause most of the serious pneumococcal disease.

The precise incidence of most forms of pneumococcal disease is unknown. Projections based on limited observations indicate that as many as 400,000–500,000 cases of pneumococcal pneumonia may occur annually in the United States. This disease continues to have an overall case fatality of 5-10% and, even with antibiotic therapy, may be particularly serious for some segments of the population such as the elderly. Appearance of some pneumococci with multiple antibiotic resistance could herald additional problems (*1*).

The incidence of pneumococcal meningitis is approximately 1.5 to 2.5 cases per 100,000 population per year (*2*). One-half of the cases occur in children between 1 month and 4 years of age. About 40% of these cases are fatal despite appropriate treatment; permanent sequelae occur in half the survivors.

Pneumococcal disease of all kinds is unusually common in persons with sickle cell anemia (3) and anatomical or functional asplenia. Pneumococcal disease is also common in patients with agammaglobulinemia, multiple myeloma, nephrotic syndrome, cirrhosis, and alcoholism. Pneumococcal meningitis has been a major complication of basilar skull fracture with cerebrospinal fluid rhinorrhea.

PNEUMOCOCCAL POLYSACCHARIDE VACCINES

Several kinds of pneumococcal vaccine were developed and tested in the 1920s, 1930s, and 1940s. A combined polysaccharide vaccine, similar to the one recently licensed, was shown to prevent pneumonia in a young male military population with a high endemic rate of disease (25 cases per 1,000 population per year) (4). A trivalent vaccine appeared to be effective in one elderly population (5). A combined polysaccharide vaccine was licensed and produced in this country from 1945-1947. However, with the availability of effective antibiotics, this vaccine was given infrequently, and the manufacturer voluntarily discontinued production.

The 14-valent polysaccharide vaccine now licensed for use in the United States contains purified capsular material of pneumococci extracted separately from those types of organisms to be combined in the final vaccine. Each dose of the vaccine contains 50 μg of each polysaccharide. The 14 particular types of pneumococci in the vaccine available in the United States—American types 1, 2, 3, 4, 6, 8, 9, 12, 14, 19, 23, 25, 51, and 56 (6)—cause at least 80% of all bacteremic pneumococcal disease seen in this country.

The majority of adults respond to vaccine with a several-fold rise in antibody measured by radioimmunoassay. Immunity is provided only against the pneumococcal types in the vaccine, although, theoretically, there might be some degree of cross-protection among immunologically similar types. There appears to be no booster effect with additional doses; further studies are underway to clarify this observation.

Nasopharyngeal acquisition of the pneumococcal types included in the vaccine appears to be reduced by immunization. Furthermore, there has been no evidence among the immunized of any increase in diseases caused by other Gram-positive or Gram-negative microorganisms. The duration of protection is as yet unknown, but elevated antibody levels appear to persist for at least 2 years after immunization.

Field tests of pneumococcal vaccine among young adult recruit gold miners in South Africa (who have consistently had a high incidence of bacteremic pneumococcal pneumonia—200 cases per 1,000 population per year) have shown that a single dose of vaccine is highly effective (7). Several other trials in various age groups are currently under way. One involving older age adults has produced preliminary results suggesting effectiveness against pneumococcal disease.

There has been only limited vaccine evaluation in children. Preliminary trials showed that children under 2 years of age responded poorly to the vaccine. However, in a small group of older children with sickle cell anemia and splenectomy, bacteremic pneumococcal disease appeared to be less common after immunization with an 8-valent vaccine (8).

In trials with the currently available vaccines, about half of the recipients had erythema and mild pain at the injection site for about a day. No serious adverse reactions have been reported.

VACCINE USAGE

Because there is as yet a limited amount of information available concerning the efficacy of pneumococcal vaccine, definitive recommendations for its use cannot be formulated at the present time. Those responsible for the health of communities and of individual patients should, therefore, evaluate each possible use of pneumococcal vaccine according to the following general concepts:

Use in Communities

1. Mass immunization of healthy people is *not* currently recommended.
2. Special populations, particularly closed groups such as those in residential schools, nursing homes, and some institutions, can be at enhanced risk of systemic pneumococcal disease, either in endemic or in epidemic form. When such is the case, immunization of the entire closed population might be an effective control measure.
3. Geographically localized outbreaks in the general population can sometimes be due to the spread of a single pneumococcal type. When this is observed, selective immunization of groups in the community epidemiologically believed to be at particular risk may be useful.
4. In view of the risks of influenza to some segments of the population, consideration should be given to vaccinating patients at high risk of influenza complications (particularly pneumonia) with pneumococcal vaccine (see below).

Use in Selected Individuals

1. On the basis of preliminary evidence, persons over 2 years of age who have splenic dysfunction (due to sickle cell disease or other causes) or who have anatomical a-splenia should benefit from being immunized.

2. Persons over 2 years of age with certain chronic illnesses where there is an increased risk of pneumococcal disease, such as diabetes mellitus and functional impairment of cardiorespiratory, hepatic, and renal systems, might benefit from immunization. Because the risk of and case-fatality rate from pneumococcal disease increase with increasing age, the benefits of vaccination should increase with increasing age.

Use in Pregnancy

There is no specific information on the safety of pneumococcal vaccine administered during pregnancy. Theoretically, it should not be harmful. However, in view of recommendations that unnecessary drugs and vaccines should not be given during pregnancy, pneumococcal vaccine should only be used when there is substantial risk of infection.

SUMMARY

1. Despite antibiotic therapy, morbidity and mortality from pneumococcal disease remain problems; the emergence of pneumococcal strains that are resistant to antibiotics further emphasizes the value of effective vaccine prophylaxis.
2. Evidence from studies done several decades ago and those in recent years leads to the following conclusions:
   a. Pneumococcal vaccine induces satisfactory antibody response in persons over 2 years of age.
   b. Antibody titers are likely to remain high for several years.
   c. Vaccination reduces by 80% or more the incidence of bacteremic pneumococcal pneumonia caused by the bacterial types included in the vaccine. Since these types account for about 80% of the pneumococcal disease in the United States, there is a resulting potential for reducing pneumococcal disease by 60-65%.
   d. In experience to date, the vaccine has proved to be safe; side effects, although frequent, are not severe.

References

1. MMWR 26:285-286, 1977
2. Fraser DW, Darby CP, Koehler RE, Jacobs CF, Feldman RA: Risk factors in bacterial meningitis: Charleston County, South Carolina. J Infect Dis 127:271-277, 1973
3. Eeckels R, Gatti F, Renoirte AM: Abnormal distribution of haemoglobin serotypes in Negro children with severe bacterial infections. Nature 216:382, 1967
4. MacLeod CM, Hodges RG, Heidelberger M, Bernhard WG: Prevention of pneumococcal pneumonia by immunization with specific capsular polysaccharides. J Exp Med 82:445-465, 1945
5. Kaufman P: Pneumonia in old age. Arch Intern Med 79:518, 1947
6. Lund E: Laboratory diagnosis of *Pneumococcus* infections. Bull WHO 23:5-13, 1960
7. Austrian R: Vaccines of pneumococcal capsular polysaccharides

and the prevention of pneumococcal pneumonia in the role of im-
munological factors in infectious, allergic and autoimmune process.
No. 8, Beers RF, Bassett EG (eds), New York, Eighth Miles International Symposium, Raven Press, 1976, pp 79-91

8. Ammann AJ, Addiego J, Wara DW, Lubin B, Smith WB, Mentzer
WC: Polyvalent pneumococcal-polysaccharide immunization of pa-
tients with sickle-cell anemia and patients with splenectomy. N Engl
J Med 297:897-900, 1977

MMWR 28:225 (5/18/79)

Isolation of Drug-Resistant Pneumococci — New York

Streptococcus pneumoniae type 6B, partially resistant to penicillin, was recently
isolated from the tracheobronchial tree of a 15-month-old female with a persistant pulmonary infiltrate, pancytopenia, and hepatosplenomegaly.

The patient was admitted to Downstate Medical Center in Brooklyn, New York, on
October 22, 1978, for the therapy of a right upper lobe infiltrate that had been present
for at least 45 days. During a previous admission the child had been treated for the same
pulmonary infiltrate with ampicillin and nafcillin. Upon readmission she was treated with
cephalothin and gentamicin for 10 days. When she responded poorly, she was given
penicillin, 200,000 units/kg. She also failed to respond to this therapy. A culture of a
bronchoscopy specimen, taken on November 8, grew 2 strains of *S. pneumoniae* type 6B,
partially resistant to penicillin. One strain was optochin sensitive, and the other was
optochin resistant. After erythromycin and high-dose penicillin therapy was initiated,
the infiltrate partially cleared, and her condition improved. No other drug-resistant organisms were isolated. *Mycoplasma* complement-fixation titers were less than 1:4.

Both organisms had similar sensitivity patterns. The minimal inhibitory concentration (MIC) levels of the pneumococci to penicillin were 0.25 μg/ml; to ampicillin,
$\leqslant$0.125 μg/ml; and to methicillin, 2-4 μg/ml (Table 1). The organisms were resistant to

TABLE 1. Minimal inhibitory concentrations (μg/ml) of partially resistant pneumococci
in New York patient, 1978

	Optochin-sensitive strain	Optochin-resistant strain
Penicillin	.25	.25
Ampicillin	$\leqslant$.125	.125
Kanamycin	32	32
Gentamicin	4	4
Tetracycline	64	16
Cephalothin	.5	.5
Chloramphenicol	1	2
Erythromycin	.06	$\leqslant$.06
Methicillin	4	2
Clindamycin	.06	$\leqslant$.06
Tobramycin	8	16
Nalidixic acid	>128	64
Colistin	>128	>64
Carbenicillin	2	4
Oxacillin	2	2
Sulfa-Trimethoprim	4.8/.25	4.8/.25
Amikacin	16	32
Vancomycin	.25	.25
Cefamandole	.5	.5

amikacin, kanamycin, and tetracycline. They were sensitive to erythromycin, clindamycin, chloramphenicol, cephalothin, rifampin, and vancomycin. Both organisms were beta-lactamase negative when tested by the chromogenic cephalosporin method.

Nasopharyngeal cultures were taken from the patients and staff of the ward where the patient resided. Although several pneumococci were isolated, none was found to be penicillin-resistant. Repeat cultures are being taken on staff and patients.

Reported by S Landesman, MD, V Ahonkahai, MD, M Sierra, PhD, H Bernheimer, PhD, R Goetz, A Josephson, G Pringle, G Schiffman, PhD, P Steiner, MD, Downstate Medical Center, Brooklyn; JS Marr, MD, New York City Epidemiologist, Bur of Preventable Diseases, New York City Dept of Health; Special Pathogens Br, Bacterial Diseases Div, Bur of Epidemiology, CDC.

Editorial Note: Reports of pneumococci with intermediate or partial resistance to penicillin (MIC=0.1 to 0.9 µg/ml) have appeared with increasing frequency in this country. A study of the penicillin susceptibility of 6,000 pneumococcal isolates submitted to a laboratory in Alberta, Canada, suggested that 2.4% may demonstrate these levels of resistance (1). The response to therapy in infections with partially resistant organisms is incompletely characterized, although the MICs are considerably less than serum levels obtainable during penicillin therapy. Peak cerebrospinal fluid levels, however, may reach only 1 µg/ml (2), which could possibly result in difficulty treating meningitis caused by these organisms. To date, pneumococci more highly resistant to penicillin (MIC >1 µg/ml)—such as those reported from South Africa (3)—have been documented in the United States only in 1 case from Minnesota (4). CDC is coordinating a national study of susceptibility to penicillin in pneumococci isolated from selected hospitals, including those participating in the National Nosocomial Infections Study.

References
1. Dixon JMS, Lipinski AE, Graham MEP: Detection and prevalence of pneumococci with increased resistance to penicillin. Can Med Assoc J 117:1159-1161, 1977
2. Hieber JP, Nelson JD: A pharmacologic evaluation of penicillin in children with purulent meningitis. N Engl J Med 297:410-413, 1977
3. Jacobs MR, Koornhof HJ, Robins-Browne RM, Stevenson CM, Vermaak ZA, Freiman I, et al: Emergence of multiply resistant pneumococci. N Engl J Med 299:735-740, 1978
4. Cates KL, Gerrard JM, Giebink GS, Lund ME, Blecker EZ, Lau S, et al: A penicillin resistant pneumococcus. J Pediatr 93:624-626, 1978

MMWR 27:271 (8/4/78)

Acute Respiratory Illness — Wisconsin

Two outbreaks of respiratory disease occurred in Wisconsin in June and July—one in campers and staff members of a boys' camp in the northern part of the state, the other in members of a national singing group that was touring the Midwest. Details of the investigations follow.

Oneida County: Ninety-two of 155 campers (59%) and 15 of 49 older staff (31%) at a boy's camp in Oneida County experienced an illness characterized by non-productive cough (100%), sore throat (35%), headache (32%), and temperature of ≥37.7 C (28%). No myalgia or pleuritis was noted. Rash, conjuctivitis, and bullous myringitis were not seen on physical examination. Chest radiographs were taken on 75 of the cases; 38 were positive (25 with unilateral discrete infiltrates, 9 with bilateral discrete infiltrates, and 4 with bilateral diffuse infiltrates). No pleural effusions were seen. Some of the campers had been ill 8 days at the time of investigation. None of the children required hospitalization, but all ill children were sent home.

Small numbers of cases occurred throughout the 2 weeks after the camp session began on June 25, but new cases increased markedly by July 6 (Figure 1). In the last 2 weeks new cases have continued to occur; documentation of these cases is in progress. Disease

FIGURE 1. Cases of respiratory illness in a boys' camp, by date of onset, Wisconsin, June 20-July 15, 1978*

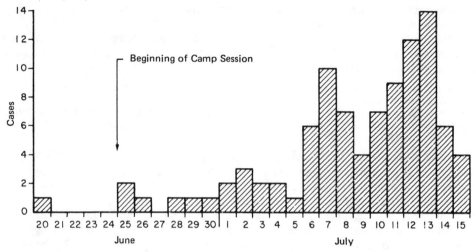

*In 6 cases the date of onset is unknown.

was limited to the camp under investigation; no other camps in the area, including a girls' camp which had participated on July 4 in a picnic with the involved camp, had any cases. Attack rates of illness, which decreased with increasing age, ranged from 88% in the 8-year-old campers to 38% in the 15-year-old campers to 32% in the 17- to 22-year-old counselors.

Campers slept in cabins with 9-11 other boys of the same age. Attack rates of illness, by cabin, ranged from 20% to 100%. Campers were confined to their cabins July 1 and 2 because of rain. The boys all ate together in a large mess hall, although residents of each cabin sat together at separate tables.

Laboratory studies to determine an etiologic agent are inconclusive, to date.

Two Rivers: On July 15 the Wisconsin State Department of Health and Social Services was notified of 9 cases of acute respiratory disease occurring in members of a singing group scheduled to perform in Two Rivers. Retrospectively, it was determined that cases had been occurring in the group, composed of 80 men and women 17-24 years of age, since June 26. A total of 29 persons were subsequently identified as having had a respiratory disease (attack rate: 36%) characterized by cough (100%), headache (83%), fatigue (83%), pharyngitis (69%), and fever (62%). Four persons had been hospitalized overnight. Attack rates were approximately the same for both sexes. Chest radiographs on 7 of the patients demonstrated bilateral infiltrates (in 1 patient), unilateral infiltrates (3), and an interstitial pattern (1); 2 were normal. Of 9 patients seen by a physician, 1 had bullous myringitis, and 3 had rales on chest examination.

Initial laboratory studies on 9 patients who had blood specimens drawn showed abnormal cold agglutinin titers on 5 patients: 1:64 in 1 patient (the patient with bilateral pneumonia) and 1:32 in 4 patients with pneumonia on X ray. The white blood cell count was normal in all 9 patients tested. Diagnosis was not confirmed; however, *Mycoplasma pneumoniae* was suspected as the cause of the outbreak.

Neither the source of the outbreak nor the method of transmission is yet known.

The group has a very active performance schedule; it has toured 2-3 cities per week since January. The members share most meals and social activities and sleep in homes of persons in the community where they are touring. Roommates are randomly assigned, 1-3 persons per home, and change from city to city.

The group's final 2 shows on the tour were canceled, and members returned to their homes. Studies are now in progress to determine the secondary attack rate in the community contacts of the group.

Reported by A T Davis, MD, Children's Memorial Hospital, Chicago; R Golubjatnikov, PhD, IE Imm, MA, State Epidemiologist, S Inhorn, MD, M LaVenture, MPH, L Montie, Wisconsin State Dept of Health & Social Services; Respiratory Virology Br, Virology Div, Virology Training Br, Laboratory Training and Consultation Div, Bur of Laboratories, Bacterial Diseases Div, Viral Diseases Div, Bur of Epidemiology, CDC.

Editorial Note: These 2 outbreaks are similar in the season of occurrence, attack rates, and the high proportion of pneumonia. Possible etiologic agents include *M. pneumoniae,* adenovirus, parainfluenza virus, respiratory syncytial virus (more common in a $\leqslant$2-year age group), influenza virus, or *Coxiella burnetii.*

The most likely cause of epidemic pneumonia in the age groups described in these 2 outbreaks would be *M. pneumoniae,* an endemic respiratory pathogen that may be responsible for up to 20% of pneumonic illness in urban populations (*1*). The incidence of mycoplasmal pneumonia usually peaks every third year, and 1978 appears to be a peak year. In contrast to lobar pneumonia, the lowest attack rates of mycoplasmal pneumonia are in children under 5 and in older persons. Also, although it occurs all year, it accounts for a larger proportion of summer pneumonia cases. When localized outbreaks of *M. pneumoniae* pneumonia occur, they are most often associated with groups that have close contact, such as military or institutionalized persons (*2*).

Although cold agglutinins may be used to make a presumptive diagnosis, complement fixation (CF) titers are necessary to make a definitive diagnosis. Elevation of the CF titers, however, may take 2-3 weeks. Early treatment with erythromycin shortens the course of the illness but will not affect the antibody response (*3*).

References
1. Joy HM, Kenny GE, McMahan R, Mansy AM, Grayston JT: *Mycoplasma pneumoniae* pneumonia in an urban area. JAMA 214:1666-1672, 1970
2. Van der Veen J, Van Nunan MCJ: Role of mycoplasma pneumonia in acute respiratory disease in a military population. Am J Hyg 78:293-301, 1963
3. Denny FW, Clyde WA, Glazen WP: Mycoplasmal pneumonia disease: Clinical spectrum, pathophysiology, epidemiology, and control. J Infect Dis 123:74-92, 1971

CHAPTER 5

Psittacosis and Q Fever

MMWR 27:417 (10/27/78)

Psittacosis — Connecticut

A 49-year-old man became ill on March 9, 1978, with intense pain in the legs followed by severe chills and headaches and a temperature spike to 104 F (40 C). The pattern of fever was intermittent. Prior to admission to the hospital, he developed a cough, a splotchy rash over the face and neck, and intense pruritis over the legs.

He was admitted to the hospital on March 16 with a productive cough with hemoptysis, chest pain in the right lower quadrant, and diarrhea. Admission X rays showed patchy, abnormal densities in the basal segments of the right lower lobe consistent with pneumonia. No definite hilar adenopathy or pleural fluid was noted.

Because the patient was a pet store owner who gave a history of recent contact with sick birds, psittacosis was suspected. After appropriate cultures and serologic studies were obtained, the patient was treated with tetracycline. He became afebrile within 12 hours of initiation of therapy and was discharged on March 22 to complete a 14-day course of tetracycline.

Acute and convalescent serum specimens submitted to the state laboratory demonstrated >4-fold rise in psittacosis group antibodies. Sputum and blood clot specimens were submitted to CDC. *Chlamydia psittaci* was isolated from the sputum but not from the blood clot.

The Connecticut State Department of Health's Preventable Diseases Division was notified of the presumptive diagnosis on March 17. The state veterinarian inspected the pet store in question and imposed a quarantine with the following guidelines: 1) birds were to be quarantined in a closed area free from contact or communication with the public or newly acquired birds or other animals; 2) birds were to be treated with appropriate antibiotics for 45 days; 3) any birds that died were to be frozen and transported to the state laboratory for further testing at CDC; and 4) the quarantine was to remain in effect from the date imposed until 60 days after the death of the last identified avian case.

The pet store had begun selling birds in early February. All people who had purchased birds there were notified by letter of their possible exposure to psittacosis and advised of its symptoms. A questionnaire was enclosed requesting information on illness among family members or their pet birds. Through this procedure, 2 ill birds were subsequently identified and tested. *C. psittaci* was recovered from the tissues of 1 bird, a grey cockatiel that had experienced several episodes of respiratory illness between February 7 and March 13. No *Chlamydia* organisms were cultured from the second bird, a parakeet. Members of the family that owned the infected bird had experienced mild illness following the bird's death, but serologic tests for psittacosis performed on them were negative. No additional cases in humans were identified as a result of this investigation.

Review of records revealed that parakeets were purchased from 3 local Connecticut dealers who were properly certified and had no illness in their birds, and that all the other birds were purchased from a large wholesaler in New Jersey. The pet store owner received from the New Jersey distributor on February 27 a shipment of birds that contained an ill albino cockatiel. He had treated this bird for a "cold" prior to onset of his own symptoms. Although this bird, which had recuperated, was among those treated during the quarantine, no serum samples were collected. The quarantine was removed from this pet store on May 16.

During the investigation, the Connecticut Department of Health submitted 6 dead birds to CDC for attempts at isolation of *C. psittaci*. As noted previously, one of these 6 was positive. No serum specimens were taken from well birds.

When notified on March 29, the New Jersey Department of Health began an investigation of the New Jersey wholesaler's facility. Serum specimens from 18 of 250 birds and from 6 employees were examined. Although 4 birds and 1 employee had complement fixing antibody titers >1:32 for psittacosis, there were no reports of human or avian illness. The facility was quarantined, with the option to treat or sacrifice the birds, and health authorities in cities and states that received or shipped the birds from January to April were notified. In view of the expense involved in implementing the quarantine and treating all the birds, the wholesaler chose to destroy all suspect animals. Following thorough cleaning of the wholesale facility, the quarantine was lifted on April 27.

Reported by J McLaughlin, PhD, L Mullany, MD, R Quintiliani, MD, RE Rentz, MD, Hartford Hospital, Hartford, Connecticut; PJ Checko, SM(AAM), JN Lewis, MD, State Epidemiologist, Connecticut Dept of Health; R Stadler, DVM, Connecticut Dept of Agriculture; EO Gilbert, DVM, RF Goldsboro, DVM, B Kohler, New Jersey Dept of Health; Virology Div, Bur of Laboratories, Bacterial Zoonoses Br, Bacterial Diseases Div, Bur of Epidemiology, CDC.

Editorial Note: The results of this investigation are typical of recent investigations of human psittacosis traced to pet birds. Generally, a large number of people are potentially exposed, and birds from many sources are found mixed together in the pet shop and wholesale facilities. Extensive investigation is required to trace potential contacts and sources, and, in many cases, poor record-keeping by dealers makes tracing of sources and contacts impossible. Finally, the quarantine and treatment requirements constitute a considerable economic hardship for the dealers.

The number of reported cases of psittacosis in humans has risen from 35 in 1973 to 93 in 1977. Sixty percent of last year's cases are known to have had contact with pet caged birds.

MMWR 28:50 (2/9/79)

Psittacosis — Virginia

On October 1, 1978, a 24-year-old female vivarium employee at a Virginia university became ill with fever, chills, malaise, and anorexia, followed several days later by a nonproductive cough and a severe headache. Physical examination revealed a firm, nontender, left axillary lymph node and dullness over the base of the left lung. A chest X ray revealed a left lower lobe infiltrate, but sputum was not obtained for culture. The patient was treated with Doxycycline,* 200 mg daily for 2 weeks; defervescence occurred in the first 24 hours. Complement-fixation testing of serum specimens revealed a rise in titer to *Chlamydia psittaci* from 1:16 on October 10 to 1:512 on October 27.

An investigation revealed that the patient's duties included cleaning cages of pigeons (the only birds to which she was exposed), rats, mice, and cats used for research purposes. There were approximately 40 pigeons, none of which appeared ill. She had been employed at the vivarium for 4 months and denied any other exposure to birds or fowl. Medical history did reveal, however, that she was anephric and on regular renal dialysis. No other cases of human respiratory illness were observed in connection with this vivarium.

The pigeons—obtained from a squab plant in South Carolina—were sacrificed and sent to CDC for culture; *C. psittaci* organisms were recovered from the tissues of 3 of 32 birds submitted. Psittacosis had been identified in the pigeons at this squab plant years previously and has been assumed to be endemic in the birds in the loft since that time; however, no cases of human psittacosis had been documented in the employees at the time of the earlier culturing, and no excess mortality had been noted in the pigeons. Therefore, it had been decided at that time not to treat the easily re-exposed pigeons.

Reported by CA Osterman, RN, RP Wenzel, MD, University of Virginia Hospital; RA Prindle, MD, Charlottesville Health Dept; GB Miller, Jr, MD, State Epidemiologist, Virginia Dept of Health; RL Parker, DVM, South Carolina State Dept of Health and Environmental Control; Viral Zoonoses Br, Virology Div, Bur of Laboratories, Field Services Div, Bacterial Zoonoses Br, Bacterial Diseases Div, Bur of Epidemiology, CDC.

Editorial Note: During 1968-1977, wild and domestic pigeons were associated with 88 (13%) of 657 cases of psittacosis in humans reported to CDC. However, this case is the only pigeon-associated human illness to be reported from a research facility in the past 10 years. Because pigeons may become exposed to infection while in the pigeon loft, they may represent a health hazard to employees of squab plants and research facilities and to pigeon fanciers. In this instance, no cases of psittacosis were uncovered during the investigation of the squab plant by the South Carolina State Department of Health and Environmental Control.

---

*Use of trade names is for identification only and does not constitute endorsement by the Public Health Service, U.S. Department of Health, Education, and Welfare.

MMWR 27:321 (9/1/78)

Q Fever — New York

On May 25, 1978, the Suffolk County Department of Health Services was informed by an infection control nurse at the Brookhaven Memorial Hospital that 2 days earlier a 27-year-old man had been admitted with a 4-day history of fever to 104 F (40 C), severe headache, chills, malaise, and vomiting. This patient had visited West Africa in April and was an employee of an exotic bird and reptile importing company in Deer Park, New York. Within 1 week, 3 other employees of that company were admitted to the same hospital with similar symptoms. One had a non-productive cough. All were treated with oral tetracycline with rapid resolution of their symptoms and complete recovery.

These 4 persons had all been involved in unpacking and deticking a shipment of approximately 500 ball pythons (*Python regius*), which were imported on May 3 from Accra, Ghana. Examination of the hemolymph of 5 ticks removed from these snakes indicated that all contained numerous bacteria, both bacillary and coccoid forms, and that 2 contained rickettsiae which were not further characterized. Three types of ticks were identified, namely, *Amblyomma nuttalli, Aponomma latum,* and *Aponomma flavomaculatum.*

Paired serum samples examined by the New York State Department of Health Laboratory revealed rising titers against the Q fever antigen by complement fixation. Serum specimens from the 4 hospitalized patients, tested at Rocky Mountain Laboratory, National Institutes of Health (NIH), by microimmunofluorescence, showed confirmatory rises in titers to Q fever.

Seven other persons were identified who had been in contact with the pythons, ticks from the pythons, or excreta of ticks or pythons. Of these, 5 had had febrile illnesses with similar, but somewhat milder, symptoms than the hospitalized group. Four of the 5 had been seen by their family physicians and had received oral tetracycline. The fifth did not see a physician. Serologic tests in 4 of these individuals confirmed a recent Q fever infection in one and probable Q fever infections in 2 others.

Samples of python blood, spleen and liver, as well as 15 live ticks and 5 frozen ticks removed from the pythons, were processed for attempted isolation of organisms; all were negative.

The county health department has been informed that 420 of the pythons have been sold to retailers all over the United States. The distribution list is unavailable at this time.
Reported by S Kim, MD, Patchogue, New York; S Guirgis, PhD, D Harris, MD, MPH, T Keelan, RN, MPH, M Mayer, MD, MPH, M Zaki, MD, DrPH, Suffolk County Dept of Health Services; L Steinert, RN, BS, Brookhaven Memorial Hospital; J Benach, PhD, D White, MS, DO Lyman, MD, State Epidemiologist, New York State Dept of Health; R Ormsbee, PhD, Rocky Mountain Laboratory, National Institute of Allergy and Infectious Diseases, NIH; Viral Diseases Div, Bur of Epidemiology, CDC.

Editorial Note: Q fever is an acute, systemic disease caused by *Coxiella burneti*. Characterized by the abrupt onset of headache, myalgia, chills and fever, it is usually a self-limited illness of 1-3 weeks duration. Pneumonia and hepatitis are frequent manifestations *(1)*, and endocarditis has been reported *(2)*. Patients with Q fever, as opposed to those with other rickettsial diseases, do not develop Weil-Felix agglutinins and virtually never have an accompanying rash. The treatment of choice is tetracycline or chloramphenicol.

Since the first described outbreak in this country in 1946 *(3)*, numerous outbreaks usually associated with cattle, sheep, and goats have been investigated. Various species of ticks (including *A. nuttalli*) carry the rickettsial organisms, but man is usually infected by inhaling aerosolized particles containing *C. burneti*.

Reptiles have rarely been documented as potential hosts for *C. burneti* *(4)*. Nevertheless, physicians seeing patients with a compatible illness and a history of ownership of pythons or other exotic pets should consider Q fever in their differential diagnosis, obtain suitable acute and convalescent blood specimens for serologic diagnosis, and report the illness to local and state health authorities.

References
1. Hoeprich PD (ed): Infectious Diseases: A Modern Treatise of Infectious Processes. New York, Harper and Row, 1977, pp 288-289
2. Freeman G, Hodson ME: Q fever endocarditis treated with trimethoprim and sulphamethoxasole. Br Med J 1:419-420, 1972
3. Irons JV, Topping WH, Shepard CC, Cox HR: Outbreak of Q fever in the United States. Public Health Rep 61:784-785, 1946
4. Tendeiro J: Nota previa sobre febre Q. Gaz Med Portuguesa 5:645-649, 1952

MMWR 28:230 (5/25/79)

Q Fever — United Kingdom

From 1967 to 1974, laboratories in the United Kingdom reported between 48 and 78 cases of Q fever annually, an average of about 59 cases a year. In the last 3 years the numbers have been somewhat greater: 104 cases in 1975, 117 in 1976, and 98 in 1977.

Improved diagnostic facilities and case reporting probably accounted for much of this increase. The 215 cases reported in 1976 and 1977 are reviewed here.

As in previous years, cases tended to be reported mostly in the summer months, and this tendency was more apparent in the long, hot summer of 1976 than in the cooler, wetter one of 1977. The preponderance of male cases in 1976 and 1977 was slightly less than in 1974-1975. Most cases reported were in adults of working age: there were 136 men (88%) and 52 women (85%) aged 15-64 years.

Less than 15% of patients gave a history of possible exposure; most had agricultural, forestry, or abattoir exposure. The distribution of cases by region showed that most were reported by laboratories in rural areas.

Pneumonia was reported in 52% of the patients, and pyrexia without localizing signs or symptoms in a further 22%. Seventeen percent of patients developed cardiac disease.

Endocarditis was diagnosed in 31 patients, 7 of whom had a prosthetic cardiac valve; only 12% of the males had endocarditis compared with 21% of the females, a pattern similar to that found in previous years. In 2 of the patients with endocarditis, *Coxiella burnetii* was isolated. One of these patients had had Q fever and a heart-valve replacement 4 years earlier, but high complement-fixation (CF) titers persisted in the intervening period despite intensive chemotherapy; during a clinical relapse the organism was isolated from a splenic biopsy. The other patient was a 26-year-old man with severe aortic regurgitation and endocarditis; both phase 1 and phase 2 antibody titers to *C. burnetii* were greater than 1:8,192, and the organism was isolated from the aortic valve at operation.

Two patients died. One was a 51-year-old man with pneumoconiosis and chronic bronchitis; he developed myocarditis and hepatitis and died with splenic infarction and massive cerebral emboli. He was thought to have had the infection for a considerable time because CF antibody titers were 1:32,000 for phase 2 and 1:4,096 for phase 1. The other patient who died was a woman with encephalitis, a rare complication, and a CF antibody titer of 1:2,048. Although mortality from Q fever is very low, some deaths from endocarditis, which has a long and chronic course in this disease, may not have been reported.

Three small outbreaks were reported. A severe influenza-like illness affected 4 of 20 young men in a small army unit. Another outbreak occurred in a family. The mother, aged 51 years, developed a pulmonary infarction in April 1976. Her phase 2 antibody titer rose within 3 weeks from 1:8 to 1:1,024; phase 1 antibody was undetectable on both occasions. Her husband and 2 children had influenza-like illnesses in June; the diagnoses for them were made on the basis of raised, single, phase 2 antibody titers. No common source of infection was discovered. The third outbreak involved 2 members of a film crew who developed pneumonia after handling straw and peat while working on a film.

Reported by the World Health Organization's Weekly Epidemiological Record 54:45-46, 1979.

MMWR 28:261 (6/8/79)

Q Fever in a U.S. Traveler to the Middle East

In March 1979, CDC was notified of a febrile illness occurring in a 64-year-old man from Syracuse, New York, who had recently participated in a group tour of the Middle East. The patient recalled having a mild upper-respiratory infection about 8 days after he and the group rode camels at Wadi Rum in Jordan. He was downwind of bedouins' flocks of goats and sheep longer than most of the group and was exposed to large amounts of dust blown from the direction of the animals. He noted no other potential exposure. He took tetracycline for 3 days and recovered.

One month later the patient was hospitalized with high fever, chills, malaise, and lethargy. Multiple non-caseating granulomas discovered by liver biopsy, a positive PPD* skin test, and inflammatory apical lung disease (indicated by radioactive isotope scan) led to an initial diagnosis of tuberculosis. Since chest X rays were normal, and cultures of liver and gastric washings did not yield mycobacteria, Q fever was suspected and later confirmed by significant rises in antibody titers to *Coxiella burnetii*. The patient recovered spontaneously and was subsequently treated with tetracycline. Upon request, the travel agency contacted the other 107 members of the tour. Twenty-five returned health questionnaires. None reported serious illness, although one noted symptoms of a mild upper-respiratory infection.

Reported by H Feldman, MD, Dept of Preventive Medicine, D Bornstein, MD, Dept of Medicine, Upstate University, Syracuse, New York; JS Marr, MD, New York City Epidemiologist, Bur of Preventable Diseases, New York City Dept of Health; R Rothenberg, MD, State Epidemiologist, New York State Dept of Health; P Fiset, MD, PhD, Univ of Maryland School of Medicine, Baltimore; Field Services Div, Respiratory and Special Pathogens Br, Viral Diseases Div, Bur of Epidemiology, CDC.

Editorial Note: Since Q fever was first described in 1937 in Australia, it has been recognized throughout the world, including in Jordan (*1,2*). *C. burnetii*, a rickettsia, is the infectious agent of Q fever. It may be harbored, inapparently, in reservoirs of cattle, sheep, goats, camels, wild animals, and ticks (*2,3*). This disease is commonly transmitted to humans in 2 ways: 1) by airborne dissemination in dust contaminated with rickettsia from placental or birth tissues or from excreta of infected animals, or 2) by processing infected animal products. The incubation period depends on the infecting dose but usually varies from 2 to 3 weeks. The severity of illness ranges from subclinical disease to a febrile pneumonia with sudden onset, retrobulbar headache, weakness, malaise, and diaphoresis. Mortality of untreated cases is less than 1%, but chronic endocarditis, hepatitis, and generalized infections can complicate the course. Diagnosis is usually made by noting a 4-fold complement-fixing, microagglutinating, or indirect-fluorescent antibody titer rise to *C. burnetii*.

Although this patient reported that he had probably received greater rickettsial exposure than other tour members, there may be other reasons why he contracted disease and others did not. However, it is possible that some members experienced mild or subclinical illness which was not reported. Q fever should be considered as a possible cause of acute illness in persons having contact with livestock in endemic areas of the world.

References
1. Hart RJC: The epidemiology of Q fever. Postgrad Med J 49:535-538, 1973
2. Kaplan MM, Bertagna P: The geographical distribution of Q fever. Bull WHO 13:829-860, 1955
3. American Public Health Association: Q fever, in Benenson AS (ed): Control of Communicable Diseases in Man. 12th Ed. Washington D.C., American Public Health Association, 1975, pp 248-250

---

*Purified protein derivative of tuberculin.

MMWR 28:333 (7/20/79)

Q Fever at a University Research Center — California

During the first 3 months of 1979, 11 confirmed and more than 30 presumptive cases of Q fever occurred among researchers and employees of the University of California, San Francisco (UCSF). One person died. Most, if not all, of the infections were introduced by pregnant sheep used in research. In the preceding 15 years, only 4 cases had been recognized at UCSF.

Preliminary results of a serologic survey of 580 employees revealed that 114 (19.6%) had complement-fixing (CF) antibodies (≥1:8) to *Coxiella burnetii*. This compares with only 4 positives (0.2%) among 2,200 specimens submitted to the Microbiology Laboratory of the San Francisco Department of Public Health (SFDPH) since routine testing of patients with respiratory infections began 2 years ago. At UCSF the highest prevalence of CF antibodies was in animal technicians and cage cleaners, and in those who worked on the floors where sheep were studied. Five of 9 employees who worked with soiled linen in the campus laundry had positive titers. Many other employees with positive titers had no direct contact with the research sheep, but used corridors and elevators where sheep were transported in open carts.

Approximately 600 pregnant ewes are supplied annually to UCSF researchers. In November 1978, 47% of 122 sheep in the supplier's flock were positive for Q fever antibodies. After the outbreak was recognized in April 1979, the sheep were removed to a separate building, which is in the process of being brought up to the National Institutes of Health's third level of containment ("P3") standards through the addition of negative air pressure, air locks, and high-efficiency particulate filters on exhaust ducts.

Editorial Note: Q fever is a rickettsial zoonosis readily transmitted by the airborne route in areas contaminated by tissues, such as the placenta, or by excreta of infected animals. Sheep, goats, and cattle are natural reservoirs; their infections are usually inapparent. In humans, the infection generally produces mild, influenza-like respiratory disease but sometimes pneumonia, hepatitis, or endocarditis, and, rarely, death.

This outbreak was recognized because the SFDPH routinely tests for Q fever in patients with respiratory infection or obscure hepatitis. Since few laboratories outside California do this (*1*), the incidence of Q fever in other medical centers remains largely unknown.

Animal vaccines, antibiotics, and improved animal husbandry are being investigated, but no means now exist to produce or maintain a flock free from Q fever and still large enough for research needs. It was therefore recommended that medical research centers using sheep take measures to minimize transmission of Q fever such as 1) monitoring the prevalence of Q fever antibodies in sheep; 2) housing sheep in containment quarters that preclude exposure of persons who do not work with sheep (*2*); 3) limiting access to persons who must work with sheep or perform essential maintenance services; 4) using acceptable microbiologic techniques to process sheep tissues; 5) sterilizing potentially contaminated fomites; 6) doing periodic serologic surveillance on investigators, animal handlers, and others potentially exposed to sheep; 7) informing persons exposed to sheep of the risks of Q fever and screening them for evidence of valvular heart disease; and 8) considering Q fever as a diagnosis in compatible illnesses.

References
1. CDC: Q fever in the United States, 1948-1977. J Infect Dis 139:613-615, 1979
2. Schachter J, Sung M, Meyer KF: Potential danger of Q fever in a university hospital environment. J Infect Dis 123:301-304, 1971

Reported by S Dritz, MD, MPH, A Back, DrPH, SFDPH; C Hine, MD, PhD, J Spinelli, DVM, R Morrish, DVM, UCSF; R Wade, PhD, MPH, State of California Occupational Safety and Health Administration; R Roberto, MD, California State Dept of Health Services, in California Morbidity Weekly Report, No. 23, June 15, 1979; Field Services Div, Bur of Epidemiology, CDC.

CHAPTER 6

Rocky Mountain Spotted Fever and Typhus

MMWR 28:181 (4/27/79)

Rocky Mountain Spotted Fever — United States, 1978

A provisional total of 1,011 cases of Rocky Mountain spotted fever (RMSF) were reported to CDC for 1978. This is a 12% decrease from 1977, when 1,153 cases (the highest recorded annual total) were reported. The incidence also dropped, from 0.53 to 0.46 cases/100,000 population, for the first time since 1970 (Figure 1).

The southeastern states accounted for 539 or 53% of all reported cases. North Carolina had the most cases, 203, for an incidence of 3.63 cases/100,000. Tennessee (114 cases) and Virginia (110) had the next highest rates, 2.62 and 2.14/100,000 population, respectively.

Case-report forms have been submitted on 946 cases or 94% of all reported cases. Of these, 537 (57%) have been confirmed by Weil-Felix agglutination, complement fixation, or microimmunofluorescent techniques. While the age distribution of cases (563 or 59.5% in individuals less than 20 years old) and the ratio of males to females (1.63:1) have remained essentially unchanged, the case-fatality rate dropped to 3.7% (35 fatalities out of 946 cases) from 4.9% (42 fatalities out of 856 cases) in 1977. In the group at highest risk, persons over the age of 40, the previous case-fatality rate of 12% also dropped—to 10%. However, the fatality rate for blacks rose to 16.4%, from 15.6% in 1977; for whites, this rate decreased from 4.1% to 3.1%.

Although cases occurred throughout the year, 95% of patients had onset between the 15th and 36th weeks (early April through early September).

Reported by Respiratory and Special Pathogens Br, Viral Diseases Div, Bur of Epidemiology, CDC.
Editorial Note: This is the first year since 1970 that the incidence of RMSF has decreased. Nevertheless, the incidence remains considerably higher than that recorded in 1959, when only 199 cases (0.11/100,000 population) were reported.

The data on age, sex, and race derived from case-report forms are similar to those noted in other reports (1-3). In 1978, this information was available on a higher percentage of reported cases (94%) than in previous years.

The high case-fatality rate in blacks may reflect differences in health-care availability as well as difficulties in detecting the characteristic early centripetal rash on darker pigmented skin. Fever and headache are the earliest symptoms of the disease and are often accompanied by myalgia, abdominal pain, nausea and vomiting, photophobia, and conjunctivitis. The presence of these may help in making the clinical diagnosis of RMSF, even when the rash is absent or undetected.

Therapy with tetracycline or chloramphenicol is usually begun before the diagnosis

FIGURE 1. Rocky Mountain spotted fever, reported cases per 100,000 population, by year, United States, 1950-1978*

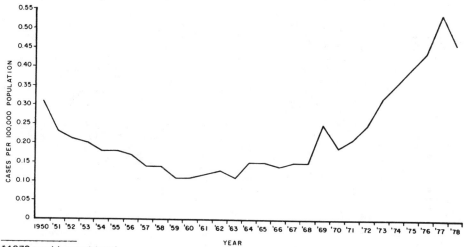

*1978 total is provisional.

is laboratory confirmed because the Weil-Felix agglutinin and complement-fixation tests are rarely positive until 10 to 14 days after onset of illness. Even though the sensitivity and specificity of these tests have been questioned recently (4), they remain the only widely available laboratory methods for confirming a suspected case.

References

1. Hattwick MAW, Peters AH, Gregg MB, Hanson BF: Surveillance of Rocky Mountain spotted fever. JAMA 225:1338-1343, 1973
2. Hattwick MAW, O'Brien RJ, Hanson BF: Rocky Mountain spotted fever. Epidemiology of an increasing problem. Ann Intern Med 84:732-739, 1976
3. D'Angelo LJ, Winkler WG, Bregman DJ: Rocky Mountain spotted fever in the United States, 1975-1977. J Infect Dis 138:273-276, 1978
4. Hechemy KE: Laboratory diagnosis of Rocky Mountain spotted fever. N Engl J Med 300:859-860, 1979

MMWR 27 (A.S., 1978): 72

Typhus Fever, Tick-Borne (Rocky Mountain Spotted Fever)

In 1978, 1,063 cases (0.49 cases/100,000) of Rocky Mountain spotted fever were reported to CDC, a decrease from the 1,153 cases (0.53 cases/100,000) reported in 1977. This was the first drop in case reporting since 1970, interrupting an otherwise steadily increasing trend. Again, the South Atlantic states accounted for the majority of reported cases (53.3%). Most cases continued to occur from May through September, most commonly in children and young adults. Less than 5% of reported cases are fatal. The disease is more serious in those older than 40.

TYPHUS FEVER, TICK-BORNE (Rocky Mountain Spotted Fever) — Reported Cases by County, United States, 1978

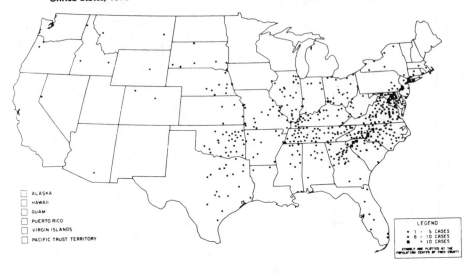

MMWR 27:215 (6/30/78)

Laboratory-Acquired Endemic Typhus — Maryland

Three cases of serologically confirmed typhus fever occurred in personnel assigned to the Rickettsial Division of the Naval Medical Research Institute, Bethesda, Maryland, during the period March 12-21, 1978. An epidemiologic investigation to identify the source of infection revealed that all 3 cases resulted from breaks in prescribed technique, 2 of which were unrecognized at the time they occurred.

Patient 1: A 32-year-old female reported ill on March 15 after 3 days of headache, neck pain, fever of 37.5-39.4 C (99-103 F), recurrent chills, and chest discomfort. Sixteen days before, she had harvested *Rickettsia typhi* from infected eggs. She had used a mask only intermittently during the purification process, several steps of which involved the risk of aerosol generation. She was treated with tetracycline (TCN) and became afebrile within 48 hours. Her antibody titers for *R. typhi*, as determined by the microagglutination technique (1), were 1:64 on March 15 and > 1:512 12 days later. Proteus OX 19 agglutinins rose from an undetectable level to 1:640 on the same samples.

Patient 2: A 29-year-old male laboratory technician reported ill on March 16 with an oral temperature of 39 C (102 F) and a 2-day history of headache and nausea, which had progressed to fever and sweats. On March 3, he had accidentally stuck his finger with a needle used to inject steroids into mice infected with *R. typhi*. He had not obtained medical advice until March 15, however, 2 days after onset of symptoms. He was treated with TCN and became asymptomatic within 48 hours. His antibody titers on March 16 and March 29 were 1:32 and >1:512, respectively, by microagglutination using *R. typhi* antigen, and 0 and 1:1280 for Proteus OX 19.

Patient 3: On March 9, a 30-year-old female laboratory technician assisted in conducting metabolic studies, performed in open vessels, of whole *R. typhi* organisms. During the 6-hour experiment, she wore her gown, mask, and gloves only when she was directly over the vessels. Although much of the experiment was conducted in a biologic safety cabinet, the vessels had been removed and placed on an open bench top for a period during the experiment. She presented sick on March 22 with a 2-day history of fever and malaise. Physical examination showed a temperature of 37.4 C (99.4 F) and pharyngeal injection. She was treated symptomatically when no history of exposure was obtained. She did not improve and returned on March 26 with fever of 38.3-40 C (101-104 F), chills, and frontal headache. Examination showed a scanty macular rash on her back, and she was hospitalized and treated with TCN. She became afebrile within 72 hours. Her disease was confirmed serologically with titers to *R. typhi* antigens rising from 1:16 on March 27 to 1:256 by April 4, as determined by microagglutination. Proteus OX 19 agglutination titers rose from 0 on March 27 to 1:640 on April 2.

All people working in the Rickettsial Division were bled, and antibody titers for *R. typhi*, *R. prowazeki*, and *R. tsutsugamushi* were performed on the serum samples. Nineteen individuals, including the 3 cases, had no pre-existing antibody to these rickettsiae. These cases represented an attack rate of *R. typhi* infection among susceptibles of 15.8%. Excluding 4 individuals who worked solely with formalin-killed organisms, the attack rate among exposed susceptibles was 3/15 or 20%. Corrective measures taken included the re-emphasis of all routine laboratory procedures and re-education of the technical staff in proper techniques for handling such organisms.

Reported by J Bellanca, MD, MPH, P Iannin, MD, B Hamory, MD, WF Miner, MD, MPH, J Salaki, MD, M Stek Jr, MS, MD, DTMH, National Naval Medical Center, Bethesda, Md; Office of Biosafety, Office of the Center Director, and Viral Diseases Div, Bur of Epidemiology, CDC.

Editorial Note: These cases resulted from unrelated exposures in which the routine safety precautions and reporting systems for laboratory accidents were not followed. As Class 3 agents (2), all rickettsiae should be handled in special containment laboratories, which routinely use proper microbiologic techniques and biologic safety cabinets. Moreover, all laboratory accidents involving these organisms should be promptly reported, and individuals involved should be evaluated by a physician. Under no circumstances should self-evaluation and self-treatment bypass these more formal mechanisms.

Unfortunately, laboratory-associated infections with organisms of the rickettsial groups are not uncommon (3-5). Since adequate immunoprophylaxis for *R. typhi* and *R. rickettsiae* is not now available, prevention of laboratory-associated infection rests on scrupulous care in handling and containing these organisms.

References
1. Fisel P, Ormsbee RA, Silberman R, Peacock M, Spielman SH: A microagglutination technique for detection and measurement of rickettsial antibodies. Acta Virol 13:60-66, 1969
2. Classification of Etiologic Agents on the Basis of Hazard. U.S. Department of Health, Education, and Welfare, 1975
3. Pike RM: Laboratory-associated infections: Summary and analysis of 3,921 cases. Health Lab Sci 13:105-114, 1976
4. Oster CN, Burke DS, Kenyon RH, et al: Laboratory-acquired Rocky Mountain spotted fever: The hazard of aerosol transmission. N Engl J Med 297:859-863, 1977
5. MMWR 26:84, 1977

MMWR 27 (A.S., 1978): 72

TYPHUS FEVER, FLEA-BORNE (ENDEMIC, MURINE) — Reported Cases per 100,000 Population by Year, United States, 1930–1977

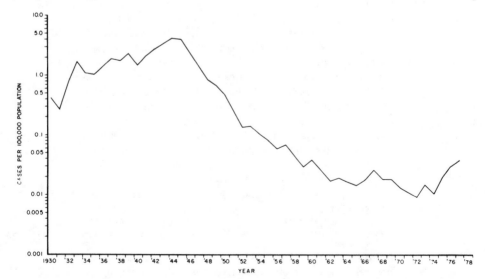

TYPHUS FEVER, FLEA-BORNE (Endemic, Murine) —
Reported Cases by Year, United States, 1969—1978

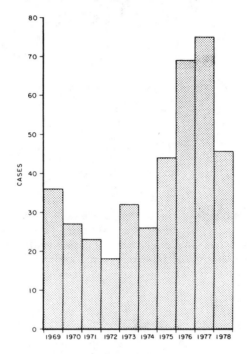

CHAPTER 7

Typhoid Fever

MMWR 27:231 (7/7/78)

Typhoid Vaccine

INTRODUCTION

The incidence of typhoid fever has declined steadily in the United States in the last half century, and in recent years fewer than 400 cases have been reported annually. The continuing downward trend is due largely to better sanitation and other control measures; vaccine is not deemed to have played a significant role. An increasing proportion of cases reported in the United States (about 50% in 1976) were acquired by travelers in other countries.

TYPHOID AND PARATYPHOID A AND B VACCINES

Although typhoid vaccines* have been used for many decades, only recently has definitive evidence of their effectiveness been observed in well-controlled field investigations. Several different preparations of typhoid vaccine have been shown to protect 70-90% of recipients, depending in part of the degree of their subsequent exposure.

The effectiveness of paratyphoid A vaccine has never been established, and field trials have shown that usually small amounts of paratyphoid B antigens contained in "TAB" vaccines (vaccines combining typhoid and paratyphoid A and B antigens) are not effective. Knowing this and recognizing that combining paratyphoid A and B antigens with typhoid vaccine increases the risk of vaccine reaction, one should use typhoid vaccine alone.

VACCINE USAGE

Routine typhoid vaccination is no longer recommended for persons in the United States. Selective immunization is, however, indicated for:

1. Persons with intimate exposure to a documented typhoid carrier, such as would occur with continued household contact.

2. Travelers to areas where there is a recognized risk of exposure to typhoid because of poor food and water sanitation. It should be emphasized, however, that even after typhoid vaccination there should be careful selection of foods and water in these areas.

There is no evidence that typhoid vaccine is of value in the United States in controlling common-source outbreaks. Furthermore, there is no reason to use typhoid

---

*Official name: Typhoid Vaccine

vaccine for persons in areas of natural disaster such as floods or for persons attending rural summer camps.

Primary Immunization

On the basis of the field trials referred to above, the following dosages of typhoid vaccine available in the United States are recommended:

Adults and children 10 years and older: 0.5 ml subcutaneously on 2 occasions, separated by 4 or more weeks.

Children less than 10 years old*: 0.25 ml subcutaneously on 2 occasions, separated by 4 or more weeks.

In instances where there is not sufficient time for 2 doses at the interval specified, it has been common practice to give 3 doses of the same volumes listed above at weekly intervals, although it is recognized that this schedule may be less effective. When vaccine must be administered for travel overseas under constraint of time, a second dose may be administered en route at the more desirable interval.

Booster Doses

Under conditions of continued or repeated exposure, a booster dose should be given at least every 3 years. Even when more than a 3-year interval has elapsed since the prior immunization, a single booster injection is sufficient.

The following alternate routes and dosages of booster immunization can be expected to produce comparable antibody responses. Generally less reaction follows vaccination by the intradermal route, except when acetone-killed and dried vaccine is used. (The latter vaccine should not be given intradermally.)

Adults and children 10 years and older: 0.5 ml subcutaneously or 0.1 ml intradermally.

Children 6 months to 10 years: 0.25 ml subcutaneously or 0.1 ml intradermally.

PRECAUTIONS AND CONTRAINDICATIONS

Typhoid vaccination often results in 1-2 days of discomfort at the site of injection. The local reaction may be accompanied by fever, malaise, and headache.

SELECTED BIBLIOGRAPHY

Ashcroft MT, Singh B, Nicholson CC, et al: A seven-year field trial of two typhoid vaccines in Guyana. Lancet 2:1056-1059, 1967

Cvjetanovic B, Uemura K: The present status of field and laboratory studies of typhoid and paratyphoid vaccine: With special reference to studies sponsored by the World Health Organization. Bull WHO 32:29-36, 1965

Hejfec LB, Levina LA, Kuz'minova ML, et al: Controlled field trials of paratyphoid B vaccine and evaluation of the effectiveness of a single administration of typhoid vaccine. Bull WHO 38:907-915, 1968

Hornick RB, Woodward TE, McCrumb FR, et al: Typhoid fever vaccine—yes or no? Med Clin North Am 51:617-623, 1967

Hornick RB, Greisman SE, Woodward TE, et al: Typhoid fever: Pathogenesis and immunologic control. N Engl J Med 283:686-691, 739-746, 1970

Mallory A, Belden EA, Brachman PS: The current status of typhoid fever in the United States and a description of an outbreak. J Infect Dis 119:673-676, 1969

Polish Typhoid Committee: Controlled field trials and laboratory studies on the effectiveness of typhoid vaccines in Poland, 1961-64: Final report. Bull WHO 34:211-222, 1966

Schroeder S: The interpretation of serologic tests for typhoid fever. JAMA 206:839-840, 1968

Typhoid vaccines. Lancet 2:1075-1076, 1967

Yugoslav Typhoid Commission: A controlled field trail of the effectiveness of acetone-dried and inactivated and heat-phenol-inactivated typhoid vaccines in Yugoslavia: Report. Bull WHO 30:623-630, 1964

Published in MMWR 15:247, 1966; revised 18(43 Suppl):26, 1969; revised 21(25 Suppl):38-39, 1972

---

*Since febrile reactions to typhoid vaccine are common in children, an antipyretic may be indicated.

MMWR 28:201 (5/4/79)

Typhoid Fever — New York

In the last week of July 1978, the New York City Department of Health was notified that severe febrile illnesses requiring hospitalization had occurred among members of a religious group in Brooklyn. An epidemiologic investigation revealed that 9 of approximately 40 people who had attended a party on June 30 were hospitalized for typhoid fever, diagnosed by blood culture.

The illness occurred 7 to 23 days following that party. The patients ranged in age from 4-49 years (mean age, 29.2 years; median age, 32 years). Six patients were male; 3 were female. None gave a history of foreign travel in the preceding month. Symptoms included fever (100%), chills or sweats (67%), fatigue and weakness (44%), headache (33%), vomiting (33%), cough (33%), anorexia (33%), and diarrhea (22%). Blood isolates were positive for *Salmonella typhi*, phage-type F3, and were sensitive to ampicillin. All 9 patients were treated with either ampicillin or chloramphenicol and recovered without sequellae.

In early August a food questionnaire was distributed to the party guests. A cake served at the party was statistically associated with illness (p<.03, Fisher's exact test). Stool culturing of the bakery employees failed to uncover a carrier.

In November 1978, 2 more hospitalized cases of typhoid fever from this community were reported. One patient had *S. typhi*, phage type F3, isolated from his blood, and the other was diagnosed by a typical clinical course of typhoid fever and by elevated antibody titers to H antigen (1:320 initially and 1:160 1 week later). The latter patient had no history of typhoid immunization. The patients had onset of symptoms 21 and 27 days, respectively, after attending a second party with approximately 70 guests in late September. Neither patient had a recent history of foreign travel.

A questionnaire was distributed to the guests at the second party. No single food or beverage was statistically incriminated.

No guest had attended both parties, but the second party was held in the home of one of the food handlers from the first party. Although no *S. typhi* organisms were found in 4 stool samples from this person, stools from 1 member of his family, a 72-year-old man, grew *S. typhi*, phage type F3. This person denied any history of typhoid fever or prolonged febrile illness, but he did have mild diarrhea that had begun approximately 4 weeks after the second party. He denied eating, preparing, or serving any food at the second party. He also denied helping prepare food for the first party. The most recent stool culture from this man, taken in mid-March 1979, remained positive; thus, he has been culture positive for at least 3½ months and may be a chronic carrier. However, repeated cultures over the course of a year will be needed to verify chronic-carrier status. This presumptive carrier has agreed not to serve food to individuals outside his immediate family.

Investigation, including a dye study, of the plumbing at this family's home showed no back siphonage. Water samples were negative for *S. typhi*. The mechanism of contamination of food at the parties is unknown.

Another person with typhoid fever was identified in this community in January 1979. The patient was a 26-year-old female cousin of the presumptive carrier. She had eaten food at his home in November and had onset of symptoms approximately 5 weeks later. She gave no history of foreign travel. The organism from her stool has not been phage typed.

Over the past 10 years, there have been 17 confirmed cases of typhoid fever in addition to those described above, in members of this same community in Brooklyn. The presumptive carrier was related by marriage to a 1976 patient. No direct association between the earlier patient and the infection of the presumptive carrier could be made since the isolate from the earlier patient was not phage typed.

Reported by WF McKinley, ET Melvin, MD, D Mildvan, MD, JW Winter, PhD, S Yancovitz, MD, Beth Israel Medical Center; EJ Bottone, PhD, Mt. Sinai Hospital; G Schlanger, PhD, Maimonides Hospital; J DeZuane, PhD, S Friedman, MD, M Gellman, MPH, EB Harvey, RN, JS Marr, MD, New York City Epidemiologist, W Mansdorf, MPH, B Neal, RN, J Payne, RN, H Vogel, PhD, JC Welton, MPH, New York City Dept of Health; Enteric Diseases Br, Bacterial Diseases Div, Bur of Epidemiology, CDC.

Editorial Note: Typhoid fever is now uncommon in the United States. In 1942, there were 5,595 reported cases *(1)*; in 1976, the number of reported isolations (cases and carriers) was only 529 *(2)*.

Most cases of typhoid fever in the United States are not associated with known outbreaks. In 1975 and 1976, 87% of typhoid cases acquired in the United States were reported as single cases; the remaining 13% of cases occurred in connection with the only 3 outbreaks reported to CDC on surveillance questionnaires *(3)*.

The F3 phage type found in this outbreak is uncommon. In New York City from 1974 through 1978, none of approximately 200 reported isolations of *S. typhi* were of the F3 phage type. Similarly, in the United States in 1975 and 1976, none of the *S. typhi* isolates reported to the CDC from cases were of the F3 phage type *(3)*.

References

1. Rubin RH, Weinstein L: Salmonellosis. Microbiologic, Pathologic and Clinical Features. New York, Stratton Intercontinental Medical Book Corp, 1977, p 13
2. CDC: Salmonella Surveillance Report (No. 127). Atlanta, CDC, 1976
3. Ryder RW, Blake PA: Typhoid fever in the United States, 1975 and 1976. J Infect Dis 139: 124-126, 1979

MMWR 28:521 (11/9/79)

Laboratory-Associated Typhoid Fever

In early 1979, CDC was informed that a case of typhoid fever had occurred in a microbiology laboratory technician who had worked with a *Salmonella typhi* culture as part of a laboratory-proficiency exercise. Subsequent investigation and review revealed 2 other cases associated with that exercise, 1 of several nationwide programs for proficiency testing of microbiology laboratory personnel for the purpose of licensure or continuing education. To determine if this was an ongoing problem, all reported cases of typhoid fever since January 1977 were reviewed. In addition, state epidemiologists were alerted to the situation and asked to report any laboratory-associated cases.

As a result of this investigation, a total of 19 cases of laboratory-associated typhoid fever were identified that had occurred since January 1977. None was fatal. The exposure for 6 of these cases was national or state proficiency exercises from 4 different programs. (The organisms were provided as lyophilized cultures.) Laboratory stock strains were the source for 11 patients, and routine laboratory isolates from clinical specimens accounted for the other 2 cases.

All 19 laboratory exposures to *S. typhi* occurred within 3 weeks of onset of illness. For 13 patients the bacteriophage type of the strain to which they were exposed in the laboratory is known to have been the same as the strain isolated from them. In the remaining 6 patients a culture of the isolated strain is not yet available for typing.

The 19 patients were from 14 states; 7 were medical technology or medical students, and 12 were non-students whose laboratory experience ranged from 2 to 16 years. The exposure for 11 patients occurred during exercises to identify unknown organisms; for

4 patients it was due to laboratory accidents; and for 3 patients there was no known direct contact, but co-workers in the laboratory had been working with *S. typhi* as an unknown. Five of the patients had current *S. typhi* immunizations. Further investigations are ongoing.

Reported by Enteric Diseases Br, Bacterial Diseases Div, Bur of Epidemiology, Enteric Section, Enterobacteriology Br, Bacteriology Div, Bur of Laboratories, and Office of Biosafety, CDC.

Editorial Note: Laboratory-associated typhoid fever was well-recognized 30 years ago *(1)*, but recently there has been little mention of this problem. The cases discussed here represent 5% of the domestically-acquired cases of typhoid fever in the United States reported for the period January 1, 1977 to August 31, 1979. These cases further demonstrate the ever-present need for all laboratory personnel to be aware of, and to diligently practice, laboratory safety. Instructors of medical and clinical microbiology students should emphasize the necessity for strict adherence to safety procedures. It is prudent to avoid hand-to-mouth activities while working with *S. typhi* and other enteric pathogens. Since all but 2 of the cases reported here were associated with the voluntary introduction of *S. typhi* into the laboratory environment, this problem should be preventable in most cases.

Typhoid immunization is recommended, but not necessarily required as a condition of employment, for individuals who are exposed to *S. typhi* on a daily basis *(2)*. It is urged that state and local health departments be notified whenever a laboratory infection is suspected.

References
1. Sulkin SE, Pike RM: Survey of laboratory-acquired infections. Am J Public Health 41:769-781, 1951
2. CDC: Laboratory Safety at the Center for Disease Control. Atlanta, Office of Biosafety, CDC, 1974

MMWR 28:593 (12/21/79)

Follow-up on Laboratory-Associated Typhoid Fever

In a previous article *(1)*, 19 cases of laboratory-associated typhoid fever that had occurred since January 1977 were identified. Further investigation has identified 6 more cases. Nine of these 25 cases were in students conducting laboratory exercises in medical technology or microbiology courses; 2 cases were in technologists working with cultures isolated from clinical specimens; the remainder were associated with strains provided through proficiency exercises. While these 25 cases constitute only 2% of all reported typhoid cases in the United States since January 1977, they represent 10% of the reported domestically acquired cases that were not associated with outbreaks or carriers.

Reported by the Office of Biosafety, Office of the Center Director, Bur of Laboratories, and Bur of Epidemiology, CDC.

Editorial Note: The problem of laboratory-associated typhoid fever serves as a marker for other, less well-described, laboratory-acquired enteric infections, and suggests that such infections may not be uncommon. Laboratory infections with salmonellae and other Class 2 pathogens *(2)* are most commonly associated with ingestion or accidental self-inoculation of the infectious agent. Less frequently, infections in laboratory personnel may result from exposure to aerosols generated by such activities as grinding, loop-flaming, centrifuging, and blending, and from aerosols resulting from forceful pipetting or spills.

Most of these 25 laboratory-acquired infections of typhoid fever presumably resulted from poor safety practices, and thus could have been avoided by adherence to proper microbiological technique, personal hygiene, and good safety practices. Mouth pipetting should not be permitted under any circumstances. Eating, drinking, and smoking must be prohibited in the laboratory. Hands should be washed after handling potentially infectious materials, and work surfaces should be decontaminated with an acceptable germicide after completion of bench activities and immediately after spills. All laboratory wastes should be decontaminated by experienced personnel, and accidents or exposures should be reported immediately to supervisors for appropriate medical appraisal and surveillance. Non-laboratory workers should not be present in a microbiology laboratory.

Potential pathogens have been included in proficiency exercises and proficiency-testing programs on the grounds that trained microbiologists charged with the responsibility for isolation and identification of pathogenic agents should be tested on their ability to do so. The need for inclusion of such agents in a general microbiology course is less clear. When possible, microorganisms for testing and teaching purposes should have low virulence for humans. Bacteria with multiple or unusual antibiotic-resistance patterns should be avoided unless this characteristic is an essential part of the learning exercise. An atypical antibiotic-resistant strain may complicate treatment in the event of an accidental infection and may potentiate transmission.

The Bacteriology Division in the Bureau of Laboratories at CDC is currently evaluating 3 strains of *Salmonella typhi* reported to have reduced virulence. Such strains must be otherwise typical if they are to be used for teaching purposes. Several potentially useful nontoxigenic strains of *Vibrio cholerae* will be similarly evaluated. The results of these evaluations and the procedure for distributing suitable teaching strains will be reported, when available. Such strains should decrease the likelihood of laboratory-acquired infections or decrease the severity of disease, but they cannot be used as a substitute for laboratory safety. Adherence to adequate safety practices is just as essential with strains of diminished virulence as with a fully virulent strain.

References
1. MMWR 28:521-522, 1979
2. U.S. Public Health Service: Classification of Etiologic Agents on the Basis of Hazard. Atlanta, Center for Disease Control, 1974

MMWR 27 (A.S., 1978): 70

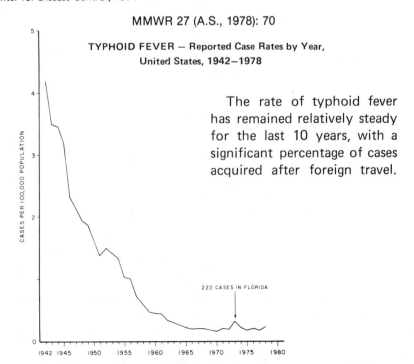

TYPHOID FEVER — Reported Case Rates by Year, United States, 1942—1978

The rate of typhoid fever has remained relatively steady for the last 10 years, with a significant percentage of cases acquired after foreign travel.

222 CASES IN FLORIDA

CHAPTER 8

Salmonellosis

MMWR 27:315 (8/25/78)

Salmonellae in Precooked Roasts of Beef — New York

The U.S. Department of Agriculture (USDA) has issued a recall of precooked roasts of beef associated with 3 outbreaks of salmonellosis in New York that have involved a total of 41 persons, to date. *Salmonella* organisms have been isolated from the implicated beef.

The first outbreak was associated with a luncheon buffet in Oswego County, New York, on July 21, 1978. Within 48 hours of this luncheon, 30 of the 78 persons who attended had developed gastrointestinal illness; 2 were hospitalized. A *Salmonella* group C1 organism was isolated from 1 patient, and *Salmonella* C1 and C2 from another. Since the initial outbreak, 11 other cases of salmonellosis in this and a neighboring county have been traced to precooked roast beef.

Investigation by the county and state health departments determined that 1 of 2 whole, unopened roasts, produced on the same date as the beef used at the luncheon, was positive for a *Salmonella* C2 organism. Cultures by the USDA of 4 of 12 whole, unopened roasts from production dates later than those associated with the initial outbreak have also been found to contain isolates of *Salmonella* groups C1, C2, and E organisms. On August 11, the New York State Department of Agriculture initiated seizure of the implicated product, which was produced by a New Jersey company and distributed in New York and northern New Jersey.

Serotyping of the human and beef isolates from the outbreak is in progress at CDC.

Reported by DO Lyman, MD, State Epidemiologist, New York Dept of Health; R Altman, MD, State Epidemiologist, New Jersey Dept of Health; USDA; Epidemiologic Investigations Laboratory Br, Enteric Diseases Br, Bacterial Diseases Div, Bur of Epidemiology, CDC.

Editorial Note: This is the fourth consecutive year in which precooked roasts of beef have been associated with outbreaks of salmonellosis *(1-3)*. All of these outbreaks have occurred in the summer. As a result of the outbreak last year, when cases due primarily to *S. newport* occurred in 7 northeastern states, the USDA issued regulations that precooked roast beef be cooked to an internal temperature of 145 F (62.7 C) to eliminate salmonellae. However, when beef is cooked to this temperature, it no longer has the rare appearance preferred by many consumers. Consequently, roast beef producers in collaboration with independent laboratories presented to the USDA data supporting various time and temperature formulas that eliminate salmonellae from beef but maintain its rare appearance. Subsequently, beginning July 18, the USDA has allowed 15 alternative time and temperature formulas for production of beef *(4)*.

USDA tests have determined that the producer of the beef associated with the current outbreak did not follow the USDA regulations.

References
1. MMWR 25:34, 1976   3. MMWR 26:277, 1977
2. MMWR 25:333, 1976   4. Federal Register 43:30793, July 18, 1978

MMWR 28:117 (3/16/79)

Salmonella Gastroenteritis Associated with Milk — Arizona

An outbreak of *Salmonella typhimurium* var *copenhagen* gastroenteritis epidemiologically linked to a commercial milk supplier occurred October 2-16, 1978, in 2 northern Arizona cities (population 8,135 and 10,750, respectively) located 60 miles apart.

The increased number of cases due to this organism was first noted in mid-October. Public announcement and contact with primary-care physicians and local laboratories identified 66 primary cases of diarrhea. Fifteen patients were hospitalized. Cultures of stools from 23 patients grew *S. typhimurium* var *copenhagen*, 1 grew *S. anatum*, 1 grew *S. oranienburg*, 1 grew salmonellae that were not typed, 20 were negative, and 20 were not cultured. Only 1 additional isolate of *S. typhimurium* var *copenhagen* was identified from other areas of Arizona in October.

Demographic data and food histories were obtained by means of 2 questionnaire surveys administered October 17-26 to most persons known to have had diarrhea and, where possible, to age-matched neighborhood controls. A case was defined as a person with diarrhea with onset from October 1-26. Twenty-three confirmed cases and 23 controls were surveyed. In families where there was more than 1 case, only data on the earliest case were analyzed.

The 23 patients ranged in age from 6 months to 59 years (median 11 years). Sixteen were female, 7 male. Thirteen lived in 1 city, 9 in another, and 1 in an area midway between the other 2 cities. Twelve of the patients attended school, but no school had more than 4 cases. In addition to diarrhea, patients reported fever (91%), abdominal pain (87%), nausea (57%), and vomiting (52%).

The first questionnaire requested a history of consumption of selected foods during the previous 3 days. Nineteen of 23 (83%) cases and 7 of 23 (30%) controls had consumed 1 brand of milk (p<.001*). Of the 19 who recalled drinking this milk in the 72 hours before illness, 16 had drunk whole milk and 1 low-fat milk; 2 did not specify.

The second questionnaire asked about the use of 100 food items in the month before onset of illness. Milk available to the communities was listed by brand. The same brand of milk implicated in the first questionnaire was found to be significantly associated with illness: 22 of 23 (96%) of patients but only 11 of 23 (48%) controls had drunk the milk (p<.01*). None of the other food items, which included 7 other brands of milk, showed significant differences between cases and controls.

The implicated brand of milk is produced in a local dairy, which distributes homogenized, low-fat, and chocolate milk to both of the affected cities and several smaller surrounding communities. A review of routine samples submitted to the state laboratory on October 3 showed a sample of pasteurized whole milk with a coliform count of 230 colonies per ml. The accepted coliform count in Grade A pasteurized milk is ≤10 colonies per ml. However, the absence of phosphatase in this sample indicated adequate pasteurization had occurred. (This enzyme, normally present in raw milk, is inactivated by the

---

*McNemar's matched pair test

high temperatures used in this process.) Inspections of the dairy on October 16 and October 24 revealed no major breaks in technique. All pasteurized samples taken on October 16 were free of coliforms; 1 sample of raw milk, however, grew S. typhimurium var copenhagen. Stool specimens from all dairy employees were negative. There were no coliform organisms found in the water from the well supplying the plant.

Control measures included recall of all milk that had been produced by the dairy before October 16 and biweekly culturing of samples of the dairy's pasteurized milk products.

Reported by LB Dominguez, BS, A Kelter, MD, FJ Marks, BA, WB Press, MS, KM Starko, MD, Acting State Epidemiologist, Arizona Dept of Health Services; Field Services Div, Bacterial Diseases Div, Bur of Epidemiology, CDC.

Editorial Note: The association of pasteurized milk with enteric infection is now uncommon in the United States. Since 1970, 7 milkborne outbreaks with confirmed bacterial etiologies have been reported to CDC. *Salmonella* organisms have been responsible for 4 of these. Two have been caused by consumption of certified raw milk contaminated with S. dublin (1), 1 was linked to ingestion of raw milk containing S. typhimurium (2), and 1 was associated with pasteurized milk contaminated with S. newport (3).

S. typhimurium var copenhagen is differentiated from S. typhimurium by the absence of O antigen 5. Although S. typhimurium is the serotype most frequently isolated from humans in the United States, S. typhimurium var copenhagen was responsible for only 1.4% of the total Salmonella isolates reported to CDC from humans in 1978.

The exact mechanism of contamination of the milk in this outbreak is unclear. Contamination after pasteurization is 1 possibility, supported by the fact that phosphatase was inactivated. Inadequate or incomplete pasteurization could also have occurred, however. The finding of the epidemic strain of Salmonella in the raw milk would support this conclusion. The high coliform count in the pasteurized milk is compatible with either hypothesis.

References
1. MMWR 23:175, 1974
2. MMWR 26:239, 1977
3. MMWR 24:413, 1975

MMWR 28:129 (3/23/79)

Salmonellosis Associated with Consumption of Nonfat Powdered Milk — Oregon

One symptomatic case of salmonellosis and 2 asymptomatic *Salmonella* infections have occurred in Oregon in association with consumption of 1 brand of nonfat powdered milk. Implicated lots of this milk have been voluntarily recalled.

The case occurred in a 14-month-old infant, who developed an acute illness consisting of diarrhea and fever on January 15, 1979. A stool culture from the patient yielded S. agona and S. typhimurium, as did a culture of a previously opened box of nonfat powdered milk taken from the patient's home. Stool cultures of the patient's family detected S. typhimurium and S. agona infections in an asymptomatic 3-year-old sibling.

A laboratory worker who was aware of the first case and had nonfat powdered milk of the same brand in his home submitted stool cultures for testing for salmonellae from himself and his wife. His wife had not consumed the nonfat powdered milk, but he had. His stool culture was positive for S. typhimurium and S. agona; his wife's was negative. S. agona and S. typhimurium organisms were isolated from the open box of powdered

TABLE 1. Reported *Salmonella typhimurium* and *S. agona* isolates, by state, November 1977-January 1978 and November 1978-January 1979

State	*S. typhimurium* isolates		*S. agona* isolates	
	November 1977- January 1978	November 1978- January 1979	November 1977- January 1978	November 1978- January 1979
Oregon	48	52	1	2
Washington	43	57	7	4
California	170	131	48	42
Utah	10	5	1	2
Idaho	10	7	0	0

milk taken from their home.

In an effort to detect other cases of salmonellosis associated with consumption of the product, the Oregon Department of Human Resources and local health departments conducted a telephone survey of 55 persons in Oregon who had had salmonellosis caused by *S. typhimurium* or *S. agona* after June 1978. None of these patients gave a history of having consumed the implicated milk.

Investigation by the Food and Drug Administration (FDA) has determined that the lot of nonfat powdered milk consumed by all 3 infected persons was packaged on October 26, 1978, and was distributed to Oregon. On February 14, 1979, the state health division released information concerning the problem. The lots of the implicated brand packaged between May 1 and November 1, 1978, were voluntarily withdrawn from the market.

Cultures by the FDA of the only 6 available unopened packages of nonfat powdered milk from the same lot as that consumed by the infected persons were negative for *Salmonella* organisms.

Oregon reported 11 isolations of *S. typhimurium* for January 1978 and 28 for January 1979. However, a review of reported *S. typhimurium* and *S. agona* isolations in Oregon and 4 other western states for the periods November 1977-January 1978 and November 1978-January 1979 revealed no significant variations (Table 1).

Reported by JD Furlong, W Lee, Multnomah County Health Division; LR Foster, MD, Deputy State Epidemiologist, LP Williams, DVM, DrPH, Oregon State Health Div; FDA; USDA; Enteric Diseases Br, Bacterial Diseases Div, Bur of Epidemiology, CDC.

Editorial Note: Pasteurization as a routine procedure with milk significantly reduced the problem of milk as a vehicle for transmitting *Salmonella* and other infections (*1,2*). Nonfat powdered milk has only occasionally been shown to be a vehicle of salmonellosis (*3,4*). The U.S. Department of Agriculture (USDA), which monitors plants producing nonfat powdered milk, has detected *Salmonella* contamination in up to 1.9% of product samples tested since 1970. The 3 most commonly found serotypes have been *S.anatum*, *S. cubana*, and *S. tennessee*. Culture-positive lots are reprocessed.

References
1. Wilson GS: The pasteurization of milk. London, E. Arnold & Co., 1942
2. Marth EH: Salmonellae and salmonellosis associated with milk and milk products: A review. J Dairy Sci 52:283-315, 1969
3. MMWR: Lactose-fermenting salmonella infection. 16:18-24, 1967
4. Collins RS, Treger MD, Goldsby JB, Boring JR, Coohon DB, Barr RN: *Salmonella* infection traced to powder milk. JAMA 203:838-844, 1968

MMWR 28:145 (4/6/79)

Salmonella heidelberg Gastroenteritis Aboard a Cruise Ship

An outbreak of gastrointestinal illness occurred aboard the *T.S.S. Festivale*, a Caribbean cruise ship of Panamanian registry owned and operated by Carnival Cruise Lines, on its February 17-24 cruise. The outbreak was detected when several passengers who were ill aboard ship notified the Dade County Health Department and the U.S. Quarantine Office after they disembarked in Miami. On the evening of February 26, a Quarantine Officer in San Juan, where the ship was docked, reviewed the ship's medical log and noted that the outbreak had begun on February 22 and that 32 (3%) of the 1,149 passengers had been seen by the physician for a diarrheal illness during the cruise (Figure 1). An outbreak was also apparently occurring on the present cruise (February 24-March 3): 26 (2%) of the 1,160 passengers and 18 (3%) of the 540 crew had reported having diarrhea to the ship's physician by February 26, and many more passengers were complaining of a gastrointestinal illness. A Public Health Service (PHS) quarantine officer and a PHS sanitarian boarded the ship in St. Martin on February 28 to begin an epidemiologic and environmental investigation.

A questionnaire survey was conducted on March 1; of the 1,129 (97%) passengers responding, 379 (34%) reported a gastrointestinal illness defined as either watery diarrhea or severe cramps and vomiting; 108 passengers became ill within 48 hours of boarding the ship on February 24. Stool cultures previously obtained from 4 passengers ill during the earlier cruise and from 14 ill crew members, removed from the ship when it docked in St. Thomas on February 27, grew *Salmonella* group B.

A sanitation inspector for the Quarantine Division inspected the ship on March 2. The water was found to have adequate levels of residual chlorine and to be negative for coliforms. Multiple deficiencies in sanitation were found, particularly in food handling and preparation. Records revealed that the ship had not passed earlier sanitation inspections conducted by the Quarantine Division.

On March 3 a second questionnaire was distributed concerning food consumed during the cruise of February 24-March 3. The survey, completed by 93% of passengers, implicated turkey and macaroni salad from the evening buffet on February 24 as vehicles of transmission. Stool cultures were obtained from 21 ill passengers and 6 well passengers before landing; *S. heidelberg* was isolated from 17 (81%) of the ill and 4 (67%) of the well passengers. The same *Salmonella* serotype was cultured from 7 of 35 different food specimens taken from the ship's galley on March 1 and 2; however, the original turkey and macaroni salad from the evening buffet of February 24 were no longer available. Stool specimens were taken from 269 food handlers and tested for salmonellae; more than 60 have been positive for *Salmonella* group B, to date. The food handlers are the employees of Apollo caterers, a Miami-based firm that caters cruise ships.

The following recommendations were made: 1) remove and destroy leftover foods, 2) completely clean and sanitize the galley, 3) screen food handlers for *Salmonella* and remove all those who are positive, 4) make structural improvements in the kitchen's refrigeration systems and dishwashing areas, and 5) provide better supervision and education of galley crew to improve food handling practices. Since these changes would take at least 1 week to implement, the PHS recommended that the company cancel the March 3-10 cruise. The company accepted and agreed to implement these recommendations.

On March 10, the *T.S.S. Festivale* sailed again with a large number of new galley crew members replacing those who had positive *Salmonella* cultures. A small outbreak of gastrointestinal illness occurred during this cruise (Figure 1), and *S. heidelberg* was isolated from 1 new passenger. During the subsequent cruise, which began March 17, only

FIGURE 1. Clinic visits for diarrheal illness among passengers and crew on 4 cruises of the *T.S.S. Festivale*, **February 10-March 24, 1979**

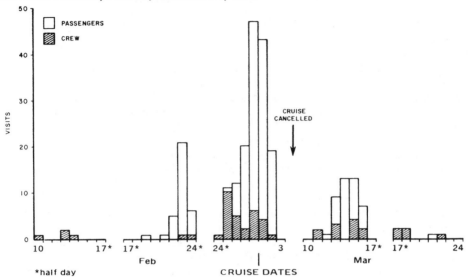

1 of more that 1,100 passengers reported to the ship's doctor with diarrhea.

Reported by DR Pinks, MD, BH Sierra, MD, South Shore Hospital, Miami; MB Enriquez, MD, R Morgan, MD, N Sokoloff, Dade County Dept of Health; Quarantine Div, Epidemiologic Investigations Laboratory Br, Enteric Diseases Br, Bacterial Diseases Div, Bur of Epidemiology, CDC.

Editorial Note: While shipboard outbreaks of gastrointestinal illness occur yearly (*1-2*), this is the first time since 1973 that CDC has recommended that a cruise be cancelled because of an outbreak (*3*). The epidemiologic data and the isolation of *S. heidelberg* from food handlers and food specimens suggested that the ship's principal problems were in the preparation and storage of food.

According to quarantine regulations, the master of a vessel is required to report to the Quarantine Station, within 24 hours before arriving in port, the number of passengers and crew who were seen by the ship's physician for the treatment of diarrhea. CDC usually conducts an epidemiologic and environmental investigation when 3% or more of passengers and crew members experience a diarrheal illness.

The Quarantine Division routinely inspects and scores cruise ships for their adherence to sanitation codes. The results of sanitation inspections on individual cruise ships as well as a monthly summary of the results of the most recent inspections of all cruise ships sailing from or calling at a U.S. port may be obtained from the U.S. Public Health Service, 1015 North American Way, Room 107, Miami, Florida 33132.

References
1. Merson MH, Hughes JM, Lawrence DN, Wells JG, D'Agnese JJ, Yashuk JC: Food and waterborne disease outbreaks on passenger cruise vessels and aircraft. Journal of Milk and Food Technology 39:285-288, 1976
2. Merson MH, Hughes JM, Wood BT, Yashuk JC, Wells JG: Gastrointestinal illness on passenger cruise ships. JAMA 231:723-727, 1975
3. MMWR 22:217-218, 1973

MMWR 28:618 (1/4/80)

Human *Salmonella* Isolates — United States, 1978

In 1978, 28,748 isolations of salmonellae (including *Salmonella typhi*) from humans were reported to CDC. This number represents an increase of approximately 5% over the previous year's total.

Increases in isolates in Massachusetts and Pennsylvania together accounted for almost three-fifths of the overall 5% increase; increases in *S. enteritidis* and *S. heidelberg* together accounted for almost three-fifths of the overall increase. Almost half of the increase in *S. enteritidis* isolates occurred in Massachusetts alone, while most of the remaining increase occurred in New York and California. The increase in *S. heidelberg* isolates was not confined to any particular state or region.

The age distribution of persons from whom isolates were obtained (Figure 3) followed a well-established pattern: the rate was highest for infants approximately 2 months of age, decreased rapidly through early childhood, and then held fairly constant from approximately age 6 through the adult years. Isolation rates for those under 20 were higher for males than for females, but for persons from 20 through 69 years old, females showed a slightly higher reported isolation rate (Figure 3).

The 10 most frequently isolated serotypes accounted for almost three-fourths of the total (Table 1). The variation in median age of persons from whom a particular serotype was isolated may indicate differences in the vehicles, the infectious dose, or other variables. For most serotypes, the median age of infected patients has been consistent

FIGURE 3. *Salmonella* attack rates, by age, United States, 1978

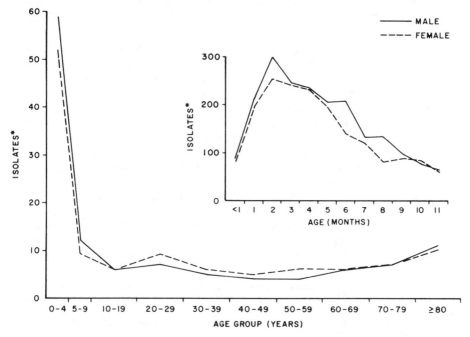

*Per 100,000 population

TABLE 1. The 10 most frequently isolated serotypes of non-typhoid *Salmonella*, United States, 1978

Serotype	Number	Percent	Median age (years)
S. typhimurium*	10,015	34.8	10
S. heidelberg	2,078	7.2	3
S. enteritidis	1,934	6.7	18
S. newport	1,879	6.5	16
S. infantis	1,225	4.3	6
S. agona	1,186	4.1	5
S. montevideo	703	2.4	15
S. typhi	604	2.1	29
S. saint-paul	602	2.1	17
S. javiana	528	1.8	9
Subtotal	20,754	72.2	11
Others	7,994	27.8	
Total	28,748	100.0	10

*Includes *S. typhimurium* var. *copenhagen*.

for the 13 years during which surveillance records have been maintained. Of the 604 isolates of *S. typhi*, 32 were obtained from carriers, 188 from infected patients, and the rest were undesignated. The median age of the carriers was 71 years; of the infected patients, 29 years; and of the unspecified, 27 years.

Reported by Statistical Servcies Br and Enteric Diseases Br, Bacterial Diseases Div, Bur of Epidemiology, CDC.
▲A copy of the report from which these data were derived is available on request from CDC, Attn: Enteric Diseases Branch, Bureau of Epidemiology, Atlanta, Ga. 30333.

MMWR 27 (A.S., 1978): 58

SALMONELLA — Reported Isolations from Humans by Week,* United States, 1974—1978

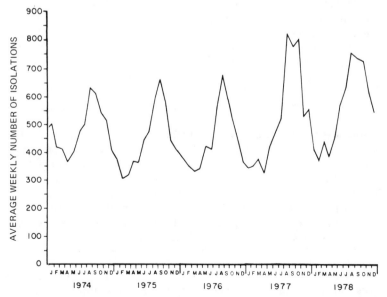

*Each point represents the weekly average number of isolates for the month.

CHAPTER 9

Shigellosis

MMWR 28:498 (10/26/79)

Shigellosis in a Children's Hospital — Pennsylvania

An outbreak of shigellosis occurred May 17-30, 1979, among hospital employees in a children's hospital in Pennsylvania. Thirty-two percent of employees reported being ill. Two hundred eighty employees and visitors with complaints of vomiting and/or diarrhea presented to the employee health service and were cultured; 142 (51%) had positive stool cultures for *Shigella sonnei*. Staffing problems during the outbreak were severe, and the hospital was closed to new admissions for a 3-day period.

Questionnaires were sent to 1,700 employees to determine the symptoms of disease and places where these persons had eaten from May 16-21; a food-specific history was obtained from those who had eaten in the hospital cafeteria. One thousand ninety-three questionnaires (64%) were returned. Analysis showed a strong association between illness and eating in the hospital cafeteria (p<.0001). Based on 78 culture-confirmed cases and 150 well controls, significant associations were found between illness and consumption of tuna salad (p≤.0001) and eating food from the salad bar (p≤.0001). A negative association between illness and consumption of hot foods was also found.

One cafeteria employee had diarrhea on May 17, the first day of the outbreak. She had been exposed to a child with severe diarrhea at home before onset of her illness. This employee was found to be culture positive for *S. sonnei*. She had worked on May 17 and May 21 and was responsible for preparing all salads and sandwiches in the employee cafeteria, where visitors also sometimes ate. The 2 peaks in the outbreak were on May 19 and May 23—consistent with the 1- to 2-day incubation period of foodborne shigellosis (Figure 2).

The organism identified from culture-positive individuals was resistant to ampicillin and tetracycline and sensitive to trimethoprim-sulfamethoxazole. All symptomatic individuals were treated with a 5-day course of the latter drug, or with furazolidone, if they were sulfa sensitive. For cafeteria employees, 3 negative rectal cultures—taken at 1-day intervals at least 48 hours after antibiotic therapy had ended—were required before a culture-positive individual could return to work. Other culture-positive hospital employees were permitted to return to work after 48 hours of therapy. No hospitalized patients became culture positive for *Shigella* as a result of the outbreak.

Reported by J Lampert, RN, S Plotkin, MD, J Campos, PhD, M Trendler, MT, D Schlagel, RN, The Children's Hospital, Philadelphia; EJ Witte, VMD, Acting State Epidemiologist, Pennsylvania State Dept of Health; Field Services Div, Enteric Diseases Br, Bacterial Diseases Div, Bur of Epidemiology, CDC.

Editorial Note: *Shigella* organisms remain a major cause of gastrointestinal illness in the

FIGURE 2. Individuals culture-positive for *Shigella*, **by date of onset, a children's hospital, Pennsylvania, May 1979***

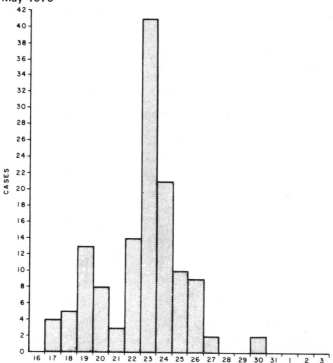

*Excludes cases in which date of onset was unknown.

United States: 15,336 isolates were reported to CDC in 1978 (*1*). Although transmission is usually from person to person, in the 18-year period from 1961 through 1978 there were 84 reported outbreaks of common-source foodborne illness due to *Shigella*. Unlike most *Salmonella* species, *Shigella* are host specific for man and generally survive poorly in the environment. When foodborne outbreaks do occur, they can almost always be traced to contamination of food by an infected food handler. As in this case, the vehicle in foodborne *Shigella* outbreaks is typically a salad or other food whose preparation requires extensive handling of ingredients. Foodborne *Shigella* outbreaks are frequently large and have a high attack rate. For foodborne *Shigella* outbreaks from 1961 to 1975, the average attack rate was 47%, with an average outbreak size of 148 persons (*2*).

The procedures used in this instance to evaluate food-service employees before their return to work follow the recommendations of the American Public Health Association— i.e., that cultures be obtained 48 hours after cessation of therapy and that they be at least 24 hours apart (*3*). More specific regulations relating to food-service employees— such as the number of cultures, the amount of time that should elapse between ceasing therapy and starting post-therapy culturing, and the time between cultures—varies from state to state, and there is no single combination of these variables which has been shown to be clearly superior in identifying infectious individuals.

No secondary spread from members of the hospital staff to patients occurred in this outbreak. This contrasts with studies in households, in which up to 35% of children present in the household have been shown to become infected with *Shigella* after an initial infection in 1 adult household member (4).

References

1. MMWR 28:486-487, 1979
2. Black RE, Craun GF, Blake PA: Epidemiology of common-source outbreaks of shigellosis in the United States, 1961-1975. Am J Epidemiol 108:47-52, 1978
3. Benenson AS (ed): Control of Communicable Diseases in Man. Washington, American Public Health Assoc, 1975
4. Thomas MEM, Tillett HE: Dysentery in general practice: A study of cases and their contacts in Enfield and an epidemiological comparison with salmonellosis. J Hyg (Camb) 71:373-389, 1973

MMWR 28:486 (10/19/79)

Shigellosis — United States, 1978

The upswing in reported *Shigella* isolates, first noted in 1977, continued last year (Figure 1).

The highest rate of reported *Shigella* isolations in 1978 was in 2-year-old children (Figure 2). A higher isolation rate was reported in females than males for the age group 20-29; otherwise, the isolation rates by sex were similar. Isolations peaked in the fall months.

Of the reported isolates last year,* 73.6% were *S. sonnei*; 23.5%, *S. flexneri*; 1.5%, *S. boydii*; and 0.9%, *S. dysenteriae*. *S. flexneri* 2a and 3a comprised 50.5% of the total *S. flexneri* isolates. These figures were similar to those reported in the period 1970-1975, when 77.6% were *S. sonnei*; 20.4%, *S. flexneri*; 0.7%, *S. boydii*; and 0.6%, *S. dysenteriae*. In that period, *S. flexneri* 2a and 3a comprised 52.7% of *S. flexneri* isolations.

Because of recurrent problems with shigellosis in certain population groups, available national data were tabulated separately for institutions and Indian reservations. Forty-nine percent of reports included data on residence of the patient at the time of onset; of these, 1.6% lived in institutions, 2.9% on Indian reservations, and the remainder in other communities. Forty-eight percent of the isolates from residents of institutions were *S. sonnei*, and the remainder, *S. flexneri*. By contrast, 62% of the isolates from residents of Indian reservations were *S. sonnei*, and the remainder, *S. flexneri*. Seventy-four percent of the isolates from residents of other communities were *S. sonnei* and 23%, *S. flexneri*.

From 1969 through 1976, data from California were not available for the annual tabulations. For 1977 and 1978, the numbers of reported isolates, including those from California, were 14,019 and 15,336, respectively.

Reported by the Statistical Services Br and the Enteric Diseases Br, Bacterial Diseases Div, Bur of Epidemiology, CDC.

---

*Excluding California.

FIGURE 1. Reported isolates of *Shigella* in the United States,* 1968-1978

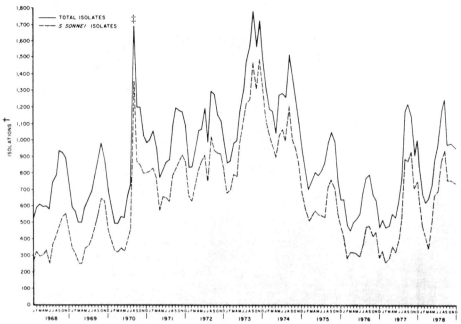

*No reports from California or the Virgin Islands after 1969.
†Adjusted to 4-week month.
‡Approximately 400 isolations in August 1970 due to common-source outbreak in Hawaii.

FIGURE 2. Shigellosis rates, by age, United States,* 1978

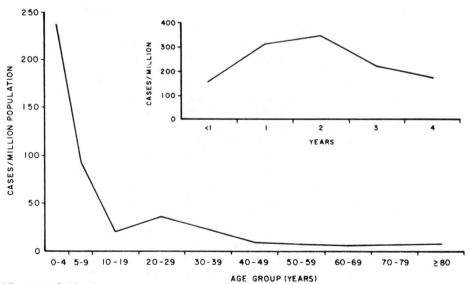

*Excluding California.

CHAPTER 10

Campylobacter Enteritis

MMWR 27:207 (6/23/78)

Waterborne Campylobacter Gastroenteritis — Vermont

A large outbreak of acute gastroenteritis occurred in Bennington, Vermont, during the 2-week period beginning May 28, 1978. An estimate from a household survey indicates that as many as 2,000 out of the town's 10,000 residents may have been affected by the illness. The number of cases peaked on June 4, and no new cases are being reported at this time. Epidemiologic investigation showed a strong association between illness and the consumption of water from the town supply (p = <.005).

The illness was characterized by abdominal pain or cramps (88%), diarrhea (83%), malaise (76%), headache (54%), and fever (52%). Symptoms generally lasted from 1-4 days. All age groups and both sexes were affected equally. All areas of the town, including those along the main supply line, had similar attack rates, ranging from 14.4% to 23%. There was no evidence of secondary spread in households.

Initial laboratory studies in a Bennington hospital for all common bacterial and parasitic pathogens did not identify the organism. Subsequently, rectal swab specimens from 5 of 9 cases cultured at CDC were positive for *Campylobacter fetus* sub. *jejuni.* None of 20 rectal swab specimens from non-ill controls from the Bennington area were positive.

Bennington has a new water treatment plant under construction, but its present main water supply comes from surface water east of the town. This water is chlorinated but not filtered. There are 2 supplementary sources of water that are used when there is low pressure in the main system; neither is chlorinated. One of these sources had not been used since February; the other turns on automatically when pressure is low. Records show that throughout the period of the outbreak, water specimens from several areas of the town had no residual chlorine.

Studies are in progress to determine if the *Campylo-*

bacter organism can be isolated from town water and from wild and domestic animals within the watershed area of the town water supply.

Reported by W Tiehan, MD, Putnam Memorial Hospital, Bennington; RL Vogt, MD, Acting State Epidemiologist, Vermont State Dept of Health; Environmental Protection Agency; Enteric Diseases Br, Bacterial Diseases Div, Bur of Epidemiology, CDC.

Editorial Note: This is the first outbreak of campylobacter diarrhea described in the United States, although isolates of what is now called *Campylobacter fetus* sub. *jejuni* have been made occasionally from blood specimens obtained from individuals in the United States with diarrhea (*1,2*). Formerly called *Vibrio fetus,* this organism has been found previously in domestic livestock and fowl.

In 1973, isolation of these organisms from stools was described in Belgium (*3*). A study in England in 1977 described a routine procedure for isolation of *Campylobacter* bacteria requiring a microaerophilic culture technique, incubation at 43 C (110 F), and a culture medium including vancomycin, polymyxin B, and trimethoprim. This method was used in studying material in the Vermont outbreak.

Campylobacter gastroenteritis has recently been described in persons with diarrhea in Rwanda and in Canada (*5,6*). As the techniques for isolation of *Campylobacter* organisms become routine a clearer idea of the frequency with which *Campylobacter fetus* sub. *jejuni* occurs with diarrhea in the United States should emerge.

References

1. King EO: Human infections with *Vibrio fetus* and a closely related *Vibrio*. J Infect Dis 101:119, 1957
2. King EO: The laboratory recognition of *Vibrio fetus* and a closely related *Vibrio* isolated from cases of human vibriosis. Ann NY Acad Sci 98:700, 1962
3. Butzler JP, Dekeyser P, Detrain M, Dehaen F: Related *Vibrio* in stools. J Pediatr 82:493-495, 1973
4. Skirrow MB: Campylobacter enteritis: A "new" disease. Br Med J 2:9-11, 1977
5. DeMol P, Bosmans E: Campylobacter enteritis in Central Africa. Lancet 1:604, 1978
6. Laboratory Centre for Disease Control: Campylobacter enteritis—Ontario. Canada Diseases Weekly Report 4:57-58, 1978

MMWR 27:226 (7/7/78)

Campylobacter Enteritis — Colorado

On June 24, 1978, the first U.S. outbreak of waterborne *Campylobacter* gastroenteritis—involving an estimated 2,000 persons in Vermont—was reported (*1*). An additional small outbreak due to *Campylobacter* organisms has now been reported in Colorado.

On June 7, 1978, 3 of 5 family members in Colorado ranging in age from 20 to 60 became ill with malaise, myalgias, and nausea. Within the next 24 hours, the illness was marked by severe cramping, lower abdominal pain, and explosive diarrhea which in 1 case became bloody. All had fever (ranging up to 40 C [104 F]), which lasted for 2 days. In 2 of the patients all symptoms remitted within 4 days with symptomatic treatment that included oral and intravenous fluid therapy. The patient with bloody diarrhea continued to have diarrhea and abdominal pain for 6 days. Erythromycin was started, and the patient subsequently improved.

Stool cultures from all 3 patients yielded *C. fetus* sub. *jejuni*. No salmonellae, shigellae, or protozoans were found. Stool cultures from the 2 asymptomatic family members were negative.

The family operates a small farm with chickens, swine, sheep, calves, and a cow. Raw milk from the cow was consumed by all 3 patients and one of the other family members. On June 13, raw milk, eggs, and all animals from the farm were cultured for *Campylobacter* organisms. All were negative with the exception of the stool culture of the cow, which yielded *C. fetus* sub. *jejuni*.

Reported by MJ Blazer, MD, J Cravens, P Riepe, B Powers, WL Wang, PhD, VA Hospital, Denver; TA Edell, MD, Acting State Epidemiologist, Colorado State Dept of Health; Enteric Diseases Br, Bacterial Disease Div, Bur of Epidemiology, CDC.

Editorial Note: *Campylobacter* is the generic name proposed in 1963 (*2*) for a group of microaerophilic organisms that clearly differed from *Vibrio* organisms. The type species is *C. fetus* (*Vibrio fetus*), which had been known as a cause of abortion in cattle and sheep; other members of the new genus have been associated with diseases of domestic animals, including enteritis of calves and pigs.

Although evidence from the outbreak reported here is incomplete, it is compatible with the transmission of *Campylobacter* organisms by unpasteurized milk. Unpasteurized milk has been previously suggested as a vehicle for such infections (*3,4*).

A recent review of the clinical and epidemiologic features of persons in England from whose feces *Campylobacter* organisms were isolated reveals that 94% had diarrhea (15% with blood, pus, or mucus), 8% had persisting or recurring diarrhea for 2 weeks or more, and 13% had severe abdominal pain. Sixty-six percent were individuals 15 years of age or older (*5*).

References
1. MMWR 77:207, 1978
2. Sebald M, Vernon M: Teneur en bases del l'ADN et classification de vibrions. Ann Institut Pasteur 105:897-910, 1963
3. Levy AJ: A gastroenteritis outbreak probably due to a bovine strain of *Vibrio*. Yale J of Biol and Med 18:243-258, 1946
4. Communicable Disease Surveillance Centre: Outbreaks of *Campylobacter* infection. Communicable Disease Report 78(20), May 19, 1978
5. Communicable Disease Surveillance Centre: Reports of *Campylobacter* isolates in 1977. Communicable Disease Report 78(13), March 31, 1978

MMWR 28:565 (11/30/79)

Campylobacter Enteritis — Iowa

On August 13, 1979, the Microbiology Laboratory at Mercy Health Center in Dubuque, Iowa, in order to improve its diagnostic capabilities, began to culture routinely all diarrheal stool specimens for the presence of *Campylobacter fetus*. Through November 14, 11 isolates were made from 238 patients at this 525-bed community hospital—a rate of

4.6%. Ten cultures were ssp. *jejuni* and 1, ssp. *intestinalis*. During this time, 5 isolates of *Salmonella* and none of *Shigella* were made.

Isolates were from 9 males and 2 females; 7 patients were less than 7 years old, and 3 were infants. Six patients were hospitalized, although no extraintestinal complications occurred. Diarrhea (in 2 instances, bloody) occurred in all these patients. The following case reports illustrate some of the clinical and epidemiologic characteristics encountered.

On August 6, 4 days after plucking chickens at a farm, a 14-year-old boy developed watery diarrhea with mucus and abdominal pain. When admitted to the hospital on the fifth day of illness, the patient was afebrile but dehydrated. Intravenous fluids were administered, and the diarrhea slowly resolved over the ensuing 2 weeks. *C. fetus* ssp. *jejuni* was identified in the stool on the fourth day of hospitalization, but no antimicrobial therapy was administered. Fecal cultures from chickens and pigs from the farm yielded *C. fetus* ssp. *jejuni*.

On September 30, 11 or more persons attended a barbecue at which chicken was eaten. The following day, 1 of those attending, a 24-year-old man, developed watery diarrhea and abdominal pain. These symptoms persisted for more than 2 weeks, and treatment with oral doxycycline, after *C. fetus* ssp. *jejuni* was identified, was of little help. Two other persons also developed watery diarrhea within 4 days of the barbecue; stool cultures were not taken from them, however. Two of the 3 ill persons recalled eating chicken that was not well cooked. Although chicken was not available for culture, *C. fetus* ssp. *jejuni* has previously been cultured from dressed, refrigerated chickens from the distributor where these chickens were obtained.

On October 26, a 35-year-old man had onset of watery diarrhea with mucus and crampy abdominal pain. His illness began 2 days after the onset of a similar sickness in his 6-year-old son. Although the son had no extraintestinal symptoms, his father had severe anorexia, chills, mild fever, and arthralgia of the hips and lower back. Cultures taken on the third day of illness in the child and the sixth day of illness in the father yielded *C. fetus* ssp. *jejuni*. Both patients received oral erythromycin. Within several days, the stools had lessened in frequency, but remained loose, and the cramping had significantly abated. A potential source of infection was undercooked, barbecued chicken that had been served 4 days before the son became ill. Two other family members who ate the same meal did not become ill and had negative stool cultures; the mother, however, was taking cephalexin for another illness at the time.

Watery diarrhea, without blood or mucus, and a fever (up to 38.8 C) developed in an 8-month-old infant on August 7. Oral ampicillin was administered, but in the ensuing week symptoms persisted. Vomiting occurred, and the dehydrated infant was hospitalized on August 14. Intravenous fluids were administered, and in the next few days, the fever disappeared and the stools became normal. A stool culture taken on admission yielded *C. fetus* ssp. *intestinalis*. Three weeks after discharge the patient was asymptomatic, and a repeat stool culture was negative. This patient also lived on a farm. No other family members had been ill, and all had negative stool cultures for *Campylobacter*. Cultures of a pet dog, raw milk, well water, frozen chicken, several cats kept in a barn, and several cows did not yield *Campylobacter*.

Reported by JR Schaefer, MS, SM (ASCP), EV Conklin, MD, DFM Bunce, DO, RD Storck, MD, FK Arnold, MD, JP Viner, MD, FB Merritt, MD, Dr. Krish, AJ Roth, MPH, Dubuque, Iowa; RW Currier, DVM, LA Wintermeyer, MD, State Epidemiologist, Iowa Dept of Health; JP Davis, MD, State Epidemiologist, Wisconsin Dept of Health and Social Services; Bacterial Zoonoses Br, Bacterial Diseases Div, Bur of Epidemiology, CDC.

Editorial Note: The importance of *C. fetus* as a human enteric pathogen has only been recognized in the past several years. Isolation rates of 1.9% and 7.1% from patients with diarrhea have been reported in Australia and Great Britain, respectively (*1,2*). In several recent studies, *C. fetus* ssp. *jejuni* was the most common bacterial pathogen isolated from stools from patients with diarrhea.

The epidemiology of diarrhea caused by *C. fetus* ssps. *jejuni* and *intestinalis* is still incompletely understood. Poultry (alive or dressed), dogs, raw milk, and contaminated water have all been implicated as sources of human infection due to *C. fetus* ssp. *jejuni*. Ssp. *jejuni* is commonly found in swine and poultry feces. In the absence of a reliable typing schema, transmission is difficult to prove. However, in the first report, the presence of infected poultry on the farm suggests these animals were the source of the boy's infection.

C. fetus ssp. *jejuni* can persist in carcasses during the preparation of chickens for commercial marketing (*3*). Thus, eating undercooked barbecued chicken may have been the source of infection for several of these patients. Person-to-person transmission probably occurs but has not been conclusively shown.

Illness due to *C. fetus* ssp. *intestinalis* is much less common than that due to ssp. *jejuni*. This may be due, in part, to culture techniques: a commonly used procedure to isolate ssp. *jejuni* includes the incubation of culture plates at 42 C, which markedly diminishes the yield of ssp. *intestinalis*.

As illustrated in this report, culturing for *Campylobacter* can be done in a community hospital at a minimum of expense. The additional cost of culturing for *Campylobacter* in this hospital is estimated to be $2.50 ($0.19 for materials and $2.31 for labor).

References
1. Steele TW, McDermott S: *Campylobacter* enteritis in South Australia. Med J Aust 2:404-406, 1978
2. Skirrow MB: *Campylobacter* enteritis: A new disease. Br Med J 2:9-11, 1977
3. Simmons NA, Gibbs FJ: *Campylobacter* ssp. in oven-ready poultry. Journal of Infection 1:159-162, 1979

CHAPTER 11

Cholera

MMWR 27:341 (9/8/78)

Vibrio cholerae — Louisiana

Vibrio cholerae (serogroup O-1) has been isolated from a person with diarrheal illness in Louisiana.

The patient, a 44-year-old man, became ill on August 10 with watery diarrhea, chills, fever of 101 F (38.3 C), and nausea. He treated himself at home with Lomotil,* Donnagel,* and paregoric, and was hospitalized on August 13 because of dehydration. He recovered and was discharged on August 19. An isolate from a stool obtained on August 18 was confirmed as *Vibrio cholerae* on August 29 at the state laboratory. CDC further characterized it as biotype El Tor, serotype Inaba, on September 4. The patient had neven been out of the country nor had he recently traveled out of the state. He had not had any raw seafood but had recently eaten boiled shrimp and boiled crab. His water source is a private well in his backyard.

An epidemiologic investigation is underway.

Reported by CT Caraway, DVM, State Epidemiologist, Louisiana Dept of Health and Human Resources; Enteric Diseases Br, Bacterial Diseases Div, Bur of Epidemiology, and the Enteric Section, Enterobacteriology Br, Bacteriology Div, Bur of Laboratories, CDC.

Editorial Note: There are many *V. cholerae* serogroups. Only toxigenic isolates of serogroup O-1 and its 2 biotypes—the classical and El Tor—have been associated with worldwide outbreaks. Non-toxic strains, not associated with disease, have been identified. Laboratory tests to determine if the Louisiana isolate produces toxin are in progress.

There have been 2 other apparently indigenous *V. cholerae* O-1 strains isolated from persons in the United States in the past decade. One was isolated from the gallbladder of a man without a diarrheal illness in Alabama in 1977 (*1*); the isolate was non-toxigenic. The other was isolated from a man with a severe diarrheal illness in Texas in 1973 (*2*).

Fever is an unusual finding in cholera, and it is possible that the diarrheal illness of this patient was not cholera; chronic, asymptomatic excretion of *V. cholerae* is highly unusual, but has been reported (*3*).

References
1. MMWR 26:159-160, 1977
2. Weissman JB, DeWitt WE, Thompson J, et al: A case of cholera in Texas, 1973. Am J Epidemiol 100:487-498, 1974
3. Azurin JC, Kobari K, Barua D, et al: A long-term carrier of cholera: Cholera Dolores. Bull WHO 37:745-749, 1967

---

*Use of trade names is for identification only and does not constitute endorsement by the Public Health Service, U.S. Department of Health, Education, and Welfare.

MMWR 27:367 (9/29/78)

Follow-up on *Vibrio cholerae* Infection — Louisiana

A fourth person clinically ill with cholera has been identified in Louisiana. The patient, a 19-year-old woman who lives near Abbeville, had onset of diarrhea on September 18. She was hospitalized on September 21, treated with tetracycline, and has recovered. Isolates from this case, the other 3 clinically ill persons, and 1 asymptomatic case have all been confirmed as *Vibrio cholerae*, biotype El Tor, serotype Inaba.

The 4 clinically ill persons had a history of ingesting steamed or boiled crab in the 2- to 5-day period before onset of illness; the asymptomatic case had also recently eaten such food. For each of the 4 ill cases, 2 matched controls were questioned about eating seafood. None of these 8 controls had recently eaten steamed or boiled crab.

An isolate of *V. cholerae*, serotype Inaba, has been made from a sample of shrimp collected in the area where crabs eaten by 1 patient were collected.

Reported by HB Bradford, PhD, Director, Bur of Laboratories, CT Caraway, DVM, State Epidemiologist, Louisiana Dept of Health and Human Resources; Enteric Diseases Br and Epidemiologic Investigations Laboratory Br, Bacterial Diseases Div, Quarantine Div, Bur of Epidemiology, CDC.

Editorial Note: These 5 persons come from 2 adjacent towns and have no single common contact or water supply. The seafoods eaten by these persons came from different locations along 60 miles of the Louisiana Gulf Coast. If the steamed crabs were a vehicle, they were insufficiently cooked to destroy *V. cholerae* organisms or they were re-contaminated after cooking. Until further information is available, residents of the area should take extra care with the preparation of crabs to insure that they are adequately cooked and not subsequently contaminated.

Since the United States will now be listed by the World Health Organization as having a cholera-infected area, the following countries will now require International Certificates of Vaccination against Cholera from travelers arriving from Vermilion Parish, Louisiana: Albania, Angola, Brunei, Cape Verde, China (People's Republic), China (Republic of), Egypt, Fiji, Iran, Iraq, Lao People's Democratic Republic, Libyan Arab Jamahiriya, Madagascar, Mali, Nauru, Pakistan, Panama, Pitcairn Island, Qatar, Ryukyu Islands, Saint Helena, Seychelles, Swaziland, Yemen, and Zambia. Five countries that always require cholera vaccination from all travelers are Malawi, Maldives, Mozambique, Papua New Guinea, and Saudi Arabia. The following countries will require a Certificate only from travelers proceeding to a country with a cholera requirement: Burma, India, and Nigeria.

An area is considered infected until 10 days has passed "since the last case identified has died, recovered, or been isolated, and there is no epidemiological evidence of spread of that disease to any contiguous area."(*1*)

Reference
1. World Health Organization: International Health Regulations (1969). 2nd ed. Geneva, World Health Organization, 1974

MMWR 27:388 (10/6/78)

Follow-up on *Vibrio cholerae* Serotype Inaba Infection — Louisiana

Four more cases of cholera and 2 asymptomatic infections have been identified in Louisiana, bringing the total number of persons known to be infected in August and September to 11. The 6 most recent infections were discovered after a 58-year-old woman from Lafayette had onset of a diarrheal illness on September 24, was hospitalized,

FIGURE 3. Locations where crabs eaten by patients with cholera were obtained, Louisiana, August-September, 1978

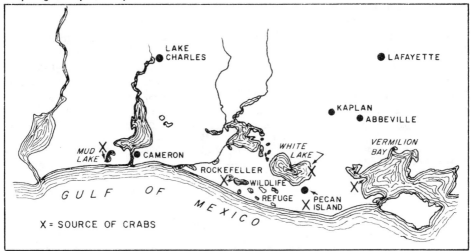

and had *Vibrio cholerae*, serotype Inaba, isolated from her stool. On September 22, she had eaten crabs that had been caught in White Lake, boiled, and then held without refrigeration for approximately 6 hours (Figure 3). Investigation found that 5 of 9 other persons who had eaten the crabs at the same time had also developed diarrheal illnesses; *V. cholerae*, serotype Inaba, organisms have been isolated from the stools of 3 of these ill persons. Some of the boiled crabs left over after the meal had been refrigerated, and *V. cholerae*, serotype Inaba, organisms were isolated from one of them. Other crabs, caught in White Lake at the same time by the same man, were boiled separately on September 22 and eaten at once by 6 persons; none became ill, but *V. cholerae*, serotype Inaba, organisms were isolated from the stools of 2 of the 6 persons. All previously reported isolates of *V. cholerae* from Louisiana in August and September were also of this serotype. The biotype of the most recent isolates has not yet been determined.

The 8 infected persons with symptoms had eaten boiled or steamed crab within 5 days before onset of illness. A case-control study of foods eaten by the first 5 symptomatic patients and 10 age- and sex-matched neighbor controls found that none of the controls had eaten crabs during comparable periods (p=0.007). The 3 asymptomatic infected persons had eaten crabs within 9 days before culture. As mentioned above, *V. cholerae*, serotype Inaba, was isolated from a boiled crab. The organism was also isolated from raw shrimp caught south of Pecan Island (1). These epidemiologic and laboratory data indicate that crabs collected in Louisiana in the area between Mud Lake, west of Cameron, and Vermilion Bay, south of Abbeville, have been the vehicles of infection for the cases of cholera (Figure 3). Crabs prepared in large lots by commercial establishments have not been implicated.

Preliminary results of studies on the effect of boiling on crabs artificially infected with *V. cholerae*, serotype Inaba, from 1 of the Louisiana cases have shown that the organism can be isolated from iced crabs individually boiled after 2, 4, 6, and 8 minutes of boiling, but not after 10 minutes. At 8 minutes the crab shell was red and the meat was firm, so these criteria are not adequate to determine if crabs are safe to eat. In actual practice, crabs are cooked in varying numbers and using a variety of methods and containers. The crabs eaten by the persons with cholera were reportedly steamed for up to 35 minutes or boiled for 10-20 minutes.

Surveillance for cases, culture of seafoods, and monitoring of sewage from 21 cities and towns will continue in Louisiana to determine if a larger coastal area than the one designated is infected, and if other seafoods from the area are causing cholera. Parrish sanitarians will visit all commercial establishments that use crabs to give them information on proper cooking and handling of crabs, including the recommendation that crabs be immersed in vigorously boiling water for at least 15 minutes, and that steaming of crabs be discontinued until studies of the efficacy of steaming have been carried out.

Reported by HB Bradford, PhD, Director, Bur of Laboratories, CT Caraway, DVM, State Epidemiologist, Louisiana Dept of Health and Human Resources; U.S. Food and Drug Administration; Enteric Diseases Br, Epidemiologic Investigations Laboratory Br, Bacterial Diseases Div, Quarantine Div, Field Services Div, Bur of Epidemiology, CDC.
Reference
1. MMWR 27:367, 1978

MMWR 27:412 (10/20/78)

Follow-up on *Vibrio cholerae* serotype Inaba Infection — Louisiana

No new confirmed environmental, seafood, or human *Vibrio cholerae* isolates have been identified in Louisiana in the past week. Subsequent culturing of the Gueydan sewerage system, triggered by the positive isolate last week (1), yielded no cholera organisms, and review of the area's hospital and physician records disclosed no recent cases of severe diarrhea.

Air-transported shipments of unprocessed crabs from Louisiana were received by 4 states last week, and their public health officials are being kept apprised of the developments in Louisiana. Monitoring of these air shipments by the U.S. Food and Drug Administration (FDA)—including culturing crabs and noting distribution sites—continues.

Reported by HB Bradford, PhD, Director, Bur of Laboratories, CT Caraway, DVM, State Epidemiologist, Louisiana Dept of Health and Human Resources; FDA; Enteric Diseases Br, Epidemiologic Investigations Laboratory Br, Bacterial Diseases Div, Quarantine Div, Field Services Div, Bur of Epidemiology, CDC.

Editorial Note: Although Louisiana has been removed from the World Health Organization's list of cholera-infected areas, travelers should be aware that because of possible delays in communication, some countries may require evidence of cholera immunization. A single dose of vaccine is sufficient to satisfy International Health Regulations (2).

Each of the Louisiana cholera patients was treated with tetracycline. The recommended dose in adults is 3 to 4 gm of tetracycline orally over 2 to 3 days (3). For pediatric cholera, the dosage is 30 to 60 mg/kg/day for 2 to 3 days, an amount believed unlikely to cause staining of teeth (4). For moderate or severe cholera cases, antibiotic therapy is merely an adjunct to the primary objective of rapidly replacing fluid and electrolyte losses. Ringers lactate with 10 mEq potassium added to each liter, or a comparable solution, is the treatment of choice (2).

The finding of 3 asymptomatic persons among the 11 cholera infections in Louisiana underscores the fact that El Tor cholera produces a high percentage of symptomless infections (5).

References
1. MMWR 27:402, 1978
2. MMWR 27:173, 1978

3. Barua D, Burrows W (eds): Cholera, Philadelphia, WB Saunders Company, 1974, p 245
4. Grossman ER, Wallchek A, Freedman H: Tetracyclines and permanent teeth: The relation between dose and tooth color. Pediatrics 57:567-570, 1971
5. Hornick RB, Music SI, Wencel R, et al: The Broad Street pump revisited, in Kahill KM (ed): Clinical Tropical Medicine, Vol II, Baltimore, University Park Press, 1972, pp 225-235

MMWR 27:442 (11/10/78)

Follow-up on Cholera — Louisiana

Vibrio cholerae O1 (serotype Inaba) has been isolated from a Moore swab (*1*) that had been in 1 of 2 main divisions of the sewerage system of Franklin, a town in the southern Louisiana parish of St. Mary, between October 20-23. State and local investigators are attempting to find the source of contamination through extensively surveying the sewerage system using Moore swabs and by culturing persons in Franklin who have recently had diarrheal illnesses.

No cases of cholera have been identified in Louisiana during the past month, despite extensive surveillance of diarrheal illnesses. The state has extended its surveillance of diarrheal illness and sewerage systems to include all of the coastal areas of Louisiana.

Reported by HB Bradford, PhD, Director, Bur of Laboratories, CT Caraway, DVM, State Epidemiologist, Louisiana Dept of Health and Human Resources; Food and Drug Administration; Enteric Diseases Br, Epidemiologic Investigations Laboratory Br, Bacterial Diseases Div, Quarantine Div, Field Services Div, Bur of Epidemiology, CDC.

Editorial Note: Moore swabs in sewerage systems have been an effective means of surveillance for *V. cholerae* O1 in Louisiana and thus far have been complimentary to and more sensitive than culturing persons seeking medical attention for diarrheal illnesses. Each surveillance method offers advantages. Culturing persons with diarrhea identifies infected persons even if their homes are not connected to municipal sewerage systems (6 of the 11 infected persons identified in Louisiana had septic tanks), and permits epidemiologic investigation to determine the mode of transmission. Moore swabs in sewage can indicate that there are infected persons in a community who may not have sought medical assistance; in Louisiana, 3 sewage isolates of *V. cholerae* O1 have not been linked with known cases. Because the 2 surveillance methods are complementary, CDC recommends that other states initiating surveillance for cholera use both methods.

Reference
1. Moore B: Detection of paratyphoid carriers in towns by means of sewage examination. Monthly Bulletin Ministry of Health (Great Britain) 7:241-248, 1948

MMWR 28:571 (12/7/79)

Non-01 *Vibrio cholerae* Infections — Florida

Since November 8, 1979, non-01 *Vibrio cholerae* organisms have been isolated from the stools of 3 persons who presented to a single hospital in northern Florida. Raw oysters harvested from or near Oyster Bay, Wakulla County, Florida, have been epidemiologically incriminated as the vehicle of transmission.

The first patient, a 24-year-old woman, became ill with nausea, vomiting, abdominal cramps, and bloody diarrhea on November 8, 30 hours after consuming raw oysters harvested at Mashes Sand near Oyster Bay. She was admitted to the hospital on November 9, was treated with intravenous fluids, and recovered.

On November 12, a 25-year-old man developed watery diarrhea, vomiting, and abdominal cramps 15 hours after he had eaten raw oysters harvested at Purify Creek on

Oyster Bay. He was seen in the hospital emergency room, but he was not clinically dehydrated and was discharged after receiving symptomatic therapy.

The third patient, a 23-year-old man, became ill with nausea, vomiting, abdominal cramps, and bloody diarrhea on November 18, 12 hours after consuming raw oysters obtained from a supplier in Wakulla County. These oysters were thought to have been harvested from Oyster Bay. He was admitted to the hospital on November 18. He was mildly dehydrated and was discharged after 24 hours of intravenous fluid therapy.

The raw oysters were consumed by these 3 patients at family and social gatherings. Another 8 persons were identified who had onset of diarrheal illness within 48 hours after eating raw oysters at these occasions.

Investigation of 11 adult control patients with diarrhea, admitted to the same hospital during November 8-24, but with stool cultures negative for *V. cholerae* non-01, revealed that none had consumed raw oysters within 48 hours prior to admission ($p < .01$). Water and oyster samples collected from the areas where oysters were harvested by the first 2 patients had elevated fecal coliform counts. These areas have been temporarily closed to oyster harvesting by state regulatory authorities, and the open and closed areas in and around Oyster Bay are being monitored for fecal coliform bacteria twice a week.

Reported by C Lewis, J Harris, MD, Tallahassee Regional Medical Center, Tallahassee; K Hausfeld, MD, Health Unit Director, Leon and Wakulla Counties, EC Prather, MD, Health Program Supervisor, District II, AE Roberts, Tallahassee Branch Laboratory, RA Gunn, MD, State Epidemiologist, H Janowoski, S Lieb, Florida Dept of Health and Rehabilitative Services; E Gissendanner, DVM, Florida Dept of Natural Resources; U.S. Food and Drug Administration; Enteric Section, Enterobacteriology Br, Bacteriology Div, Bur of Laboratories, Epidemiologic Investigations Laboratory Br, Enteric Diseases Br, Bacterial Diseases Div, and Field Services Div, Bur of Epidemiology, CDC.

Editorial Note: The species *V. cholerae* now includes not only the strains that cause cholera epidemics (*V. cholerae* 0 group 1) but also organisms that are similar biochemically and by DNA homology to the epidemic strains but which have not been associated with epidemic disease (*V. cholerae* of other 0 groups, or non-01 *V. cholerae*). The latter were formerly referred to as non-agglutinating vibrios (NAGs) or non-cholera vibrios (NCVs).

Sporadic cases of disease associated with isolation of non-01 *V. cholerae* do occur in the United States (*1*). Although some such cases have been anecdotally associated with eating raw shelltish, in this instance raw oysters were epidemiologically incriminated. In the first 2 cases reported here, the incriminated oysters came from areas with elevated fecal coliform counts, suggesting that there was fecal contamination of the areas. Consumption of raw shellfish from contaminated waters carries a significant risk to health. Other diseases, including hepatitis and viral gastroenteritis, have occurred after consumption of contaminated shellfish (*2*). In Florida and other states, regulatory authorities monitor, under the National Shellfish Sanitation Program, the fecal coliform counts of oyster beds harvested for commercial distribution. At the federal level, this program is administered by the U.S. Food and Drug Administration.

References
1. Hughes JM, Hollis DG, Gangarosa EJ, Weaver RE: Non-cholera vibrio infections in the United States: Clinical, epidemiologic and laboratory features. Ann Intern Med 88: 602-606, 1978
2. Earampamoorthy S, Koff RS: Health hazards of bivalve-mollusk ingestion. Ann Intern Med 83: 107-110, 1975

MMWR 28:311 (7/6/79)

Cholera — Worldwide, 1978

A total of 74,632 cases ot cholera were reported, worldwide, for 1978, compared with 58,087 cases in 1977 and 66,020 in 1976. Cholera was more widespread in 1978, affecting 40 countries; this number is the maximum recorded since the beginning of the present pandemic in 1961.

Eight new countries were infected in 1978—the highest number in any 1 year since 1970 and 1971, when cholera first spread to the African continent. The newly infected countries were Burundi, Congo, Rwanda, Zaire, Zambia, the Maldives, Nauru, and the United States.

Eighteen countries in Africa reported 23,317 cases, as compared with 12 countries reporting 8,388 cases in 1977. Nearly two-thirds of the reported cases were from Burundi and the United Republic of Tanzania, where large outbreaks occurred. Ten of these 18 countries did not report cholera in 1977. A marked decrease in the number of cases from 1977 was noted in Ghana, Liberia, Malawi, and Togo.

In Asia, 50,765 cases (22 of them imported) were reported by 19 countries. Although this situation appears very similar to that of 1977, when 48,937 cases were reported by 20 countries, in fact, most countries showed considerably decreased figures when compared with the previous year. On the other hand, 5 Asian countries that reported cholera in 1978 had not been infected in 1977. A large outbreak of 11,336 cases in the Maldives was rapidly brought under control by measures which included purifying the drinking water and establishing careful epidemiologic surveillance of cases. For the first time since 1973, a large outbreak, which involved 906 cases, occurred in Bahrain; this outbreak was unique in that the highest attack rates were in children under 1 year of age, especially those who were bottle-fed. Outbreaks also occurred in India and Thailand associated with post-monsoon flooding.

As in 1977, a small number of cases occurred in Japan (1). A small outbreak also occurred in the United States—the first on the North American Continent during the present pandemic (2). Nontoxigenic *Vibrio cholerae* organisms with some atypical characteristics were also isolated from the sewerage system of Santos, Brazil, where no cholera cases or carriers were identified. Cholera spread to yet another country in Oceania: a small outbreak of 38 cases occurred on Nauru.

Editorial Note: In at least 1 country where cholera vaccination was required from all travelers on entry, this measure failed to prevent the introduction of cholera. Consideration should be given to the cost-effectiveness of using medical and paramedical personnel to establish diarrheal disease surveillance—even if it is of the most elementary form—in preference to assigning such personnel to recognized ports of entry for the ritualistic examination of cholera vaccination certificates.

Reported by the World Health Organization in the Weekly Epidemiological Record 54(17), April 27, 1979.

References
1. MMWR 28:98, 1979
2. MMWR 27:402, 1978

CHAPTER 12

Food Poisoning

MMWR 27:164 (5/12/78)

Clostridium perfringens Food Poisoning — California

An outbreak of *Clostridium perfringens* food poisoning in Ojai, California, traced to the consumption of bean-filled burritos,* illustrates that foods other than meat, poultry, or gravy contain the essential amino acids to support growth of this organism.

The burritos were one of many Mexican-style foods offered for sale at an outdoor fund-raising event on September 18, 1977, in Ojai. On September 19, the Ventura County Environmental Health Division began receiving reports of illness and initiated an investigation. To identify cases, hospital and community doctors, school nurses, and the event-organizers were contacted, and press releases were distributed to the local media. By these means, 181 ill persons who had attended the event were identified. Information from 40 other persons who ate at the event but did not become ill was also obtained. It is not known how many persons consumed burritos at this event, although sales receipts showed that about 1,200 had been sold.

Symptoms consisted primarily of diarrhea (96.2%) and cramps (79.7%). Only 3 (1.7%) of those ill reported vomiting. The mean incubation period was 11 hours, with 87% reporting illness from 8-22 hours after eating. The majority of ill persons were free of symptoms within 24 hours of onset. No one was hospitalized. Analysis of food histories incriminated the bean-filled burritos ($p < .01$).

Containers of leftover bean-burrito filling, green chili sauce, taco sauce, and shredded longhorn cheese refrigerated at 5 C (40 F) were sampled by county investigators 3 hours after closing of the food stand. Samples of 1

---

*burrito: a flour tortilla filled with either meat or beans and generally garnished with hot sauce and cheese frozen burrito, another held at room temperature, and a frozen enchilada were also obtained. All of the food samples were examined for the presence of *Salmonella, Shigella, Staphylococcus,* and *C. perfringens* and for total aerobic colony counts. The bean-burrito filling and the unrefrigerated whole burrito were found to contain 4.0×10^6 and 7.1×10^6 *C. perfringens* bacteria per gram, respectively. None of the other food specimens contained more than 30,000 *C. perfringens* organisms per gram. No *Shigella, Salmonella,* or staphylococcal organisms were found in food specimens.

The bean-burrito filling contained no meat or meat extracts. It was prepared from dried pinto beans that had been boiled with water in metal pots, mashed, and stored in cafeteria refrigerators overnight. The pots of beans were kept refrigerated while they were being transported the following morning. They were transferred to smaller open containers and reheated for an undetermined period of time before being served in the burritos. Several persons throughout the day reported that the beans were not heated and the burritos were served at ambient temperature. During that day, shade temperatures reached 29.4 C (85 F). There was no evidence of cross contamination with meat products.

Reported by S Matson, BS, County of Ventura Health Dept, Ventura; EH Rau, RS, County of Ventura Environmental Resource Agency; J Chin, MD, State Epidemiologist, California Dept of Health; Bur of Training, Enteric Diseases Br, Bacterial Diseases Div, Bur of Epidemiology, CDC.

Editorial note: Pinto beans and other legumes provide an excellent substrate for *C. perfringens* (1). If beans are not served immediately after cooking, they should be held at $\geqslant$60 C (140 F) or rapidly cooled in shallow containers in refrigerators and reheated to 74 C (165 F) before being served.

Reference
1. Rockland LB, Gardiner BL, Pieczarka D: Stimulation of gas production and growth of *Clostridium perfringens* type A (No. 3624) by legumes. J Food Sci 34:411-414, 1969

MMWR 27:345 (9/15/78)

Vibrio parahaemolyticus Foodborne Outbreak — Louisiana

An outbreak of *Vibrio parahaemolyticus* food poisoning occurred the last week of June affecting approximately two-thirds of 1,700 persons from a 4-parish area who attended a dinner at Port Allen, Louisiana, on June 21, 1978.

A questionnaire survey to obtain information concerning the illness was administered to a sample of 122 people. Of this sample 82 (67.2%) reported illness. The mean incubation period was 16.7 hours, with a range of 3 to 76 hours. The duration of illness ranged from less than 1 day to over 8 days, with a mean of approximately 4.6 days. Physicians were seen for treatment by 32 patients (26.2%), and 9 (7.4%) required hospitalization.

Symptoms of the illness included diarrhea (95.1%), cramps (91.5%), weakness (90.2%), nausea (71.9%), chills (54.9%), headache (47.7%), fever (47.5%), and vomiting (12.2%). Both sexes were equally affected; ages ranged from 13 to 78 years.

Foods served included boiled shrimp, hogshead cheese, boiled potatoes, boiled corn, boiled salt meat, bread, butter, and watermelon. Eighty-one (68.1%) of the 119 individuals consuming shrimp became ill while only 1 of 3 who did not eat shrimp became ill. Although this difference in attack rates is not statistically significant, 99% of the ill people ate shrimp while no other food was consumed by more than two-thirds of those ill.

Laboratory analysis yielded positive cultures for V. parahaemolyticus from the leftover boiled shrimp, boiled potatoes, boiled corn, and hogshead cheese and from 7 of 15 stool specimens from patients. All stool isolates were Kanagawa-positive. Since the person who gathered the food for storage after the dinner placed all leftover food in 1 container, cross-contamination probably occurred.

The raw shrimp was purchased at 1 location and shipped to a second location in standard, wooden, seafood boxes. It was boiled on the morning of June 21 and placed back into the same boxes in which it had been shipped. After being covered with aluminum foil to keep the contents warm for serving, it was transported 40 miles in an unrefrigerated truck to the location of the dinner. It was held unrefrigerated a minimum of 7-8 hours until serving time at 7:30 PM.

An inspection of the wholesale seafood establishment where the shrimp was purchased was undertaken on June 27. Unsanitary conditions were noted. The investigation revealed that the shrimp had been boiled in 300-pound batches in the following manner. A batch was placed in a container until the water came to a "rolling boil." At this time the gas was turned off, and the shrimp allowed to soak in the hot water for 15 minutes. Boiled shrimp collected from the seafood establishment during the inspection 6 days after the outbreak was cultured and found to be positive for V. parahaemolyticus.

For preparation of boiled seafood Louisiana law requires a minimum of 7 minutes boiling to insure destruction of pathogens.

Reported by East and West Baton Rouge, East and West Feliciana, Point Coupee, and Iberville Parish Health Units; Louisiana Bur of Laboratory Services; CT Caraway, DVM, State Epidemiologist, J Gregg, BS, L McFarland, MPH, Louisiana State Dept of Health and Human Resources.

MMWR 28:45 (2/2/79)

Staphylococcal Food Poisoning — New York

In August 1978, an outbreak of staphylococcal food poisoning occurred in a county jail in New York. Of 231 inmates eating the noon meal on August 29, 104 developed nausea, vomiting, diarrhea, and/or abdominal cramps. In addition, 3 of 25 staff persons also became ill. The onset of the majority of cases was 5 to 6 hours after eating; the range was 2 to 12 hours. The disease was self-limited, and few inmates had any complaints the following morning. No one required hospitalization.

Food histories obtained from 63 persons who ate the suspect meal incriminated macaroni salad as the vehicle of spread. Bacterial cultures of leftover food items confirmed the epidemiologic findings; $>10^7$ *Staphylococcus aureus* colonies per gram, phage type 83/85A, were isolated from the macaroni salad. No patient specimens were obtained for culture. Culture of a nasal swab from one of the food handlers grew *S. aureus*, but of a different phage type from that found in the macaroni salad.

The macaroni salad had been prepared the day before it was served. It had been stored overnight in 2 large, deep containers in a walk-in cooler. Sanitary inspection of the kitchen revealed a number of violations which may have contributed to the outbreak: 1. food was refrigerated in large, deep containers which did not allow for adequate cooling; 2. most of the work performed in the kitchen was done by inmates, who were inadequately trained and not well supervised; and 3. environmental surfaces and cooking utensils were found to be dirty and contaminated with dried food. These violations have been corrected, and there have been no further outbreaks at the jail.

Reported by KM Bell, MD, JL Nitzkin, MD, MPH, DPH, K Pratt, Monroe County Health Dept; P Greenwald, MD, Acting State Epidemiologist, New York State Dept of Health; Enteric Diseases Br, Bacterial Diseases Div, Bur of Epidemiology, CDC.

Editorial Note: This outbreak is typical of staphylococcal food poisoning, with the short incubation period indicative of an intoxication. High-protein foods are generally involved, and the organism is able to grow in high salt concentrations. *S. aureus* is frequently carried on the skin and in the nares, and contamination of food is undoubtedly very common. However, contamination alone is not sufficient to cause disease. Once contaminated, only if the food is kept in a temperature range that allows the organism to reproduce will sufficient toxin be produced to lead to illness. In this outbreak it is likely that August temperatures and the storage of the macaroni salad in large containers that could not easily be cooled combined to keep the salad at a temperature conducive to the growth of the organism.

MMWR 28:153 (4/6/79)

Staphylococcal Food Poisoning — Florida

In November 1978, a Thanksgiving dinner shared by approximately 350 students, faculty, and guests at a college in Florida resulted in an outbreak of staphylococcal food poisoning. At least 54 individuals developed an illness characterized by the abrupt onset of nausea and vomiting, followed by diarrhea. None reported fever. The onset of the majority of cases was 4 to 5 hours after eating; the range was 2 to 8 hours. Two persons were hospitalized.

Food histories obtained from 64 persons who ate the meal incriminated ham as the vehicle of spread (p<0.001). Bacterial cultures of leftover food items confirmed the epidemiologic findings; $> 10^7$ *Staphylococcus aureus* colonies per gram were isolated from the ham and turkey. Phage typing was not done, and no specimens from patients or food handlers were cultured.

Because of the holiday, the dinner was prepared by a large number of students instead of the usual kitchen personnel. Interviews with these students indicated that hams and turkeys had been partially thawed at room temperature and that the temperature controls on the ovens used for cooking were not functioning properly. The sliced ham and turkey had been stored at temperatures favorable for the growth of *S. aureus* (<60 C; <140 F) for as long as 8 hours before serving.

Reported by JA Barstow, JS Coles, A McCallister, RA Miller, MSEH, JS Rayl, MA Weise, Martin County Health Dept; RM Yeller, MD, State Epidemiologist, Florida State Dept of Health; Enteric Diseases Br, Bacterial Diseases Div, Bur of Epidemiology, CDC.

Editorial Note: Improper thawing of meat and storing of prepared foods provided the conditions necessary for this outbreak to occur. This incident serves as a reminder of the importance of having trained, supervised personnel involved in the preparation of food for the public—a consideration overlooked by some institutions and establishments during holiday seasons.

MMWR 28:179 (4/20/79)

Staphylococcal Food Poisoning Associated with Genoa and Hard Salami — United States

Since January 1, 1979, 8 incidents of staphylococcal food poisoning associated with salami products produced by the Patrick Cudahy, Inc. plant, Establishment 28, Cudahy, Wisconsin, have been reported. The reports came from Pennsylvania (4), Virginia (2), Minnesota (1), and Wisconsin (1). Nineteen persons have become ill with symptoms compatible with staphyloenterotoxicosis after an average incubation period of 4 hours. At least 7 persons were hospitalized.

Although laboratory analysis of remaining specimens of the implicated salami did not reveal staphylococcal enterotoxin or high counts of *Staphylococcus aureus*, investigation found that the procedure used by the company to manufacture the salami did not provide adequate controls to prevent staphylococcal growth and concomitant enterotoxin production. In addition, analysis of other products with the same establishment code and lot numbers as the salami associated with illness revealed counts of coagulase-positive staphylococci ranging from 16,000 to 930,000 organisms per gram; staphylococcal enterotoxin was identified in 1 lot.

On March 9, the U.S. Department of Agriculture (USDA) announced a voluntary recall of 4 implicated lots of 4 oz., sliced, vacuum-packaged Genoa salami with labels marked "sell by" 1 of 4 dates: February 25, March 9, March 30, and April 20. Since that announcement, 4 more outbreaks have occurred associated with products not involved in the initial recall; Genoa and hard salamis, sliced to order from whole sticks sold in groceries and delicatessens, were implicated. Analysis of random sticks of these 2 types of salami from Establishment 28, found in marketing channels, revealed counts of coagulase-positive staphylococci ranging from 0 to $>10^6$ organisms/g. Independent laboratory testing of company-supplied samples of Genoa salami, obtained by USDA at Establishment 28 after the recall, revealed counts of coagulase-positive staphylococci ranging from 2,600 to $>10^6$ organisms/g. One specimen also contained staphylococcal enterotoxin C. On April 13, on the basis of these findings, the manufacturer voluntarily recalled its Genoa salami and hard salami produced at Establishment 28.

Editorial Note: In the production of fermented sausage, lightly salted meat is intentionally temperature-controlled to allow lactobacilli to grow; these usually inhibit the growth of other organisms. However, if the procedure is not adequately monitored, *S. aureus* organisms may multiply on the surface of the sausage and produce enterotoxin. The typical 1- to 2-month curing period for sausage will eventually cause these staphylococcal organisms to die off, but the enterotoxin—which causes human illness—will remain. Detection of enterotoxin is difficult because: (1) it is found only in the outer, one-eighth inch surface of the salami and then only in random locations (it varies from salami to salami and within individual sticks); and (2) the *in vitro* tests used to detect its presence are not sufficiently sensitive to detect small amounts.

Reported by Epidemiology Br, Food Safety and Quality Services, USDA.

MMWR 28:445 (9/21/79)

Staphylococcal Food Poisoning — Delaware

On March 10, 1979, 64 cases of acute gastrointestinal disease occurred among 107 guests at a wedding reception in Sussex County, Delaware.

Symptoms included vomiting (85%), nausea (74%), abdominal cramps (61%), and diarrhea (39%). Thirty-eight of those affected sought emergency room attention, although none were hospitalized. Incubation periods of the illness ranged from 1.6 to 6.5 hours, with a median of 3.5 hours.

Food histories, obtained from 103 of the guests, implicated chicken salad as the food associated with illness. The attack rate among those who ate chicken salad was 76% (62/82), while only 9% (2/21) of those not eating this salad became ill (p<.001). Coagulase-positive *Staphylococcus aureus* was subsequently isolated from the chicken salad and the food grinder used to prepare it. No skin lesions were evident on any of the 6 food handlers, but *S. aureus* was cultured from nasal swabs of 3. Phage typing, performed at CDC, demonstrated that the isolates from the chicken salad, the food grinder, and the nasal swab from the chicken salad preparer were all type 95.

The food was mostly prepared in private homes. The chicken for the salad was cooked and deboned on March 8 and refrigerated in a large, plastic washtub. The following day the chicken was ground in a meat grinder with celery and onions, mixed with mayonnaise, and then refrigerated in the same tub. On the day of the reception, the salad was not refrigerated during transport or before or during the reception—a total time period of approximately 7 hours. During serving, it was noted that the chicken salad from the central portion of the container felt warmer than that from the top, indicating uneven refrigeration.

Reported by E Connors, RN, J Tobin, MD, Naticoke Hospital; GE Bender, MD, H Chaski, P Johnson, M Shull, RN, R Tator, D Wasson, Sussex County Health Unit; B Kaza, PhD, ES Tierkel, VMD, State Epidemiologist, MP Verma, PhD, Delaware Dept of Health and Social Services; Bacteriology Div, Bur of Laboratories, Bacterial Diseases Div, Bur of Epidemiology, CDC.

Editorial Note: This classic staphylococcal outbreak underscores the need for continuing public education in proper food handling, particularly with regard to prompt and adequate refrigeration of prepared foods. Staphylococcal food poisoning has been recognized since 1914, when an outbreak in the Philippines, caused by inadequate refrigeration of milk from a cow with a chronic staphylococcal infection, was described (1). This type of food poisoning remains a major cause of outbreaks of acute gastrointestinal disease, constituting approximately 25% of all foodborne outbreaks of known etiology reported to CDC between 1972 and 1977.

The illness is caused by the presence of a heat-stable enterotoxin produced by only a few strains of *S. aureus,* often from phage group 3; phage typing alone, however, cannot determine whether a given strain will produce enterotoxin.

The vehicle of transmission in staphylococcal food poisoning is almost always a protein-containing food. Ham is the most common vehicle in the United States, where it is implicated in 28% of outbreaks. Contamination, as in this case, is usually assumed to be from food handlers; use of improper holding temperatures allows multiplication of the staphylococci and elaboration of the toxin. After ingestion, the incubation period may range from 30 minutes to 8 hours, with vomiting the predominant symptom. The illness produced may be quite severe, although short-lived; a few fatal cases have been reported (2).

Bacillus cereus may cause a similar clinical syndrome mediated by a heat-stable emetic toxin; the median incubation period is less than 6 hours, with illness characterized by vomiting and abdominal cramps (*3*). *B. cereus* is also capable of producing a heat-labile diarrheal toxin, which may mimic *Clostridium perfringens* (*4*).

References
1. Barber MA: Milk poisoning due to a type of *Staphylococcus albus* occurring in the udder of a healthy cow. Philippine Journal of Science 98:515-519, 1914
2. Currier RW, Taylor A, Wolf FS, Warr M: Fatal staphylococcal food poisoning. South Med J 66: 703-705, 1973
3. Terranova W, Blake PA: *Bacillus cereus* food poisoning. N Engl J Med 298:143-144, 1978
4. Turnbull PCB, Kramer JM, Jorgensen K, Gilbert RJ, Melling J: Properties and production characteristics of vomiting, diarrheal, and necrotizing toxins of *Bacillus cereus*. Am J Clin Nutr 32:219-228, 1979

CHAPTER 13

Botulism

MMWR 27:17 (1/20/78)

Follow-up on Infant Botulism — United States

Infant botulism, a disease apparently resulting from intra-intestinal toxin production by *Clostridium botulinum* (*1*), was first recognized as a distinct clinical entity in late 1976 (*2-4*). Since then, cases have been identified with increasing frequency—1, retrospectively, in 1975, 15 in 1976, 42 in 1977—and have been reported to CDC from 15 states throughout the country: California (37),* Pennsylvania (4), Utah (4), Washington (2), and (1 each) Arizona, Colorado, Montana, Nevada, New Jersey, New York, North Dakota, Oregon, Tennessee, Texas, and Wisconsin (Figure 1). Cases have occurred most often in the fall months, particularly in the past year; however, increased physician awareness may have accounted for this observation (Figure 2).

All patients identified thus far have had sufficient neuromuscular paralysis to need hospitalization. Constipation was the first symptom of illness in most cases, but it was frequently initially overlooked. A spectrum in the severity of symptoms has been noted (*1*). Some infants showed only lethargy, mild weakness, and slowed feeding, while others became acutely ill with obvious feeding difficulty, severe generalized weakness, and hypotonia over a 1-3 day period which, in some cases, progressed to respiratory insufficiency. One California and 1 Utah infant died following respiratory arrest.

Polyvalent antitoxin was administered to the first patient (in 1975) because the case was thought to be food-borne botulism. However, subsequent patients that received

---

*Active intensive case-finding most likely accounts for the large number of California cases.

FIGURE 1. Cases of infant botulism reported to CDC, January 1, 1975-December 31, 1977

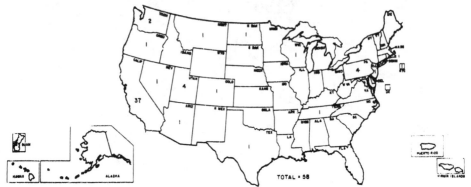

TOTAL = 58

meticulous supportive care which focused on their nutritional and respiratory needs have been successfully managed.

In general, affected infants were the product of a normal gestation and delivery. They had no congenital abnormalities and were healthy until onset of illness. Thirty-three (57%) of the 58 patients were males. The median age at onset was 10 weeks, the range 3-26 weeks.

In all cases the diagnosis was established by the identification of *C. botulinum* toxin and/or organisms in the feces of patients. Botulinal toxin was identified in the feces of 52 (90%) of the 58 cases, while in the other 6, only *C. botulinum* was found. By comparison, in an ongoing California study no botulinal toxin has been found in the feces of over 100 healthy age-matched control infants. (*C. botulinum* was isolated on 1 occasion from the feces of a control infant, but not from his subsequent specimens.)

Of the 58 cases, 33 were type A and 25 were type B. All but 1 of 8 cases east of the Mississippi were type B, while type A cases predominated in the West. This distribution reflects the known geographic distribution of type A and type B spores in American soil (5).

No source of ingestible preformed botulinal toxin has been identified for any infant, nor have the patients shared any exposure to a common food. Cases have occurred in exclusively breast-fed and exclusively formula-fed infants, although most infants have had some exposure to food items other than milk. A potential source of *C. botulinum* spores, however, has been identified for 6 cases. Vacuum cleaner dust from the home of an infant with type A illness was found to contain *C. botulinum* type A, while soil from the yard of an infant with type B illness yielded type B organisms. Three opened jars of honey taken from the homes of 3 infants with type B botulism who had been fed honey and water were found to contain type B organisms. Similarly, an unopened jar of honey of the same brand as that fed to an infant with type A illness was shown

FIGURE 2. Infant botulism cases reported to CDC, by month of
onset, January 1, 1975-December 31, 1977

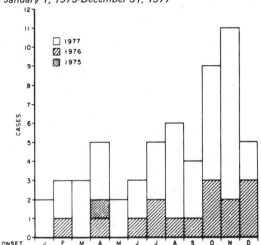

to harbor type A organisms. In contrast, *C. botulinum* was
not found in 17 other commercial honey specimens, in 1
specimen from a private beekeeper (*1*), or in over 100 other
foods tested, including cereals, baby food, formula, and
breast milk; however, testing of foods and other potential
sources of spores has not been done for all cases.

Reported by SS Arnon, MD, J Chin, MD, State Epidemiologist,
K Damus, RN, MSPH, TF Midura, PhD, S Snowden, B Thompson,
MPH, RM Wood, PhD, California State Dept of Health; appropriate
state health departments and State Epidemiologists; Enterobacteri-
ology Br, Bacteriology Div; Bur of Laboratories, Field Services Div,
Enteric Diseases Br, Bacterial Diseases Div, Bur of Epidemiology,
CDC.

Editorial Note: The identification of 57 of the 58 cases in
only 24 months in 15 states located throughout the United
States indicates that infant botulism occurs more commonly
than previously realized. In California, Pennsylvania, and
Utah, some hospitals and physicians diagnosed subsequent
cases shortly after identifying their first case. If cases are
evenly distributed in the country, then by a conservative
estimate at least 250 cases needing hospitalization may be
occurring annually. Furthermore, since botulinal spores are
found worldwide (*4,5*), there is no reason to suppose that
cases are limited to the United States. Failure to identify
cases in other countries may be explained by lack of physician awareness and limited laboratory facilities. Intensive
case-finding is needed to provide sufficient data to elucidate
the actual incidence, full clinical spectrum, mode of transmission, and other risk factors associated with this toxigenic disease.

Indications for the use of botulinal antitoxin or oral
antibiotics in the therapy of infant botulism are at present

uncertain. It is not known whether administration of either will ameliorate the disease, shorten hospitalization, or diminish the risk of serious complications.

References

1. Arnon SS, Midura TF, Clay SA, Wood RM, Chin J: Infant botulism: Epidemiological, clinical and laboratory aspects. JAMA 237: 1946-1951, 1977

2. Pickett J, Berg B, Chaplin E, Brunstetter-Shafer M: Syndrome of botulism in infancy: Clinical and electrophysiologic study. N Engl J Med 295:770-772, 1976

3. Midura TF, Arnon SS: Infant botulism: Identification of *Clostridium botulinum* and its toxins in faeces. Lancet 2:934-936, 1976

4. Black RE, Arnon SS: Botulism in the United States, 1976. J Infect Dis 135:829-832, 1977

5. Smith LDS: Botulism: The Organism, its Toxins, the Disease. Springfield, Ill., Charles C Thomas, 1977

MMWR 27:138 (4/21/78)

Botulism — New Mexico

During the week of April 9-16 an outbreak of botulism involving 32 reported cases occurred in Clovis, New Mexico, a town of 40,000 stituated close to the Texas border. There were no deaths.

On April 13, CDC was informed that a 35-year-old enlisted man had been flown from Cannon Air Force Base, located outside of Clovis, to El Paso because of a progressive neurologic syndrome that began April 10. The New Mexico State Department of Health was notified, and arrangements were made for blood and stool specimens to be sent to CDC to be tested for botulinal toxin and the presence of *Clostridium botulinum*. An investigation revealed that the patient was a part-time employee in a country club restaurant in Clovis.

Early April 15, CDC was notified by a physician in Amarillo, Texas, that 2 women with acute myasthenic syndromes had been transferred from a Clovis hospital. Clinical findings in both patients included ptosis, extraocular muscle palsies, decreased gag reflexes, and generalized weakness. Over the next few hours both patients required intubation with mechanical respiration. One patient had eaten in the country club restaurant on April 9, and the other had eaten there on April 12. They had become symptomatic on April 11 and 14, respectively.

During the next 48 hours, an additional 29 patients with objective neurologic findings were seen and admitted to hospitals in Amarillo and Lubbock, Texas, and Clovis, Albuquerque, and Sante Fe, New Mexico. The Special USAF Air Evacuation System transported 11 of the patients to Albuquerque. The patients ranged in age from 10 to 72. Twenty-one were male. Twenty patients were treated with antitoxin.

All 32 patients had eaten at the country club in Clovis on April 9, 12, or 13. Illness was significantly associated with exposure to a salad bar (p<.01) for the 3 meals. Epidemiologic analysis further identified 2 items served at the salad bar on several days, potato salad and 3-bean salad, as being associated with illness (p<.05), but neither was eaten by all patients. Incubation periods ranged from 1-3 days with a median of 2 days. Eleven patients eventually required intubation and mechanical respiration.

Type A botulism toxin has been identified by CDC in serum specimens of 2 patients and, by the Food and Drug Administration, in the potato salad obtained from the incriminated restaurant. Further epidemiologic and laboratory investigations are in progress.

Reported by M Ryan, MD, High Plains Baptist Hospital, Amarillo, Texas; Methodist Hospital, Lubbock, Texas; CR Webb, Jr, MD, State Epidemiologist, Texas Dept of Health; Clovis Memorial Hospital, Clovis; St. Joseph's Hospital, and Bernalillo County Medical Center, Albuquerque; St. Vincent's Hospital, Sante Fe; JM Mann, MD, State Epidemiologist, J Thompson, MPH, New Mexico Dept of Health and Social Services; J Begin, Major, U.S. Air Force Hospital, Cannon AFB, Clovis; RE Morrison, MD, William Beaumont Army Medical Cen *El Paso; R Brockett, PhD, G Lathrop, MD, PhD, P Moynahan, RN, Air Force School of Aerospace Medicine, San Antonio; Food and Drug Administration; Enterobacteriology Br, Bacteriology Div, Bur of Laboratories, Field Services Div, and Enteric Diseases Br, Bacterial Diseases Div, Bur of Epidemiology, CDC.*

Editorial Note: This is the second largest outbreak of botulism reported in the United States since recording began in 1899 (*1*). Although an average of 15 outbreaks occur each year in the United States, the typical outbreak has involved fewer than 3 individuals and usually has been related to home-canned products (*2*).

In the present outbreak 2 separate foods were incriminated, but neither separately accounted for all of the cases. This suggests either cross-contamination or the addition of a common contaminated ingredient.

References
1. MMWR 26:117, 1977
2. Center for Disease Control: Botulism in the United States, 1899-1973: Handbook for Epidemiologists, Clinicians, and Laboratory Workers. Issued June 1974

MMWR 27:249 (7/21/78)

Honey Exposure and Infant Botulism

Of the 43 documented cases of infant botulism reported from California since 1976, 13 have had a history of ingestion of honey before the onset of constipation, the first symptom of most cases. Of foods fed to babies who developed infant botulism in California, only honey was found to contain *Clostridium botulinum* organisms. No honey specimens containing *C. botulinum* organisms contained preformed botulinal toxin. In 3 California cases, *C. botulinum* was isolated from honey fed the affected infants; in each case the infant had type B illness, and the honey sample contained type B organisms. In a fourth California case, no honey was available for culture; however, a jar of honey of the identical brand and size as that consumed by the patient, purchased at the market where the family shopped, contained type A botulism organisms. This case was type A botulism. Of over 60 honey specimens tested in California, about 13% have contained *C. botulinum.* This finding has been confirmed independently by 4 laboratories elsewhere in the United States. In 2 other states, *C. botulinum* type B was isolated from honey fed to 2 type B cases.

Since honey ingestion occurred in less than one-third of all California cases of infant botulism, development of infant botulism involves additional risk factors. However, since honey is not an essential food for infants, the California Department of Health concurs with the recent recommendation of the Sioux Honey Association that honey not be fed to infants under 1 year of age.

Reported by S Arnon, MD, J Chin, MD, State Epidemiologist, K Damus, RN, MSPH, T Midura, PhD, S Snowden, BA, P Taylor, MD, B Thompson, MPH, and R Wood, PhD, California Dept of Health, in the California Morbidity Weekly Report, July 14, 1978; Field Services Div, Bur of Epidemiology, CDC.

Editorial Note: Much of California's data concerning honey and infant botulism have been previously discribed (1). *C. botulinum* spores are present in soil and on the surface of many vegetables. When vegetables are canned commercially, they are subjected to sufficient heat ($\geq$123 C or $\geq$253.4 F) and pressure to destroy the botulism spores. The repeated finding of botulinal organisms of the same type in infants with botulism and a history of honey ingestion and in the honey, itself, suggests that honey may have been the source of infection for these and perhaps other infants. Although ingestion of honey was recorded in only a third of the cases and was therefore not the only risk factor, it appears prudent that honey not be recommended as a food for infants. The safety of honey as a food for older children and adults remains unquestioned.

Reported by the Bacterial Diseases Div, Bur of Epidemiology, CDC.

Reference
1. MMWR 27:17-18, 23, 1978

MMWR 27:411 (10/20/78)

Infant Botulism — Arizona

Botulism toxin has been isolated from the serum and stool of a 6-week-old boy hospitalized in Phoenix, Arizona, with infant botulism. This is the first time that toxin has been isolated from the serum of an infant with the disease.

The infant was born on July 31 in California and was constipated since birth (4 stools in 6 weeks). He was breast-fed but occasionally drank some canned fruit juices. He had no known ingestion of honey. On September 17, he was noted to have decreased appetite; previously he had been described as a vigorous eater. On September 18, he was hypotonic and suffered a respiratory arrest after being hospitalized. He was noted to have pooling of secretions, poorly reactive pupils, extra-ocular muscle dysfunction, and absent deep tendon reflexes.

CDC isolated botulism toxin from the boy's serum and stool on September 23. The stool contained type A botulism toxin; insufficient serum was available to permit typing the toxin detected in it. A subsequent serum specimen obtained on September 23, 3 days after the initial specimen, was shown to contain type A toxin.

Blood chemistries and hematological studies were normal. Blood, urine, throat, and spinal fluid cultures showed no pathogens on culture. Cerebrospinal fluid pressure, cell count, and glucose and protein content were normal. An electromyogram was consistent with neuromuscular blockade, showing the BSAP pattern described in infant botulism.

The infant was initially treated with ampicillin and gentamicin for presumed sepsis. These were discontinued when cultures were negative and the diagnosis of infant botulism was made. No antitoxin has been given. As of October 16, the infant continued to require mechanical ventilation, although bowel motility was normal, and he showed increased spontaneous movements.

Reported by D Alexander, MD, A Kaplan, MD, A Lersch, MD, St. Joseph's Hospital, Phoenix; A Kelter, MD, State Epidemiologist; Bacterial Diseases Div, Bur of Epidemiology, CDC.

Editorial Note: The syndrome of infant botulism has been recognized frequently since its initial description in 1976 (*1-3*). The question of whether antibiotics and/or antitoxin are indicated in therapy, in addition to supportive care, remains to be answered, pending further studies on the natural history of this illness.

References
1. Pickett J, Berg B, Chaplin E, Brunstetter-Shafer M: Syndrome of botulism in infancy: Clinical and electrophysiologic study. N Engl J Med 295:770-772, 1976
2. Arnon SS, Midura TF, Clay SA, Wood RM, Chin J: Infant botulism: Epidemiological, clinical and laboratory aspects. JAMA 237:1946-1951, 1977
3. MMWR 27:17-23, 1978

MMWR 28:73 (2/23/79)

Botulism — United States, 1978

Cases of botulism in humans in the United States are now classified into 4 categories. Foodborne botulism, which caused the most reported cases in 1978, is an intoxication caused by ingestion of preformed botulinal toxin in contaminated food. Infant botulism, the most recently recognized form of botulism, is an intoxication caused by absorption of botulinal toxin produced *in vivo* in the intestinal tract of an infant after colonization and multiplication of *Clostridium botulinum* organisms. Wound botulism, the rarest form of botulism, results from elaboration of botulinal toxin *in vivo* after multiplication of *C. botulinum* in an infected, traumatized wound. Finally, there is an undetermined classification for those cases of botulism in individuals older than 12 months in which no food or wound source has been implicated.

Foodborne: Twelve outbreaks of foodborne botulism involving 58 cases occurred in the United States in 1978. This compares with 17 outbreaks with 80 cases in 1977 and an average of 7.9 outbreaks with 18.7 cases from 1970 through 1976. No changes from previous years were noted in the age distribution of cases in 1978 nor in the ratio of affected males to females. Of the 58 cases, 55 were due to *C. botulinum* type A toxin and 3 to type B toxin. The case-fatality rate of 5.2% (3 deaths) in 1978 approximated the 6.3% figure for 1977. In 1978 epidemiologically implicated foods, including those in which a laboratory confirmed the presence of toxin, included olives, vegetables, fish, spaghetti sauce, tamales, and pork and beans—all of which were home-processed.

Two large type A botulism outbreaks occurred in 1978. Thirty-four people contracted the disease after eating bean or potato salad at a private club in New Mexico (*1*), and 8 persons became ill after eating potato salad prepared at a restaurant in Colorado (*2*).

Infant Botulism: Since the recognition of infant botulism as a disease entity (*3,4*), 21 states have reported a total of 98 laboratory-proven cases to CDC (Figure 1). In addition, single cases have been reported from England and Australia. The single 1975 case was identified retrospectively in 1976 (*5*). Fifteen cases were reported in 1976, and 43 cases in 1977. In 1978, 12 states reported 39 infant botulism cases, and cases were reported for the first time from Arkansas, Delaware, Georgia, Maryland, Missouri, and New Mexico.

Review of the data since 1975 shows no seasonality of infant botulism cases or of toxin type. Age at onset has ranged from 22 days to 8 months, with a median age of 2½ months. The geographic distribution of infant botulism cases by toxin type parallels the distribution of *C. botulinum* toxin types in the environment. Of the 18 cases east of the Mississippi River, 17 (94%) were type B; 52 (65%) of the 80 cases west of the Mississippi River were type A.

Regarding risk factors, a case-control study of 41 cases in California (*6*) showed that in 29.2% (both type A and B) the infants had received honey before the onset of constipation, but use of honey was significantly associated with only the type B cases (p = 0.005). In the same study the source of milk was evaluated, but the numbers of infants included in each feeding category (only breast milk, mainly breast milk, half breast milk and half formula, mainly formula, and only formula) were too small to allow for definitive statistical comparison.

Wound Botulism: Fourteen cases of wound botulism were reported in the 7-year period 1970–1976; none were reported in 1977 or 1978.

Classification Undetermined: This category includes illnesses in persons over 12 months old characterized by the symptoms and signs of botulism but for which no vehicle was identified. Ten unclassifiable outbreaks involving 13 persons were reported in 1978; 4 cases were associated with 1 outbreak, and the others were single-case outbreaks. This compares with 3 outbreaks, which involved a total of 5 cases, in 1977. An average of 3.3 such outbreaks involving an average of 7.1 cases occurred from 1970 through 1976.

Nine unclassifiable cases in 1978 were caused by type A toxin, while no toxin was recovered from 4 patients. In 1977, 2 of the 5 cases were caused by type A toxin, and in 3 no toxin was recovered. From 1970 through 1976, 29 type A cases, 3 type B cases, and 1 type E case were reported; no toxin was recovered in 16 cases.

Reported by Enterobacteriology Br, Bacteriology Div, Bur of Laboratories, Enteric Diseases Br, Bacterial Diseases Div, Bur of Epidemiology, CDC.

Editorial Note: The decline in the case-fatality ratio of foodborne botulism from the 60%-70% figure seen in the first 50 years of this century to the 12.6% figure seen since 1970 is due mainly to improved supportive care, especially mechanical ventilatory assistance (*7*).

In previous years those cases classified here as undetermined were reported in the foodborne totals. Although many of these cases may be due to ingestion of preformed toxin, another possible but unproved mechanism could be toxicoinfection, the mechanism involved in infant botulism. In toxicoinfection botulinal toxin is produced *in vivo*,

FIGURE 1. Cases of infant botulism by state and toxin type, January 1975 through December 1978

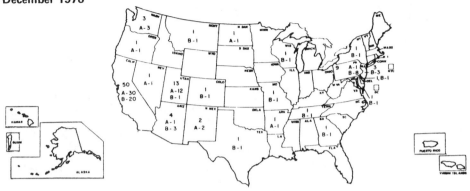

after *C. botulinum* organisms multiply in the intestine. It is possible that intoxication of an adult could develop in a manner similar to that of infant botulism if the normal host-microbial relationships were disturbed.

That no wound botulism cases have been reported in the past 2 years may be a reporting artifact. Since *C. botulinum* spores are ubiquitous in the environment and the sources of wounds seen in previous patients are not uncommon (auto, motorcycle, buckshot, handsaw, and machine part accidents), continued occurrence of cases would be expected. Search for a wound source should always be included in the evaluation of each patient with suspected botulism (*8*).

Infant botulism is now being recognized more frequently throughout the country. California, a state with a special surveillance system for infant botulism, reported all but 20% of the U.S. cases in 1976, while in 1978, 68% were reported from other states.

References
1. MMWR 27:138, 1978
2. MMWR 27:483, 1978
3. Pickett J, Berg B, Chaplain E, Brunstetter-Shafer MA: Syndrome of botulism in infancy: Clinical and electrophysiologic study. N Engl J Med 295:770-772, 1976
4. Arnon SS, Midura TF, Clay SA, Wood RM, Chin J: Infant botulism: Epidemiological, clinical and laboratory aspects. JAMA 237:1946-1951, 1977
5. MMWR 25:269, 1976
6. Arnon SS, Midura TF, Damus K, Thompson B, Wood RM, Chin J: Honey and other environmental risk factors for infant botulism. J Pediatr 94:331-336, 1979
7. CDC: Botulism in the United States, 1899-1973, Handbook for Epidemiologists, Clinicians, and Laboratory Workers. Atlanta, CDC, 1974
8. Merson MH, Dowell VR Jr: Epidemiologic, clinical and laboratory aspects of wound botulism. N Engl J Med 289:1005-1010, 1973

MMWR 27 (A.S., 1978): 19

BOTULISM (FOODBORNE)   — Reported Cases and Deaths by Year, United States, 1960—1978

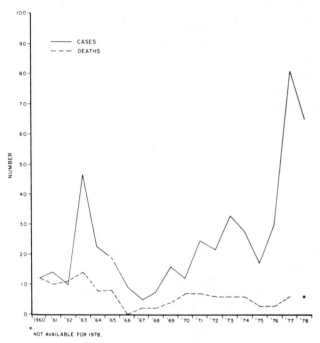

The peaks in foodborne botulism in 1977 and 1978 reflect large common-source outbreaks in Michigan and New Mexico, respectively.

CHAPTER 14

Brucellosis

MMWR 28:437 (9/21/79)

Brucellosis — United States, 1978

In 1978, 172 cases of brucellosis were reported to the Center for Disease Control. This is a decrease of 69 cases from the 241 reported in 1977, and it is also the lowest number of cases reported in any year since 1927, when brucellosis was first recognized as a common cause of human illness.

Of these 172 cases, surveillance reports were received on 161 (94%); 127 (79%) of these were classified as initial infections, and 15 (9%) were recrudescent.* No reinfections were reported with onset in 1978. There were also no fatal cases.

Onset of illness was specified as acute or insidious in 104 brucellosis cases: acute in 57 (55%) and insidious in 47 (45%). In 136 cases the month of onset was specified. Onset of illness was reported to occur more frequently in the spring and summer than in the fall and winter—a pattern observed for the period 1965-1974 (1).

As in the past, brucellosis predominantly affected adult males. Of 160 cases for which sex was specified, 134 (84%) were in males; 116 (82%) of 142 cases for which age was given were in persons between 20 and 60 years of age. This is the age category of the work force in the United States and the population at greatest risk of acquiring brucellosis in the meat-packing and livestock industries. Indeed, 58 (46%) of the 127 cases for which information was available were in individuals working in the meat-processing industry (Figure 1).

Thirty-eight states reported cases last year (Figure 2) compared with 37 states, Puerto Rico, and Guam in 1977. Two states, Iowa and Texas, reported more than 15 cases each and together accounted for 22% of the 1978 total. Idaho reported the greatest increase in total cases (5), while Virginia reported the greatest decrease (33). Virginia's

---

*A confirmed case was defined as 1). a clinical specimen culture-positive for *Brucella*, or 2). clinical symptoms compatible with brucellosis, such as any combination of fever, sweats, chills, undue fatigue, anorexia, weight loss, arthralgia, lymphadenopathy, and splenomegaly, and a ⩾4-fold change in *Brucella* agglutination titer between acute and convalescent serum specimens obtained 2 or more weeks apart and studied at the same laboratory. A presumptive case was defined as clinical symptoms compatible with brucellosis with either a *Brucella* agglutination titer positive at a ⩾1:160 dilution on a single serum specimen obtained after the onset of symptoms or a stable *Brucella* agglutination titer positive at a ⩾1:160 dilution in serum specimens obtained after the onset of symptoms. A recrudescent case is a confirmed or presumptive case in a person who, within the preceding 3 years, had an illness diagnosed as brucellosis followed by a period of apparent recovery.

FIGURE 1. Total brucellosis cases and proportion associated with abattoirs,* United States, 1967-1978

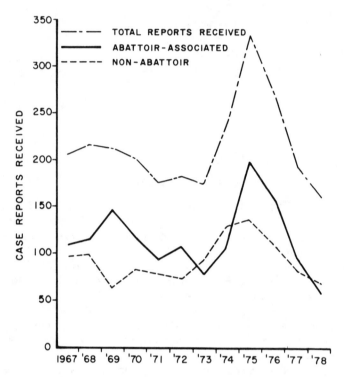

*Includes packinghouse employees, government meat inspectors, and rendering plant workers.

marked decline was because of a reduction in swine-associated cases in abattoir workers. The majority of the Idaho cases were associated with cattle.

As in the period 1975-1977, cattle were the most common source of human infection last year. Contact with infected cattle resulted in 54 (34%) human cases in 1978. Swine-associated cases were markedly reduced, due primarily to Virginia's decrease in such cases. Contact with infected domestic swine was responsible for 16 cases (10%), and feral swine for 2 cases in hunters. An additional 18 (11%) cases resulted from contact with cattle and swine. Three cases were associated with contact with dogs. Fourteen (9%) cases were attributed to the ingestion of unpasteurized dairy products—9 of these to milk produced in the United States. Five cases were attributed to foreign dairy products, including raw milk or cheese from Mexico (3 cases), Iran (1 case), and an unspecified Latin American country (1 case). Accidental injection of strain 19 *Brucella* vaccine was listed as the cause in 3 cases, all in veterinarians, and laboratory accidents resulted in 2 cases.

Reported by the Bacterial Zoonoses Br, Bacterial Diseases Div, Bur of Epidemiology, CDC.

Editorial Note: A review of brucellosis cases in the United States from 1967 to 1978 emphasizes the importance of abattoirs in the epidemiology of brucellosis. In 7 of the last 10 years, more than half of reported cases occurred in people associated with the meat-processing industry (Figure 2). Of 2,063 cases on which reports were received in this 10-year period, 1,171 (57%) were in abattoir workers.

FIGURE 2. Human brucellosis cases, by state, United States, 1978

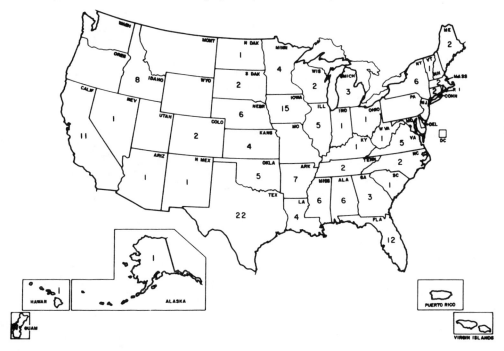

Reference
1. Fox JD, Kaufmann AF: Brucellosis in the United States, 1965-1974. J Infect Dis 136: 312-316, 1977

▲ A copy of the surveillance report from which these data were summarized is available on request from CDC, Attn: Bacterial Zoonoses Br, Bacterial Diseases Div, Bur of Epidemiology, CDC.

MMWR 27 (A.S., 1978): 21

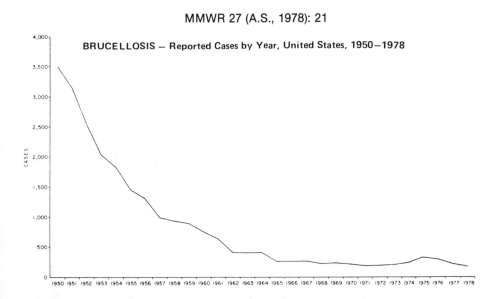

BRUCELLOSIS — Reported Cases by Year, United States, 1950—1978

BRUCELLOSIS — Reported Cases by County, United States, 1978

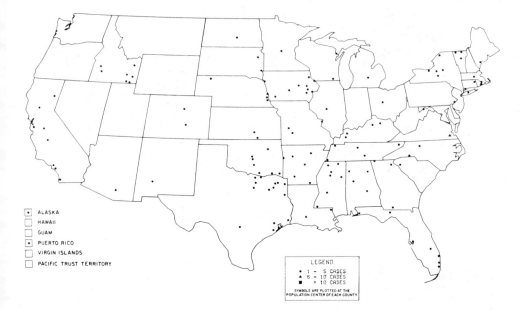

ALASKA
HAWAII
GUAM
PUERTO RICO
VIRGIN ISLANDS
PACIFIC TRUST TERRITORY

LEGEND
• 1 — 5 CASES
▲ 6 — 10 CASES
■ > 10 CASES
SYMBOLS ARE PLOTTED AT THE
POPULATION CENTER OF EACH COUNTY

CHAPTER 15

Tularemia

MMWR 27:105 (3/24/78)

Pneumonic Tularemia — Washington

On November 15, 1977, a 19-year-old King County resident went deer hunting with friends and relatives in central Washington state. While on the trail 2 days later, he found a partially dismembered dead rabbit. The hunter amputated the front paws for good luck charms, which he gave to another hunter in the party.

The rabbit had been handled with bare hands that were bruised and scratched from the hunter's work as an automobile mechanic. Festering sores on his hands, legs, and knees were noted on November 19. Spiking fevers followed 24 hours later. He was cared for at home until December 11 when his physician admitted him to a local hospital because of continued bouts of fever and a weight loss of 10 pounds.

Initial white blood counts showed 8,400 cells/mm^3 with a normal differential pattern. The chest X rays showed a right superior mediastinal mass with hilar adenopathy and no evidence of peripheral pneumonitis. Because Hodgkin's disease was suspected, a mediastinoscopy with a mediastinal needle biopsy was performed. The report indicated the presence of necrotizing granuloma. By December 14 the fevers had subsided, and the patient was discharged.

A blood specimen, drawn on December 16, was sent to the state's public health laboratory for agglutination tests for tularemia, brucellosis, and proteus OX 2, OX 19, and OX K. Because of a high positive titer for tularemia (1:20,480), an epidemiologic investigation was begun.

Despite repeated attempts to elicit a history of exposure to wild rabbits, none was obtained until after Christmas, when the grandfather remembered the rabbit paw incident. A 10-day course of tetracycline therapy (2 gms. daily) was started on December 21. On January 3 a second blood specimen showed no decline in agglutination titer. The patient has declined further blood studies. He remains well with no evidence of relapse.

The recipient of the "good luck charms" remains well. He had discarded the paws, however, so they could not be recovered.

Reported by DG Kestle, MD, Bellevue, Washington; AHB Pedersen, MD, MPH, J Spearman, RN, MN, E Tronca, MS, Seattle-King County Health Dept; J Allard, PHD, JW Taylor, MD, State Epidemiologist, Washington Dept of Social and Health Services; Bacterial Zoonoses Br, Bacterial Diseases Div, Bur of Epidemiology, CDC.

Editorial Note: It is presumed that illness resulted from exposure to the dead rabbit and that the portal of entry was primarily through traumatic skin breaks in the hands, with secondary mediastinal involvement. However, simultaneous inhalation of aerosolized *Francisella tularensis* cannot be excluded.

MMWR 27:352 (9/15/78)
Tularemia — Massachusetts

In August 1978, all 7 members of a household on Martha's Vineyard developed a febrile illness. The patients, all adults, were at their cottage on August 2-4; some had been there at various other times throughout the summer. Seven other persons present in the last week of July and one present on August 6-11 have remained well. The patients were seen by physicians on Martha's Vineyard and in Boston, Connecticut, and Colorado.

Onset of illness was between August 6 and 11 for 6 of the individuals. Illness was characterized by fever to 104 F (40 C), myalgia, headache, and non-productive cough. Chest X rays on 5 of the 7 showed pulmonary infiltrates. One patient required respiratory support. Erythromycin and tetracycline appeared to hasten recovery. All are recovering. Four of the 5 persons tested to date show seroconversion to *Francisella tularensis*.

Review of hospital records, chest X rays, and emergency room records for July and August 1978 did not show a significant increase compared with 1977 in the number of cases of pneumonia or febrile illness on the island; no respiratory illness in neighbors was found. Environmental studies are in progress.

Reported by R Hoxsie, MD, AD Langmuir, MD, MPH, Martha's Vineyard, Chilmark Board of Health; N Fiumara, MD, State Epidemiologist, Kenlock, Massachusetts, Dept of Health; J Lewis, MD, State Epidemiologist, Connecticut Dept of Health; P Moran, MD, Grand Junction, Colorado; TM Vernon, MD, State Epidemiologist, Colorado Dept of Health; Parasitic Diseases,Viral Diseases, and Field Services Divisions, Bur of Epidemiology, CDC. DR Kimloch, MD, Massachusetts Department of Health.

MMWR 28:529 (11/9/79)
Tularemia — Montana, Colorado, Alaska, and Georgia

Through October 13 of this year, 166 cases of tularemia were reported to CDC. Five recent reports exemplify several of the clinical and epidemiologic characteristics commonly observed with this disease.

Montana: From May 30 to July 3, 1979, 3 serologically confirmed* and 8 presumptive† cases of tularemia occurred on the Crow Indian Reservation in southcentral Montana. Nine cases were in children. Illness was mild, consisting primarily of fever and lymphadenopathy localized in the neck. All patients recovered; most improved before therapy with streptomycin was initiated. The presumed mode of transmission was ticks. No cases occurred after July 3, a finding consistent with the sudden decrease in free-living ticks normally observed in this area during the hot summer months. *Francisella tularensis* (type B) was isolated from 8 of 14 lots of ticks (*Dermacentor variabilis*) taken off dogs in early August, and 29 of 31 dogs from the reservation had tularemia agglutinating antibody titers ≥1:40.

Colorado: During the week of April 23, 4 of 9 members of a sheep-shearing crew working west of Rangely became ill with fever and headache. Three persons developed left axillary lymphadenopathy with lesions on the dorsum of the left hand. The other patient, who did not have adenopathy or a skin lesion, suffered a more severe illness associated with a pulmonary infiltrate. All patients consulted a physician approximately 10 days after onset of illness and recovered with tetracycline therapy. One patient had a 4-fold rise in antibody to *F. tularensis*, while the other 3 had single titers of ≥1:160. Before becoming ill, these men had sheared sheep that had appeared ill and were covered with wood ticks (*D. andersoni*). The presence of lesions on only the left hand is explained by the procedure the workers use in shearing sheep. The men part fleece with their bare left hand, while shearing with the right hand—often rupturing ticks in the process, spilling blood onto the left hand.

In late June, a 31-year-old laboratory technician was hospitalized in Grand Junction, with an illness of 2 weeks' duration that had begun several days after working with an isolate of *F. tularensis*. Symptoms included fever to 105.8 F (41 C), headache, and pleuritic chest pain; pneumonitis and pleural effusion were confirmed by X ray. A diagnosis of tularemia was made, based on a 16-fold rise in titer. The patient recovered with streptomycin therapy.

Alaska: On August 31, a 49-year-old man in Fairbanks became ill 3 days after dressing a rabbit killed by his dog. Initial symptoms were a fever of 105 F (40.5 C) and vomiting; within 2 days he developed bilateral axillary adenopathy with 2 ulcerations just proximal to a cut on his left hand. Culture of a lymph node aspirate grew *F. tularensis*, and the patient made an uneventful recovery with tetracycline therapy. A number of dead rabbits had been recently observed in the area.

Georgia: In mid-September, 2 boys aged 10 and 11, from Calhoun, became ill after handling a dead rabbit they had found. Both boys developed fever, epitrochlear and axillary adenopathy, and ulcerative lesions on their hands. When seen on October 1, both patients were still ill, and cultures of both hand lesions and 1 lymph node aspirate grew *F. tularensis* (type A). Both patients are recovering with streptomycin therapy. No evidence of a tularemia epizootic among rabbits was observed in the area.

Reported by CA Connors, MD, PR Strange, MD, MS Myers, MD, GA Ostahowski, MD, GK Call, MD, Crow Agency, Montana; JD Carney, Billings Area Office, Indian Health Service; MD Skinner, MD, State Epidemiologist, Montana State Dept of Health and Environmental Sciences; CT Frey, MD, Cedaredge, Colorado; C Lindes, MD, Paonia, Colorado; RD Schmidt, Grand Junction, Colorado; RS Hopkins, MD, State Epidemiologist, JK Emerson, DVM, MPH, Public Health Veterinarian, Colorado State Dept of Health; RJ Burger, MD, R Zeimis, MS, Fairbanks, Alaska; DF Tirador, MD, State Epidemiologist, Alaska State Dept of Health and Social Services; R Ingraham, MD, Dalton, Georgia; RK Sikes, DVM, JS Terry, MD, Acting State Epidemiologist, Georgia Dept of Human Resources; Vector-borne Diseases Div, Bur of Laboratories, Field Services Div, and Bacterial Zoonoses Br, Bacterial Diseases Div, Bur of Epidemiology, CDC.

---

*≥4-fold change in agglutinating antibody titer between acute and convalescent serum specimens, with 1 titer being ≥1:160.
†≤4-fold change with 1 titer being ≥1:160.

Editorial Note: Tularemia is an uncommon disease in the United States. An average of 157 cases were reported annually for the years 1969-1978, although in previous decades the average annual incidence was severalfold higher.

The 5 cases reported here illustrate part of the clinical spectrum of tularemia as well as at least 3 different modes of transmission. Clinical illness ranges from a mild, self-limited illness similar to that seen in the Montana cases to more severe and lingering illness, which can include pneumonia, meningitis, and death. Symptoms normally appear first at the site of inoculation and include ulceration and regional adenopathy (with cutaneous inoculation) or pneumonia (with inhalation exposure). In the case of the fourth sheep shearer, the infection probably resulted in typhoidal tularemia, with pneumonia occurring secondary to bacteremia, although inhalation as a route of infection cannot be excluded. The laboratory technician may have developed pneumonia following inhalation of infectious aerosols generated during examination of the *F. tularensis* isolate, but other modes of transmission have not been ruled out. This case illustrates the hazards associated with culturing *F. tularensis*.

In addition to factors such as host susceptibility, route of infection, and inoculum size, severity of disease is also partially dependent on the virulence of the infecting strain. Although elaborate animal inoculation tests may be done to determine virulence, strains capable of fermenting glycerol are more pathogenic than those that do not (*1*). The strains isolated in Montana were glycerol-negative (type B), while those in Georgia were glycerol-positive (type A).

Reference

1. Olsufiev NG, Emelyanova OS, Dun*yeva TN: Comparative study of strains of *B. tularense* in the Old and New World and their taxonomy. J Hyg Epidemiol Microbiol Immunol (Praha): 3:138-149, 1959

MMWR 27 (A.S., 1978): 69

TULAREMIA — Reported Case Rates by Year, United States, 1950—1978

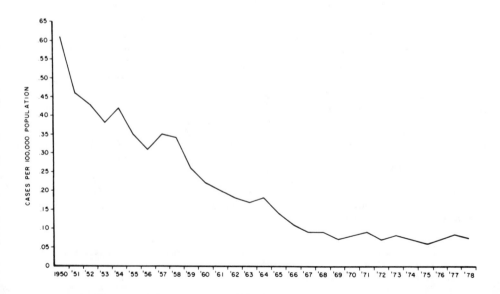

TULAREMIA — Reported Cases by County, United States, 1978

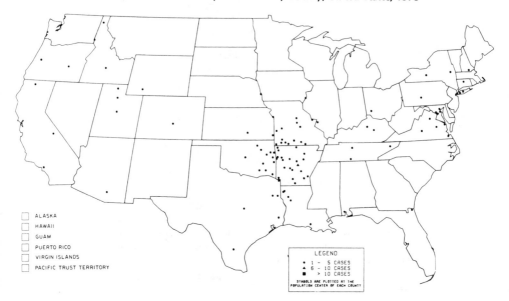

ALASKA
HAWAII
GUAM
PUERTO RICO
VIRGIN ISLANDS
PACIFIC TRUST TERRITORY

LEGEND
• 1 – 5 CASES
▲ 6 – 10 CASES
■ > 10 CASES

SYMBOLS ARE PLOTTED AT THE
POPULATION CENTER OF EACH COUNTY

CHAPTER 16

Plague

MMWR 26:337 (10/14/77)

Plague — United States

Fifteen cases of bubonic plague in humans have been reported to CDC in 1977. Seven cases were acquired in New Mexico, 3 in Arizona, 3 in California, 1 in Colorado, and 1 in Oregon (Table 1). Four patients had secondary pneumonic involvement.

TABLE 1. Reported confirmed cases of plague, United States, 1977

Patient	Age	Sex	Onset	County	State
1*	39	M	Feb	Moffat	Colorado
2*	3	M	June	McKinley	New Mexico
3*	23	F	June	Coconino	Arizona
4*	43	M	June	Rio Arriba	New Mexico
5	5	M	July	Santa Fe	New Mexico
6†	3	F	July	Placer	California
7	36	M	July	Valencia	New Mexico
8	21	M	July	Klamath	Oregon
9	15	M	Aug	Apache	Arizona
10†	55	M	Aug	Santa Clara	California
11	44	F	Aug	McKinley	New Mexico
12	48	F	Sept	Kern	California
13	6	M	Sept	Valencia	New Mexico
14	56	F	Sept	Rio Arriba	New Mexico
15	16	M	Sept	Coconino	Arizona

*Reported in MMWR 26:215, 1977
†Died

The case history of one patient (#13) is of particular interest because he apparently acquired the infection from a pet cat. On September 6 the 6-year-old boy had onset of fever, chills, vomiting, and bilateral axillary pain. He was examined by a physician, who diagnosed possible viral syndrome and prescribed erythromycin. Later that day the child was admitted to a hospital with a temperature of 104-105 F and delirium. On September 7 he had not improved and diarrhea developed. He was transferred to a hospital in Albuquerque, where admission findings included a temperature of 104 F and a white blood count of 17,400. He had multiple abrasions, scratches, and insect bites (attributed to mosquitoes) on both arms and painful bilateral non-fluctuant axillary lymphadenophathy. Cefazolin therapy was instituted after blood, throat, and cerebrospinal fluid cultures had been obtained. On September 8 one of the axillary nodes was aspirated. Results with Gram, Wayson, and fluorescent antibody (FA) stains were consistent with *Yersinia pestis* infection; therapy was changed to chloramphenicol and streptomycin. By September 17 the patient had become afebrile, but the painful axillary lymphadenopathy persisted. The nodes were incised and drained on September 19; cultures of this material were positive for *Y. pestis,* as were the original node aspirate and blood culture. The patient was discharged from the hospital on September 22 and has since completely recovered.

Epidemiologic investigation revealed that the patient lived with his parents in a mobile home in Valencia County, New Mexico. Few rodents were found in the vicinity, and the patient had had no exposure to dead animals. On September 3 he and his family had visited his grandparents on their farm in Valencia County. The farm has many outbuildings known to be infested with rodents. The grandfather periodically shoots rabbits — most recently on August 31 — in the immediate area and feeds them to his 20-30 cats and 4 dogs. The patient had taken a pet cat home with him on September 3. The cat climbed a tree and bit and scratched the boy on both upper extremities when he tried to retrieve it. The cat subsequently appeared ill, staying in its box, and was returned to the grandparents on September 4. It disappeared on September 5 and was later found dead under a woodpile; tissue specimens were FA- and culture-positive for *Y. pestis.*

Reported by F Heaton, MD, Albuquerque; J Gaskin, K Marchiando, St. Joseph's Hospital, Albuquerque; L Hughes, PhD, G Graves, J Mann, MD, State Epidemiologist, P Matzner, C Montman, A Pressman, MD, K Weeks, New Mexico Health and Social Services Dept; JM Counts, DrPH, State Epidemiologist, Arizona State Dept of Health Services; SB Werner, MD, Califiornia State Dept of Health; TM Vernon Jr, MD, State Epidemiologist, Colorado State Dept of Health; JA Googins, MD, State Epidemiologist, Oregon State Health Div; Plague Br, Vector-Borne Diseases Div, Bur of Laboratories, and Bacterial Zoonoses Br, Bacterial Diseases Div, Bur of Epidemiology, CDC.

Editorial Note: If this case represents transmission of *Y. pestis* from a domestic cat to a human, as the epidemiologic evidence suggests, it is the second such occurrence this year (1) and only the third ever reported (1,2).

References
1. MMWR 26:215, 1977
2. Isaacson M, Levy D, Te BJ, et al: Unusual cases of human plague in Southern Africa. S Afr Med J 4:2109-2113, 1973

MMWR 27:255 (7/21/78)

Plague Vaccine

INTRODUCTION

Plague is a natural infection of rodents and their ectoparasites and occurs in many parts of the world, including the western United States, where a few human cases develop each year following exposure to infected wild rodents or their fleas. Epidemic plague may result when domestic rat populations and their fleas become infected. Recently the areas of the most intensive epidemic and epizootic infection have been some countries in Africa, Asia, and South America.

PLAGUE VACCINE

Plague vaccines* have been used since the late 19th century, but their effectiveness has never been measured precisely. Extensive field experience indicates that immunization with plague vaccine reduces the incidence and severity of disease.

The plague vaccine licensed for use in the United States is prepared from *Yersinia pestis* organisms grown in artificial media, inactivated with formaldehyde, and preserved in 0.5% phenol.

VACCINE USAGE

General Recommendations

Because human plague is rare in most parts of the world, there is no need to vaccinate persons other than those at particularly high risk of exposure. Routine vaccination is not needed for persons living in plague-enzootic areas like those in the western United States. It is not indicated for most travelers to countries reporting cases,† particularly if their travel is limited to urban areas with modern hotel accommodations.

In most countries of South America, Asia, and Africa where plague is reported, the risk of exposure exists primarily in rural mountainous or upland areas. Following natural disasters and at times when regular sanitary practices are interrupted, plague can extend from its usually endemic areas into urban centers. Rarely, pneumonic plague has been reported in conjunction with outbreaks of bubonic plague, and tourist travel to those specific locations should be avoided.

Routine bacteriologic precautions are sufficient to prevent accidental infection with plague; therefore, immunization of clinical laboratory workers is unnecessary,

Ecologists and other field workers who might come in contact with wild animals and their ectoparasites in areas where plague has been known to occur should be made aware of the potential risks of plague and told how to minimize direct contact with potentially infective animals and their tissues or parasites. These precautionary measures are generally sufficient to prevent infection.

Vaccine Recipients

Vaccination should be a routine requirement for:

1. All laboratory and field personnel who are working with *Y. pestis* organisms resistant to antimicrobics;

2. Persons engaged in aerosol experiments with *Y. pestis*; and

3. Persons engaged in field operations in plague-enzootic areas where preventing exposure cannot be observed (such as some disaster areas).

---

*Official name: Plague Vaccine

†For a current listing, consult the most recent issue of the World Health Organization's *Weekly Epidemiological Record.*

Selective plague vaccination might be considered for:

1. Laboratory personnel regularly working with *Y. pestis* or plague-infected rodents;

2. Workers (for example, Peace Corps volunteers and agricultural advisors) who reside in plague-enzootic or plague-epidemic rural areas where avoidance of rodents and fleas is impossible; and

3. Persons whose vocation brings them into regular contact with wild rodents or rabbits in plague-enzootic areas.

Primary Immunization

All injections should be given intramuscularly.

Adults and children over 10 years old: The primary series consists of 3 doses of vaccine. The first 2 doses, 0.5 ml each, should be administered 4 or more weeks apart, followed by a third dose, 0.2 ml, 4-12 weeks after the second injection. When less time is available, satisfactory but less than optimal results can be obtained with 3 injections of 0.5 ml administered at least 1 week apart.

Children less than 10 years old: The primary series also is 3 doses of vaccine, but the doses are smaller. The manufacturer's guide to proportionate dosages is: infants under 1 year—one-fifth adult dose; 1-4 years—two-fifths adult dose, 5-10 years—three-fifths adult dose. The intervals between injections are the same as for adults.

Boosters Doses

When needed because of continuing exposure, boosters should be given at approximately 6-month intervals to a total of 5 doses (3 primary vaccination doses plus 2 boosters). More than 90% of vaccinees should then have a passive hemagglutination (PHA) antibody titier of 1:128 or more. Thereafter, booster doses at 1-2 year intervals, depending on the degree of continuing exposure, should provide good protection.

Booster dosages for children and adults is the same as the third dose in the primary series. The primary series need never be repeated for booster doses to be effective.

SUMMARY

The recommended doses for primary and booster vaccination are shown in Table 1.

TABLE 1. Recommended doses, by volume (ml), for immunization against plague

Dose number	Age (Years)			
	<1	1-4	5-10	>10
1 & 2	0.1 ml	0.2 ml	0.3 ml	0.5 ml
3 & Boosters	0.04 mi	0.08 ml	0.12 ml	0.2 ml

PRECAUTIONS AND CONTRAINDICATIONS

Mild pain, erythema, and side effects sucn as induration at the injection site occur frequently. With repeated doses, fever, headache, and malaise are more common and also tend to be more severe. Sterile abscesses occur, but rarely. No fatal or disabling complications have been reported.

SELECTED BIBLIOGRAPHY

Bartelloni PJ, Marshall JD Jr, Cavanaugh DC: Clinical and serological responses to plague vaccine U.S.P. Milit Med 138:720-722, 1973

Burmeister RW, Tigertt WD, Overholt EL: Laboratory-acquired pneumonic plague. Ann Intern Med 56:789-800, 1962

Cavanaugh DC, Elisberg BL, Llewellyn CH, et al: Plague immunization. V. Indirect evidence for the efficacy of plague vaccine. J infect Dis 129 (Suppl):S37-S40, 1974

MMWR 28:285 (6/22/79)

Human Plague — California

California's first case of human plague in 1979 was confirmed the week ending May 18 in a 55-year-old man who lives in Diamond Bar, a suburban community in southeast Los Angeles County. Although wild rodent plague was documented as recently as last year in Los Angeles County, this is the first human case acquired in the county since 1936.

The patient developed fever and pain in the right groin on May 9. The next day, he saw a physician who noted fever of 40.5 C, pyuria, and hematuria. The patient was treated with intramuscular penicillin and was given a prescription for oral ampicillin for presumed urinary tract infection. On May 11, he appeared flushed, toxic, and tremulous and was admitted to a hospital. His temperature at that time was 39.4 C, and his pulse, 100. He had a tender, rubbery, nonpulsatile, nonfluctuant mass in his right groin. Laboratory data included a white blood count (WBC) of 16,000/mm^3 with a marked shift to the left. Urinalysis revealed gross hematuria, 4+ proteinuria, and many granular and red blood casts. Admitting diagnosis was fever of undetermined origin with septicemia. After 3 blood cultures were drawn, parenteral treatment with ampicillin and gentamicin was started.

Massive diarrhea began on May 11, and by May 13 abdominal films suggested possible bowel obstruction. A laparotomy was performed showing only lymphadenitis near the right groin. Positive blood cultures were flown on May 16 to the state's Microbial Diseases Laboratory, where *Yersinia pestis* was identified by fluorescent-antibody and bacteriophage tests. Antibiotic treatment was switched from ampicillin to tetracycline; gentamicin was retained. The patient has been recovering satisfactorily. There have been no signs of pneumonic involvement.

The patient had not traveled or camped recently. He played golf each weekend at the Diamond Bar golf course and jogged 2 miles daily (always with long pants) around his home. He has a cat and small house dog; both animals have been well. The patient had no known insect bites or direct contact with rodents.

The patient's home is about 2½ miles from Sycamore Canyon County Park. The park was closed and treated with insecticide in late 1978 because of a plague epizootic among ground squirrels. The patient had not been in the park recently, but the above-mentioned golf course is adjacent to that park. His home site abuts on grassy, hilly, undeveloped land with chaparral. Ecologic studies in the vicinity of the house revealed abandoned rodent burrows with fleas and blowflies, suggesting a recent rodent die-off. A ground squirrel carcass found approximately 100 feet from the property was culture positive for *Y. pestis*.

Reported by J Pickleseimer, MD, T Davis, RN, Presbyterian Intercommunity Hospital, Whittier, California, and S Fannin, MD, Los Angeles County Dept of Health Services, in the California Morbidity Weekly Report, No. 20, May 25, 1979; Plague Br, Vector-Borne Diseases Div, Bur of Laboratories, and Bacterial Zoonoses Br, Bacterial Diseases Div, Bur of Epidemiology, CDC.

Editorial Note: Seven cases of human plague with onset in 1979 have been reported to CDC since January 1. For the past 5 years, the average number of cases reported during the corresponding time period was 5. In addition to 2 cases reported from California, Arizona has reported 3 cases, and New Mexico has reported 2 cases. Plague infection has been bacteriologically confirmed in 3 of the cases; confirmation is pending for the other 4.

Plague infection in the patient reported here was presumably acquired in the vicinity of his home or, possibly, the golf course. Ecologic studies suggesting a recent wild rodent die-off support the impression that this case was sylvatic in origin, even though it occurred in a suburban area.

MMWR 27 (A.S., 1978): 49

PLAGUE – Reported Cases in Humans by Year, United States, 1950—1978

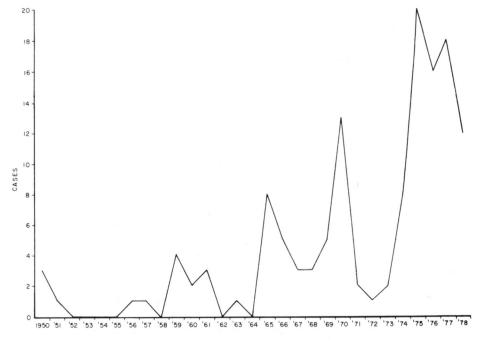

PLAGUE – Reported Cases and Deaths in Humans by Age Group, United States, 1950—1978

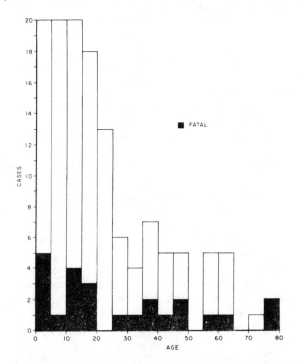

CHAPTER 17

Gonorrhea, Gonococcal Endocarditis, and Pelvic Inflammatory Disease

MMWR 28:189 (4/27/79)

Penicillinase-Producing *Neisseria gonorrhoeae* — Alaska

Alaska's second and third cases of penicillinase-producing *Neisseria gonorrhoeae* (PPNG) were identified in December 1978.

On December 14, a 60-year-old man presented to an Anchorage Health Department venereal disease clinic, giving a history of a recent urethral discharge. Examination revealed no urethral discharge so a urethral culture for gonorrhea was obtained, and he was asked to return to the clinic for the results. When he was examined on December 17, a urethral discharge was evident. At this time the patient stated he had recently traveled in the Philippines. Gram strain of the urethral discharge was positive. He was treated with 4.8 million units aqueous procaine penicillin G (APPG) intramuscularly (IM) and 1 g of probenecid orally. He named no contacts in an interview.

On December 22, still complaining of a slight urethral discharge, the patient returned to the clinic for a test-of-cure (TOC) culture. On December 26, he returned to the clinic, saying the discharge was worse. The results of penicillin-sensitivity tests were still pending on the TOC isolate of December 22. Because he had recently been in the Philippines and his infection had not responded to penicillin therapy, PPNG infection was suspected. The patient was treated with 2 g of spectinomycin, IM.

On January 2, the state laboratory confirmed that the isolate was PPNG. The patient returned to the clinic for a TOC culture, as scheduled, and he was reinterviewed. At this time, the patient indicated that he had had 2 sexual contacts: 1 on December 5 in the Philippines, the other on December 15—1 day after the urethral discharge had developed—in Anchorage.

Investigation revealed that the patient's Anchorage contact had already presented to the outpatient department of the Alaska Native Medical Center (ANMC) on December 29 with a copious vaginal and rectal discharge. She was cultured and received 4.8 million units IM of APPG plus 1 g of probenecid. She returned to the ANMC on January 2. When it was learned that she was a contact of a patient with PPNG, she was treated with spectinomycin and interviewed for contacts. Both cultures taken from her on December 29 were subsequently found positive and confirmed as PPNG.

This woman's 1 contact was her estranged husband, who lived in the remote Iliamma Lake region. He was contacted and found to be asymptomatic. However, a culture specimen was taken from his anterior urethra, and he and his 2 contacts were treated epidemiologically with spectinomycin. There was no incubator in the area, and heavy snows delayed the investigator's return to Anchorage for 3 days. No gonococci were isolated by the state laboratory. However, because of these conditions, the culture was judged unsatisfactory.

Reported by DLO Bourne, TR Kelly, TL Woodard, MD, Acting State Epidemiologist, Alaska State Dept of Health and Social Services; Program Services Br, Veneral Disease Control Div, Bur of State Services, CDC.

Editorial Note: State and local health departments reported 220 cases of PPNG during 1978 and 554 total cases during the 3-year period ending February 1979. Many cases have been identified through the nationwide PPNG surveillance network, established after the initial case was reported in March 1976. High priority contact-tracing has uncovered numerous other PPNG cases and has helped contain several potential outbreaks. The prevention of PPNG cases requires that health providers strongly encourage all gonorrhea patients to have a TOC culture 3 to 5 days following therapy. PPNG infection should be suspected in patients who are still infected or who have recently traveled in the Far East. Patients with PPNG infections as well as their sexual partners should receive 2 g of spectinomycin IM; but the drugs of choice for uncomplicated gonorrhea remain APPG, ampicillin, and amoxicillin, all with 1 g of probenecid or the oral regimen of tetracycline hydrochloride (1).

Reference
1. **MMWR** 28:13-16, 21, 1979

MMWR 28:85 (3/2/79)

Penicillinase-producing *Neisseria gonorrhoeae* — United States, Worldwide

A total of 508 cases of penicillinase-producing *Neisseria gonorrhoeae* (PPNG) from 31 states, the District of Columbia, and Guam were reported to CDC from March 1976, when the first case was detected, through December 1978 (Figure 1). California, the only state that has experienced one or more cases each month since nationwide surveillance for PPNG began in September 1976 (Figure 2), reported 289 (56.9%) of the cases.

Approximately 40% of PPNG cases in California and about one-half of the cases elsewhere in the United States were imported or linked to imported cases. All index patients, except for 1 from Ghana, came from or were infected in Southeast Asia. Military personnel or their dependents were responsible for two-thirds of the imported cases. Although the remaining PPNG cases may reflect indigenous transmission, no defined endemic focus of PPNG has been identified.

Twenty-seven countries in Europe, Asia, Africa, Oceania, and North America have reported cases of PPNG to the World Health Organization (WHO). The organism accounts for about 30% of all recent gonococcal isolates in the Philippines and 16% in the Republic of Singapore. The current incidence of PPNG in Singapore contrasts with only 3 PPNG cases in 1976 and 22 (0.24%) in 1977. Singapore and the Philippines are the only 2 countries with proven high prevalence of PPNG, but epidemiologic assessment of PPNG cases imported into Europe indicates that the organisms are also prevalent in West Africa.

The clinical spectrum of PPNG infection is similar to ordinary gonorrhea. The frequency of complications is approximately the same. Septicemia, conjunctivitis, acute salpingitis, adolescent vulvovaginitis, and asymptomatic urethral infection (in males) have been reported in association with PPNG.

Field investigations conducted in Utah, Minnesota, and New Jersey revealed 13 independent chains of transmission consisting of 2 to 8 epidemiologically linked generations of cases. Gonococcal infection occurred in 60 of the 115 sexual contacts who were located and examined. Twenty-one of these 60 infections were due to PPNG; most were

FIGURE 1. Cases of penicillinase-producing *Neisseria gonorrhoeae*, by state, March 1976 through December 1978

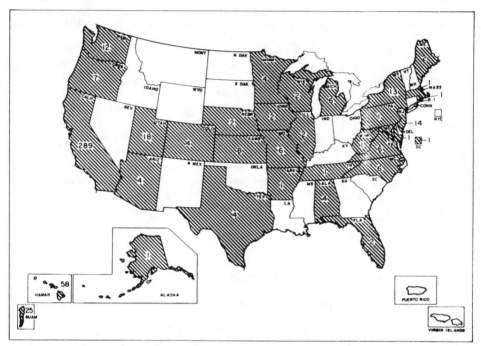

FIGURE 2. Comparison of U.S.* and California cases of penicillinase-producing *Neisseria gonorrhoeae*, by month of onset, March 1976 through December 1978

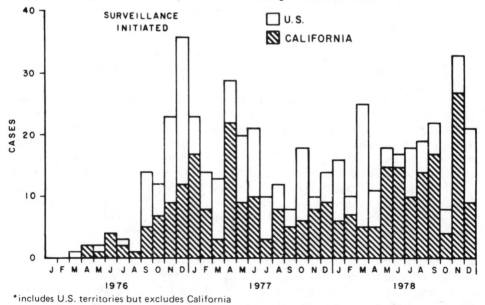

*includes U.S. territories but excludes California

seen within the first few generations of cases.

Reported by GM Antal, Venereal Disease Control Div, WHO, Geneva; EH Sng, Ministry of Health, Republic of Singapore; Venereal Disease Control Div, Bur of State Services, CDC.

Editorial Note: Among the factors thought to contribute to the high prevalence of PPNG in the Philippines and Singapore is the preventive use of oral penicillins, especially by prostitutes. Despite the continual importation of PPNG, infections due to PPNG have not yet reached significant prevalence in the United States. The limited spread here may be due to spontaneous loss of the gonococcal plasmid responsible for penicillinase production in the absence of selective antibiotic pressure, as well as to prompt tracing and treatment of contacts exposed to known PPNG infection. Until the factors that contribute to high PPNG prevalence are more clearly identified, however, it is important that effective surveillance continue.

All gonorrhea patients not successfully treated with penicillin should continue to be treated with spectinomycin, 2.0 g intramuscularly, and gonococcal isolates obtained from them should be tested for penicillinase production. Routine screening of pretreatment gonococcal isolates is also indicated in areas at high risk for importation of PPNG.

MMWR 28:290 (6/29/79)

Results of Culture Testing for Gonorrhea — United States, 1978

In the 12-month period ending December 31, 1978, a total of 8,641,188 culture specimens were taken from women as part of gonorrhea-control programs; 403,098 (4.7%) were positive (Table 1). Although the positivity rates were highest (19.5%) in venereal disease (VD) clinics, 89% of all tests were performed in other settings. In these settings, culture-positivity rates in women ranged from 1.4% in student health centers to 4.9% for women in correctional or detention centers. Among 1,866,306 women tested by private physicians, 35,573 (1.9%) cultures were positive.

Provisional data indicate that an additional 2,160,529 women were tested at all types of facilities in January, February, and March 1979, or about 720,176 per month. For this period, the overall positivity rate of cultures from all sources was 4.3%.

Reported by Venereal Disease Control Div, Bur of State Services, CDC.

Editorial Note: Total reported gonorrhea morbidity in the United States increased by 1.1% in 1978 compared to 1977. The overall positivity rate among women tested for gonorrhea was 4.7% for both 1977 and 1978. However, the number of women tested and the number and percentage with positive tests within different health facilities changed in 1978 for several reasons: more testing of high-risk groups, more emphasis on hospital and health-center testing, and changes in the actual disease incidence or prevalence.

In VD clinics, testing was less frequent in 1978 than 1977 (the number of women tested decreased by 0.9%), but the number of infections detected increased by 5.1%. Rescreening women who had been previously treated for gonorrhea in these clinics might have accounted for these changes.

Testing in health-care facilities other than VD clinics increased by 2.6% from 1977 to 1978. The greatest increases in testing were within hospital inpatient wards, manpower training centers, community health centers, and group health centers; 152,144 more tests were performed in these facilities, and 3,069 more infections were detected in 1978 compared to 1977.

By contrast, testing in private physicians' offices decreased by 0.8% and was associated

TABLE 1. Results of gonorrhea culture tests on females, United States,* 1977 and 1978

Reporting source	Number tested 1978	Number tested 1977	Percent change	Number positive 1978	Number positive 1977	Percent change	Percent positive 1978	Percent positive 1977	Percent change
Health-care providers									
(excluding VD clinics)	7694114	7501076	+ 2.6	218110	217212	+ 0.4	2.8	2.9	− 3.4
Health dept.									
Non-VD clinics	1852081	1815976	+ 2.0	61417	59254	+ 3.7	3.3	3.3	0.0
Family Planning	1310478	1280159	+ 2.4	42722	40802	+ 4.7	3.3	3.2	+ 3.1
Prenatal, ob-gyn	200444	184904	+ 8.4	6288	5582	+ 12.6	3.1	3.0	+ 3.3
Cancer detection	20108	22268	− 9.7	385	396	− 2.8	1.9	1.8	+ 5.6
Combination or other	321051	328645	− 2.3	12022	12474	− 3.6	3.7	3.8	− 2.6
Public/private hospital									
Outpatient	1381656	1365615	+ 1.2	62983	61013	+ 3.2	4.6	4.5	+ 2.2
Family planning	210269	247957	− 15.2	6542	8153	− 19.8	3.1	3.3	− 6.1
Prenatal ob-gyn	322731	323954	− 0.4	10203	10445	− 2.3	3.2	3.2	0.0
Cancer detection	11434	18334	− 37.6	448	540	− 17.0	3.9	2.9	+ 34.5
Combination or other	837222	775370	+ 8.0	45790	41875	+ 9.3	5.5	5.4	+ 1.9
Inpatient	67993	57792	+ 17.7	1628	1400	+ 16.3	2.4	2.4	0.0
Obstetric	3825	2803	+ 36.5	37	51	− 27.5	1.0	1.8	−44.4
Gynecologic	2942	812	+ 262.3	120	27	+344.4	4.1	3.5	+ 24.2
Combination or other	61226	54177	+ 13.0	1471	1322	+ 11.3	2.4	2.4	0.0
Community health centers	792411	706968	+ 12.1	22667	20776	+ 9.1	2.9	2.9	0.0
Family planning	245095	195498	+ 25.4	4845	3910	+ 23.9	2.0	2.0	0.0
Prenatal ob-gyn	79589	56595	+ 40.6	2055	1475	+ 39.3	2.6	2.6	0.0
Cancer detection	8967	7275	+ 23.3	92	45	+104.4	1.0	0.6	+ 66.7
Combination or other	458760	447600	+ 2.5	15675	15346	+ 2.1	3.4	3.4	0.0
Private physicians	1866306	1880855	− 0.8	35573	37943	− 6.2	1.9	2.0	− 5.0
Private family-planning									
groups	1077229	1032220	+ 4.4	17445	16966	+ 2.8	1.6	1.6	0.0
Group health clinics	194437	152942	+ 27.1	4101	3392	+ 20.9	2.1	2.2	− 4.5
Student health centers	204734	206377	− 0.8	2892	3496	− 17.3	1.4	1.7	−17.6
Manpower training agencies	28935	13930	+ 107.7	997	756	+ 31.9	3.4	5.4	−37.0
Industrial screening	1621	3423	− 52.6	55	75	− 26.7	3.4	2.2	+ 54.5
Military/dependents	77815	76710	+ 1.4	2357	2164	+ 8.9	3.0	2.8	+ 7.1
Correctional detention									
centers	57312	64230	− 10.8	2823	3354	− 15.8	4.9	5.2	− 5.8
Not specified	91584	124038	− 26.2	3172	6623	− 52.1	3.5	5.3	−34.0
Venereal disease clinics	947074	955334	− 0.9	184988	176093	+ 5.1	19.5	18.4	+ 6.0
Total all clinics	9641188	8456410	+ 2.2	403098	393305	+ 2.5	4.7	4.7	0.0

*Trust Territory of the Pacific Islands did not report data for January-December 1977.

with a 6.2% reduction in the number of positive tests. Although several factors might have caused these changes, the most likely explanation is that there was an actual decrease in the incidence and prevalence of gonococcal infection among women seen in private medical practice. It is possible that there has been a shift of higher-risk populations from the private to the public sector of the health-care delivery system. Less likely is that the changes were caused by the selection of lower-risk persons to be tested or by lowered quality control of the culture system.

MMWR 27 (A.S., 1978): 26

GONORRHEA — Reported Civilian Case Rates by Year, United States, Calendar Years 1941–1978

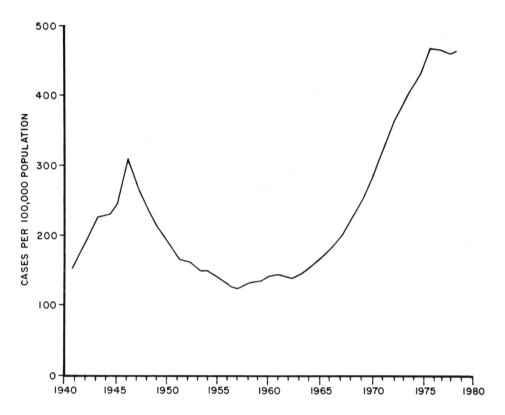

The sharp increase in the reporting of gonorrhea during the past decade appears to have leveled off. Both an actual increase in the occurrence of disease as well as improved case ascertainment are thought to be reasons for the earlier increase. The recent plateau in reported cases is thought to be due to disease-intervention activities initiated by health departments (e.g., screening high-risk populations for gonorrhea, providing sexual-partner referral services to patients with gonorrhea, and providing facts about venereal disease to people at risk to prevent exposure and to influence infected individuals to seek early medical care for themselves and their sexual partners). The geographic clustering may reflect a high incidence of disease as well as a high level of case detection. The impact of the introduction of penicillinase-producing *Neisseria gonorrhoeae* in 1976 has not been determined.

GONORRHEA — Reported Cases in Civilians per 100,000 Population by State, United States, 1978

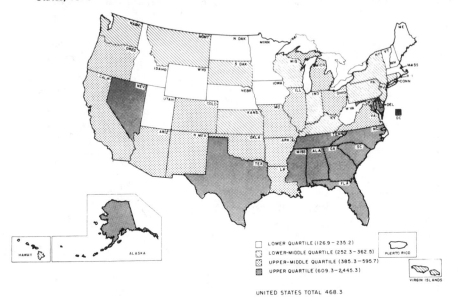

LOWER QUARTILE (126.9 – 235.2)
LOWER-MIDDLE QUARTILE (252.3 – 362.5)
UPPER-MIDDLE QUARTILE (385.3 – 595.7)
UPPER QUARTILE (609.3 – 2,445.3)

UNITED STATES TOTAL 468.3

GONORRHEA — Reported Cases in Civilians and Cases per 100,000 Population by Age and Sex, United States, 1977 and 1978

Age Group	Male			
	1977		1978	
	Cases	Rate	Cases	Rate
0-14	3,108	11.8	2,889	11.1
15-19	104,802	1005.3	101,701	977.6
20-24	232,404	2482.0	229,829	2409.9
25-29	141,309	1671.5	141,940	1648.0
30-39	87,026	657.8	91,365	660.7
40-49	20,627	188.3	21,467	196.3
50+	8,750	35.1	8,448	33.5
Total	598,026	576.8	597,639	571.8

Age Group	Female			
	1977		1978	
	Cases	Rate	Cases	Rate
0-14	8,979	35.5	9,069	36.5
15-19	148,185	1424.9	153,227	1481.7
20-24	155,407	1569.0	158,155	1568.7
25-29	59,064	665.0	60,434	669.3
30-39	26,108	185.4	27,995	190.7
40-49	4,631	39.8	4,946	42.6
50+	1,819	5.9	1,971	6.3
Total	404,193	364.1	415,797	371.5

Age Group	Total			
	1977		1978	
	Cases	Rate	Cases	Rate
0-14	12,087	23.4	11,958	23.5
15-19	252,987	1214.8	254,928	1228.9
20-24	387,811	2013.5	387,984	1977.6
25-29	200,373	1155.8	202,374	1147.0
30-39	113,134	414.2	119,360	418.7
40-49	25,258	111.8	26,413	117.1
50+	10,569	19.0	10,419	18.4
Total	1,002,219	466.8	1,013,436	468.3

MMWR 28:261 (6/8/79)

Death Due to Gonococcal Endocarditis — Washington State

The Washington Department of Social and Health Services recently reported a death secondary to gonococcal endocarditis.

In January 1979, a 54-year-old man was admitted to the psychiatric service of a local hospital because of worsening confusion and depression of approximately 4 to 6 week's duration. Before the initiation of tricyclic antidepressants, a screening electrocardiogram revealed a right bundle branch block. Seven days after admission, a cardiology consultant noted subtle heart murmurs consistent with aortic insufficiency and mitral stenosis. Shortly afterwards, the patient developed a fever of 38 C; 5 blood cultures were obtained, and he was transferred to the medical service. Within 24 hours, he developed acute left ventricular failure, and an emergency cardiac catheterization demonstrated severe aortic insufficiency and moderate mitral regurgitation. Following the cardiac catheterization, the patient had a cardiopulmonary arrest; resuscitation was unsuccessful. Autopsy showed destruction of the left coronary cusp of the aortic valve with granular vegetations extending into the left ventricle. Other findings revealed congestion of the lungs, liver, and spleen, consistent with the clinical picture. Four of the 5 blood cultures revealed *Neisseria gonorrhoeae*. No other sites were cultured on media suitable for detection of *N. gonorrhoeae*.

Reported by F Condie, MS, Veterans Administration Hospital, Seattle, Washington; HH Handsfield, MD, Seattle-King County Health Dept; JW Taylor, MD, MPH, State Epidemiologist, L Klopfenstein, Washington State Dept of Social and Health Services; Field Services Div, Bur of Epidemiology, CDC.

Editorial Note: The last reported death due to *N. gonorrhoeae* in Washington State before this case was in 1973; it also resulted from gonococcal endocarditis. Neither that patient nor the one described here had arthritis or dermatitis. In the pre-antibiotic era approximately 10% of bacterial endocarditis was due to *N. gonorrhoeae* (1,2), and the majority of such patients showed signs of the gonococcal arthritis/dermatitis syndrome (GADS). It seems likely that GADS is now diagnosed and treated relatively promptly, preventing many cases of endocarditis, and that most cases of diagnosed gonococcal endocarditis therefore result from atypical, disseminated gonococcal infection, without GADS.

References
1. Williams RH: Gonococcal endocarditis: A study of twelve cases with ten postmortem examinations. Arch Intern Med 61:26-38, 1938
2. Holmes KK, Counts GW, Beaty HN: Disseminated gonococcal infection. Ann Intern Med 74:979-993, 1971

MMWR 28:605 (1/4/80)

Pelvic Inflammatory Disease — United States

Although Pelvic Inflammatory Disease (PID) is not a reportable condition, several estimates of its occurrence in the United States are available.

Two of these sources estimate rates of visits to office-based, private physicians for PID. The National Disease and Therapeutic Index (NDTI) estimated that rates of visits to such physicians for salpingitis and PID increased from about 3,500 to about 4,500 per 100,000 female population from mid-1960s to early 1970s (Figure 1). By 1977, these estimated rates had fallen to about 2,500 per 100,000 female population according to the National Ambulatory Medical Care Survey (NAMCS), which is conducted annually by the National Center for Health Statistics (NCHS).

Both surveys are probability samples and provide essentially unbiased estimates of frequency of visits to physicians' offices by diagnosis. Extrapolation from both surveys

FIGURE 1. Total salpingitis and PID visits per 100,000 female population (age 10-50), United States, 1961-1977*

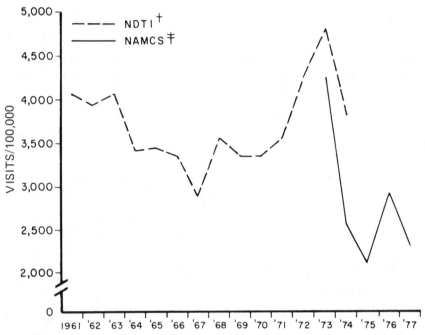

*1977 PID projected from NAMCS information available on PID as principal diagnosis among women 10-50 years of age. Total PID is defined as salpingitis (acute, ICDA #612; chronic, ICDA #613; and unqualified, ICDA #614) plus disease of parametrium and pelvic peritoneum, ICDA #616
†NDTI: National Disease and Therapeutic Index, IMS, Inc., Ambler, Penn. Population estimates from Bureau of Census
‡NAMCS: National Ambulatory Medical Care Survey (NCHS)

indicates that an estimated 7.6 million visits to private physicians' offices for PID were made for the period 1973 through 1977.

Estimates for hospitalizations for salpingitis and PID* have also been made, based upon 2 hospital data systems (Figure 2). One of these, the Professional Activities Study (PAS), is an ongoing statistical study of hospitals' patient-discharge abstracts from approximately 2,200 short-stay hospitals. These hospitals discharge about 17 million patients annually. PAS is conducted by the Commission on Professional and Hospital Activities, and although the hospitals participating in the study do not constitute a probability sample, they are a relatively stable group responsible for about half of all U.S. hospital discharges. The other basis for estimating hospitalizations for PID is the Hospital Discharge Survey (HDS), conducted by NCHS. It is a probability sampling of discharge records from U.S. short-stay hospitals. In both studies, the proportion of all women hospitalized due to salpingitis and PID slowly increased from 1970 through 1977.

Reported by the Venereal Disease Control Div, Bur of State Services, CDC.

*Using the same International Classification of Diseases Adapted (ICDA) code as above.

FIGURE 2. Total diagnoses of salpingitis and PID per 100,000 females discharged from hospitals, by data source, United States, 1970-1977

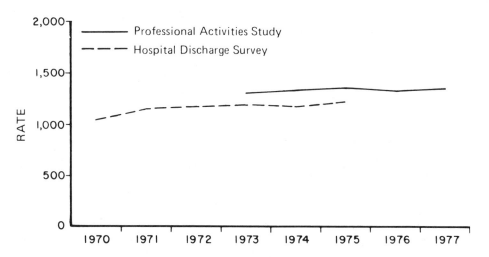

Editorial Note: Salpingitis and PID are often used synonymously in reference to upper genital-tract infections in women. *Neisseria gonorrhoeae* and possibly *Chlamydia trachomatis* are causes of PID. After an initial episode of PID, women often experience recurrences and are at high risk for infertility and ectopic pregnancy.

As reflected by the large number of visits to private physicians and hospital admissions for this disease, PID is a major health problem. Following the institution of a gonorrhea control program in 1972 (*1*), not only have reported cases of gonorrhea in men and women leveled off, but also the rate of visits to office-based, private physicians for PID has declined. However, hospitalization rates for PID did not decline. This difference in trend remains unexplained. Possibly, a larger proportion of patients now seek care for PID in health facilities other than private physicians' offices. It may also be possible that women with PID are now more likely to be hospitalized because of a better appreciation of the severity of this syndrome. Because recurrent PID accounts for a major portion of women hospitalized for PID, it may also be too early to expect a decline in the rates of hospitalization for PID. Declines in PID hospitalization rates and further decreases in PID visit rates are possible if gonorrhea prevention programs are improved and if prevention is directed at non-gonococcal as well as gonococcal PID.

Reference
1. MMWR 28:533-534, 1979

CHAPTER 18

Syphilis and Other Sexually Transmitted Diseases

MMWR 27:296 (8/18/78)

Increases in Early Syphilis

A marked reversal has occurred in the national trends of reported cases of early syphilis (primary, secondary, and early latent of less than 1 year's duration). After decreasing for 4 consecutive 6-month periods, reported cases for January-June 1978 increased 1.0% over cases reported in January-June 1977 (Table 1). When compared to the same month in the preceding year, monthly increases were first noted in March and have occurred each month since.

TABLE 1. Reported early syphilis* cases by 6-month periods, United States, January-June 1975 — January-June 1978

Reporting period	Number of cases	Percent change compared to similar 6-month period of preceding year
January-June 1975	23,060	+7.9
July-December 1975	22,822	+0.5
January-June 1976	22,101	−4.2
July-December 1976	20,442	−10.4
January-June 1977	18,535	−16.1
July-December 1977	18,278	−10.6
January-June 1978	18,726	+1.0

*Primary, secondary and early latent (less than 1 year's duration) syphilis

The reversal in national trends for the first 6 months of 1978 was primarily due to increases in 7 areas that account for 71% of the cumulative increase (Table 2). During the same time, 28 areas experienced decreases and 2 areas reported no change. The 7 areas that reported increases of 90 or more cases during the first 6 months of 1978 were Chicago (+266), Texas (+240), New York City (+216), Los Angeles (+168), Mississippi (+122), Georgia (excluding Atlanta) (+106), and Atlanta (+92). The 3 reporting the largest decreases were North Carolina (−363), San Francisco (−173), and Philadelphia (−134) (Table 2).

Reported cases of congenital syphilis among infants (<1 year of age), a disease closely related to infectious syphilis in women, have also increased slightly. In the 6-month period October 1976-March 1977, 66 cases of congenital syphilis among infants were reported, and for October 1977-March 1978 (latest period for which data are available), 70 cases were reported. Of these 70, Texas reported 21 and California, 11. The District of Columbia and 18 states reported 1 to 4 cases, and 30 states reported no cases between October 1977 and March 1978.

TABLE 2. Summary of reported primary, secondary, and early latent (less 1 year) syphilis cases, by reporting area, June 1978 and June 1977 — provisional data

Reporting Area by HEW Regions	June 1978	June 1977	Calendar Year Cumulative January-June 1978	1977
Connecticut	26	34	145	157
Maine	0	7	13	18
Massachusetts	64	95	384	500
New Hampshire	0	3	5	9
Rhode Island	5	2	39	11
Vermont	2	1	3	6
REGION I TOTAL	97	142	589	701
New Jersey	81	60	345	388
New York (Excl. NYC)	35	39	227	247
New York City	345	265	1,874	1,658
REGION II TOTAL	461	364	2,445	2,293
Delaware	2	1	13	23
District of Columbia	103	102	507	639
Maryland (Excl. Baltimore)	25	25	184	165
Baltimore	43	47	267	246
Pennsylvania (Excl. Philadelphia)	16	17	120	158
Philadelphia	37	59	202	336
Virginia	84	85	447	481
West Virginia	2	0	17	12
REGION III TOTAL	312	336	1,757	2,060
Alabama	34	18	157	120
Florida	309	249	1,731	1,723
Georgia (Excl. Atlanta)	105	105	714	608
Atlanta*	74	60	452	360
Kentucky	32	16	138	106
Mississippi	89	41	400	278
North Carolina	113	111	531	894
South Carolina	50	59	231	293
Tennessee	39	37	265	215
REGION IV TOTAL	845	696	4,619	4,597

Reporting Area by HEW Regions	June 1978	June 1977	Calendar Year Cumulative January-June 1978	1977
Illinois (Excl. Chicago)	30	25	114	197
Chicago	143	112	1,000	734
Indiana (Excl. Indianapolis)	8	15	102	94
Indianapolis*	0	1	54	39
Michigan	40	56	258	274
Minnesota	17	15	163	109
Ohio	48	57	343	424
Wisconsin	9	16	67	90
REGION V TOTAL	295	297	2,101	1,961
Arkansas	10	6	72	45
Louisiana	124	103	605	632
New Mexico	10	9	85	76
Oklahoma	19	12	96	66
Texas	345	338	2,017	1,777
REGION VI TOTAL	508	468	2,875	2,596
Iowa	10	3	42	27
Kansas	9	10	78	63
Missouri	17	18	137	151
Nebraska	4	5	20	41
REGION VII TOTAL	40	36	277	282
Colorado	12	14	103	111
Montana	0	4	10	10
North Dakota	0	0	2	2
South Dakota	0	2	1	4
Utah	7	0	19	13
Wyoming	0	0	4	3
REGION VIII TOTAL	19	20	139	143

Reporting Area by HEW Region	June 1978	June 1977	Calendar Year Cumulative January-June 1978	1977
Arizona	17	29	119	169
California (Excl. LA & SF)	189	179	1,345	1,270
Los Angeles*	219	211	1,418	1,250
San Francisco*	98	118	661	834
Hawaii	8	7	31	36
Nevada	3	4	33	20
REGION IX TOTAL	534	548	3,607	3,579
Alaska	1	8	12	41
Idaho	3	0	5	4
Oregon	19	13	126	95
Washington	36	41	173	183
REGION X TOTAL	59	62	316	323
UNITED STATES TOTAL	3,170	2,969	18,726	18,535
Puerto Rico	91	97	524	516
Virgin Islands	5	0	19	17
UNITED STATES, INCLUDING OUTLYING AREAS	3,266	3,066	19,269	19,068

Note: Cumulative totals include revised and delayed reports through previous months.

Source: CDC 9.98, HEW, PHS, CDC, BSS, VD Control Division, Atlanta, Georgia 30333

*County data

Reported by the Venereal Disease Control Div, Bur of State Services, CDC.

Editorial Note: A single explanation for reversal of disease trends in those areas experiencing large increases is not possible, but several contributing factors are being investigated. In the Southwest and West the proportion of infectious syphilis cases in seasonal farm laborers appears to have increased. Also, in some areas dramatic increases in syphilis among seasonal farm workers have been linked directly to a high incidence of syphilis in an itinerant prostitute population. Traditional control measures are frequently less effective with these populations because of frequent moves to different areas and unavailability or underutilization of health facilities. In some areas, the increase appears to be related to a decrease in the number and the timeliness of referrals, examinations, and treatment of persons exposed to infectious syphilis.

Recently a few health departments have hired and trained additional staff. When appropriate, multilingual case workers have been sought. New approaches (for example, selective mass treatment and field-screening of blood samples) are being evaluated in high-risk population groups.

Syphilis incidence is decreasing or is stable in many program areas; the national downward trend of syphilis which began in 1976 can be re-established by concentrating control resources in areas experiencing the largest increases.

MMWR 28:433 (9/14/79)

Congenital Syphilis — United States, 1978-1979

In calendar year 1978, 434 cases of congenital syphilis were reported in the United States, a 6.3% decrease in cases since 1977. Of last year's cases, 107 were among in-

TABLE 2. Congenital syphilis, United States, 1977-1978, and January-March of 1978 and 1979

State	Total all ages 1977	Total all ages 1978	Under 1 year of age 1977	Under 1 year of age 1978	Total all ages January-March 1978	Total all ages January-March 1979	Under 1 year of age January-March 1978	Under 1 year of age January-March 1979
Alabama	—	4	—	2	1	—	1	—
Alaska	—	—	—	—	—	—	—	—
Arizona	6	5	5	3	1	—	1	—
Arkansas	1	—	1	—	—	—	—	—
California	23	36	17	11	18	14	3	10
Colorado	4	3	1	1	2	—	1	—
Connecticut	5	—	5	—	—	1	—	—
Delaware	1	2	—	—	—	—	—	—
District of Columbia	4	7	1	2	2	—	—	—
Florida	8	5	7	3	1	1	1	1
Georgia	3	8	1	6	1	1	1	1
Hawaii	—	—	—	—	—	—	—	—
Idaho	1	—	1	—	—	—	—	—
Illinois	67	69	4	7	16	8	3	—
Indiana	21	17	2	4	2	1	1	—
Iowa	5	3	—	—	—	4	—	—
Kansas .	25	16	—	—	6	--	—	—
Kentucky	6	5	3	1	2	—	1	—
Louisiana	12	9	4	7	3	3	2	3
Maine	—	—	—	—	—	—	—	—
Maryland	7	7	2	3	—	2	—	—
Massachusetts	24	16	2	—	5	7	—	2
Michigan	7	5	3	3	2	1	1	1
Minnesota	2	4	—	1	—	—	—	—
Mississippi	2	6	2	1	2	2	—	—
Missouri	2	1	—	—	—	1	—	—
Montana	—	—	—	—	—	—	—	—
Nebraska	—	—	—	—	—	—	—	—
Nevada	—	—	—	—	—	1	—	—
New Hampshire	—	—	—	—	—	—	—	—
New Jersey	22	22	4	1	7	4	—	—
New Mexico	4	7	2	4	4	—	1	—
New York	24	25	15	10	4	6	1	1
North Carolina	9	5	3	3	—	4	—	2
North Dakota	—	—	—	—	—	—	—	—
Ohio	15	20	1	2	10	2	—	2
Oklahoma	4	6	1	1	1	1	1	—
Oregon	1	—	—	—	—	—	—	—
Pennsylvania	14	25	1	—	3	1	—	—
Rhode Island	1	—	—	—	—	—	—	—
South Carolina	7	5	1	3	4	—	2	—
South Dakota	—	—	—	—	—	—	—	—
Tennessee	14	5	1	—	3	2	—	—
Texas	61	39	33	21	12	4	8	2
Utah	2	—	2	—	—	—	—	—
Vermont	—	—	—	—	—	—	—	—
Virginia	25	23	6	3	6	6	—	—
Washington	1	1	1	—	—	—	—	—
West Virginia	18	16	1	1	4	4	1	—
Wisconsin	5	5	1	—	—	1	—	—
Wyoming	—	2	—	—	—	—	—	—
Total United States	463	434	144	107	122	82	31	26

*Includes proportionally distributed cases for which age had not been specified.

fants*—a figure 25.7% less than that reported for infants in the previous year. During the 3-month period January-March 1979, 26 infants were reported to have congenital syphilis, a decrease of 16.1% from the cases reported in this period in 1978 (Table 2).

During January-March 1979, infectious syphilis cases among women numbered 1,381—

*Defined as children less than 1 year of age.

an increase of 6.8% over the number reported in January-March 1978.

Reported by the Venereal Disease Control Div, Bur of State Services, CDC.

Editorial Note: Congenital syphilis among infants usually correlates with the trend of infectious syphilis cases among women. Recently, however, congenital syphilis among infants has not increased, perhaps because of ongoing surveillance programs for pregnant women. In addition, pregnant women are the first priority in contact-tracing so that they can receive adequate medical attention to eliminate the risk of congenital syphilis among their offspring.

MMWR 27 (A.S., 1978): 64

SYPHILIS (Primary and Secondary) — Reported Civilian Case Rates by Year, United States, 1941—1978*

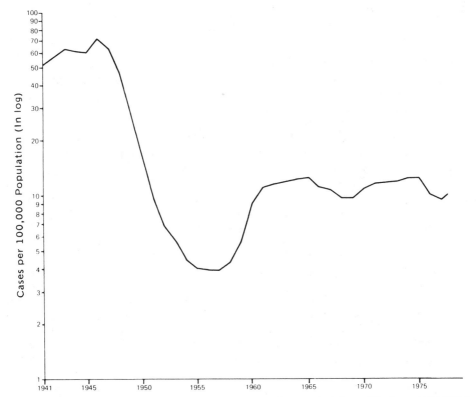

*1941-1946 Fiscal Years: Twelve month period ending June 30 of year specified. 1947-1978 Calendar Years.

MMWR 28:61 (2/16/79)

Nonreported Sexually Transmissible Diseases — United States

Only 5 sexually transmissible diseases (STD)—gonorrhea, syphilis, chancroid, lympho-granuloma venereum, and granuloma inguinale—are reported to most state health departments. In recent years, other STD such as genital herpes, nongonococcal urethritis, and trichomoniasis have received increasing attention. However, because their occurrence is not reported, very few data are available to describe their incidence and define the magnitude of the problem created by them.

In 1975, the Venereal Disease Control Division at CDC established an STD study to examine the incidence of nonreported STD in patients attending public clinics. Six STD clinics—located in New Haven, Connecticut; Detroit, Michigan; Lexington, Kentucky; DeKalb County, Georgia; Denver, Colorado; and Minneapolis, Minnesota—were linked by a common protocol to report the incidence of STD in patients attending these clinics. A Los Angeles family planning clinic was included to examine a presumably different patient population. The results and analyses of the first 9 complete months of data collection (October 1, 1976, through June 30, 1977) are presented in Tables 1 and 2.

Excluding follow-up visits, there were 40,821 visits to the 7 clinics. Men accounted for 67.7% of visits. Female patients were younger than male patients. Most women (79.8%) seen in STD clinics were 16-30 years old (median, 23.0 years); the majority of women seen in the family planning clinic were 21-30. The median age of men seen in the 6 STD clinics was 25.1 years.

Most men (64.5%) voluntarily came to these clinics because they were symptomatic. Women were twice as likely to have been referred to the clinic by sex partners.

For male patients, the nongonococcal urethritis case rate was approximately equal to the gonorrhea case rate in all clinics except those in Lexington and Detroit (Table1). For women in the STD clinic population, gonorrhea accounted for almost one-fourth of all STD; trichomoniasis and nonspecific vaginitis were the most common diseases seen in the population attending the family planning clinic (Table 2). Case rates of genital herpes, venereal warts, and nonspecific vaginitis varied considerably. The combined total of cases of STD other than gonorrhea far exceeded the total of gonorrhea cases alone.

Reported by Venereal Disease Control Div, Bur of State Services, CDC.

Editorial Note: Many of the STD clinics in the United States restrict diagnostic and treatment services to syphilis, gonorrhea, chancroid, granuloma inguinale, and lympho-granuloma venereum. However, other sexually transmissible diseases are more prevalent in both men and women attending STD clinics than the 5 historically defined venereal diseases. All STD clinics need to broaden the spectrum of their service to include additional sexually transmissible diseases (*1-3*). Differences in clinics are probably due to 2 factors: varying prevalence of diseases in different areas and lack of objective diagnostic criteria, i.e., cultures, for some diseases such as herpes, trichomoniasis, and nonspecific vaginitis. These results do not reflect disease prevalence in the general community. The data are applicable only to the proportion of the population seeking care in an STD clinic.

References
1. Armstrong JH, Wiesner PJ: The need for problem-oriented venereal disease clinics. Am J Vener Dis Assoc 1:23-28, 1974
2. Dans PE: The establishment of a university-based venereal disease clinic. I: Description of the clinic and its population. J Am Vener Dis Assoc 1:70-78, 1974
3. Dans PE, Klaus B, Owen M: A problem-oriented approach to the venereal disease clinic patient. J Am Vener Dis Assoc 1:158-162, 1975

TABLE 1. Sexually transmissible diseases (STD) in men, STD clinics, October 1, 1976–June 30, 1977

Diagnoses	Cases per 100 visits by men						
	New Haven	Detroit	Minneapolis	Denver	DeKalb County	Lexington	Total
Gonorrhea	22.3	44.4	20.9	20.1	22.4	36.7	24.0
Nongonococcal urethritis	29.5	25.1	24.6	27.6	24.4	4.2	24.8
Genital herpes	2.7	0.1	4.3	3.0	7.3	1.7	3.4
Venereal warts	1.0	0.1	4.6	5.5	6.5	2.2	4.3
Syphilis	2.5	2.2	1.8	1.2	1.3	3.3	1.7
Scabies	2.2	0.0	1.8	1.0	2.4	0.6	1.3
Pediculosis pubis	4.5	0.4	2.1	4.3	1.8	2.5	2.9
All other*	0.8	0.3	0.3	2.1	2.2	0.1	1.2*
Total	65.5	72.6	60.4	64.8	68.3	51.3	63.6
Total visits	1,900	2,178	6,811	8,919	2,455	1,535	23,798

*Includes (cases per 100 visits): molluscum contagiosum (1.0), chancroid (0.1), lymphogranuloma venereum (<0.1), and granuloma inguinale (0.0).

TABLE 2. Sexually transmissible diseases (STD) in women, STD clinics, October 1, 1976–June 30, 1977

Diagnoses	Cases per 100 visits by women								
	New Haven	Detroit	Minneapolis	Denver	DeKalb County	Lexington	Total STD Clinics	Los Angeles Family Planning	Total
Gonorrhea	23.0	36.2	21.7	20.4	23.0	27.2	23.5	0.3	15.7
Genital herpes	1.9	0.0	2.5	2.1	3.2	0.3	2.1	0.3	1.5
Venereal warts	1.0	0.0	7.0	3.8	5.3	1.2	4.0	1.0	3.0
Syphilis	1.6	1.8	0.9	0.9	1.0	2.1	1.1	1.8	1.4
Trichomonal vaginitis	8.7	25.3	8.5	9.4	11.9	12.1	11.5	8.5	10.4
Candida vaginitis*	12.0	4.8	4.2	12.1	5.9	5.8	7.9	2.5	6.1
Nonspecific vaginitis	3.0	8.6	14.6	4.9	31.5	0.6	12.3	9.5	11.3
Scabies	0.6	0.1	0.5	0.4	1.0	0.1	0.5	0.3	0.4
Pediculosis pubis	2.3	0.6	3.5	2.5	1.5	2.7	2.3	<0.1	1.6
Other**	0.0	0.0	0.1	0.8	0.6	0.0	0.4	0.2	0.3†
Total	54.1	77.4	63.5	57.3	84.9	52.1	65.6	24.5	51.7
Total visits	700	1,082	2,318	3,845	2,352	967	11,264	5,742	17,006

*Although candida vaginitis is a sexually transmissible disease, it is not usually transmitted in this manner.

†Includes molluscum contagiosum (0.3 cases per 100 visits), chancroid (0.1 per 100), lymphogranuloma venereum (0.0), and granuloma inguinale (0.0).

CHAPTER 19

Meningitis and Meningococcemia

MMWR 27:327 (9/1/78)

Meningococcal Polysaccharide Vaccines

INTRODUCTION

Polysaccharide vaccines against diseases caused by *Neisseria meningitidis* serogroups A and C are now licensed in the United States. They are prepared as monovalent and as bivalent antigens. The purpose of this statement is to summarize available information on these antigens and to offer general guidance regarding their role in the control of epidemics of meningococcal disease in the civilian population of the United States.

MENINGOCOCCAL DISEASE

Meningococcal disease is endemic in the United States and throughout the world. It caused serious epidemics approximately every 10 years from 1900 to 1945 in this country. The fact that it also regularly caused outbreaks among military recruits was a catalyst for the development of serogroup-specific vaccines.

During the last decade an estimated 3,000-6,000 cases a year of meningococcal disease occurred in the United States. From 1964 to 1968 and since 1972, the serogroup most often isolated from patients has been serogroup B. From 1969 through 1971 serogroup C was most common in the civilian and military populations. Serogroup A was only rarely identified until the occurrence recently of small outbreaks in several cities of the Pacific Northwest. In 1971 the Armed Forces began administering serogroup C meningococcal polysaccharide vaccine routinely to all recruits. Since then, the incidence of meningococcal disease in the military has declined sharply, and serogroup C disease has been virtually eliminated in that population.

Sulfa-sensitive serogroup B strains currently cause the majority of U.S. cases. Highest attack rates are in infants. Serogroup C strains account for about one-third of cases. Although the highest age-specific attack rate for serogroup C is also in infants, about 70% of serogroup C cases occur in persons over 2 years old. More than two-thirds of all meningococcal disease occurs in patients less than 20 years old.

In recent years meningococcal disease in civilians has occurred primarily as single isolated cases or, infrequently, as small, localized clusters. Secondary cases occur more frequently in household contacts than in the general population, and appropriate antibiotic prophylaxis has been the principal means of reducing the risk for immediate contacts of cases.

MENINGOCOCCAL VACCINES

Three meningococcal polysaccharide vaccines, monovalent A, monovalent C, and bivalent A-C vaccine,* are licensed for selective use in the United States. These vaccines are chemically defined antigens consisting of purified bacterial capsular polysaccharide, each inducing specific serogroup immunity. The duration of immunity conferred by each vaccine is unknown.

Serogroup A vaccine was evaluated in 62,000 Egyptian schoolchildren 6-15 years old and appeared to be highly effective and not to induce any serious side effects. When used to control an outbreak in Brazil, it appeared to be effective in all age groups beyond the first year of life. Further confirmation of effectiveness was found in children of ages 3 months-5 years in a vaccine trial carried out in Finland. Serogroup A vaccine has also been used to control outbreaks in the United States in Portland, Seattle, Anchorage, and Fairbanks.

Serogroup C vaccine has been given routinely to American military recruits since October 1971. More than 500,000 young adults have been vaccinated without significant adverse reactions. Serogroup C vaccine has been studied in infants, preschool and school-age children, and adults. It elicited antibody in all age groups, although older children and young adults had the highest levels. Serogroup C vaccine does not appear to be effective in children less than 2 years of age.

VACCINE USAGE
General Recommendations

Routinely vaccinating civilians with meningococcal polysaccharide vaccines is **not** recommended because of insufficient evidence of its value when the risk of infection is low. The serogroup-specific monovalent vaccines should be used, however, to control outbreaks of meningococcal disease caused by N. meningitidis serogroup A or C.

Vaccine may be of benefit for some travelers planning to visit countries recognized as having epidemic meningococcal disease. Although cases among Americans traveling in such areas are rare, prolonged contact with the local populace could enhance the risk of infection and make vaccination a reasonable precaution.

Vaccination should be considered an adjunct to antibiotic chemoprophylaxis for household contacts of meningococcal disease cases caused by serogroups A or C. This is because half the secondary family cases occur more than 5 days after the primary case— long enough to yield potential benefit from vaccination if the antibiotic chemoprophy-laxis has not been successful.

Primary Immunization

For both adults and children, vaccine is administered parenterally as a single dose in the volume specified by the manufacturer.

PRECAUTIONS AND CONTRAINDICATIONS
Reactions

Adverse reactions to meningococcal vaccine are infrequent and mild, consisting princi-pally of localized erythema lasting for 1-2 days.

Pregnancy

The safety of meningococcal vaccines in pregnant women has not been established. On theoretical grounds, it is prudent not to use them unless there is a substantial risk of in-fection.

EPIDEMIC CONTROL

In an epidemic of meningococcal disease due to serogroups A or C, the population at

---

*Official names: Meningococcal Polysaccharide Vaccine, Group A; or , Group C; or , Groups A & C

risk should be identified. It should be delineated by neighborhood, census tract, or other reasonable boundary. If there is ample vaccine, all residents in that area should be vaccinated. If not, persons expected or known to be at highest risk of disease by virtue of age, socioeconomic status, or area of residence should receive priority vaccination.

SELECTED BIBLIOGRAPHY

Artenstein MS, Winter PE, Gold R, et al: Immunoprophylaxis of meningococcal infection. Milit Med 139:91-95, 1974

Peltola H, Mäkelä PH, Käyhty H, et al: Clinical efficacy of meningococcus group A capsular polysaccharide vaccine in children three months to five years of age. N Engl J Med 297:686-691, 1977

Wahdan MH, Rizk F, el-Akkad AM, et al: A controlled field trial of a serogroup A meningococcal polysaccharide vaccine. Bull WHO 48:667-673, 1973

Revision of MMWR 24:381-382, 1975

MMWR 28:249 (6/1/79)

Nosocomial Meningitis Caused by
Citrobacter diversus — Connecticut, Florida

Five cases of hospital-related meningitis due to *Citrobacter diversus* have recently occurred in 2 institutions.

Connecticut: A 37-week infant boy, weighing 1,930 grams, was born August 29, 1978, by cesarean section 36 hours after the mother's membranes ruptured. He was discharged when he was 10 days old. Two days later, he became febrile and lethargic; he also fed poorly. When he was readmitted to the hospital, he was found to have sepsis and meningitis due to *C. diversus.* Computerized tomographic scan of the head showed multiple brain abscesses. After a prolonged hospitalization he died.

The second patient, a full-term infant boy, was born September 20 after a normal pregnancy, labor, and delivery. Discharged at 3 days of age, he was readmitted September 26 with sepsis and meningitis due to *C. diversus.* A subdural empyema was present. He died after a short illness.

No isolates of *C. diversus* from children had been identified in the hospital during the preceding 12 months. However, when nasal, throat, rectal, and umbilical cultures were obtained from all newborns born in the period October 10-29, 1978, 9 infants with umbilical colonization by *C. diversus* of the same antibiogram as the isolates from the 2 described cases (resistant to ampicillin and carbenicillin only) were identified.

Colonized infants did not differ from controls in respect to sex, maternal room number, exposure to nursery personnel, obstetrician, pediatrician, internal monitoring, method of feeding, or care of their umbilicus. Multiple environmental cultures, 109 throat and rectal cultures from all patient-care personnel in contact with the infants or their mothers, and rectal and vaginal cultures from the mothers of the 2 patients were negative for *C. diversus.* A culture of the hands of 1 nurse yielded *C. diversus* and *Klebsiella pneumoniae,* however, and she was sent home on medical leave. She had a dermatitis, aggravated by frequent handwashing and low humidity; for this condition, she applied an emollient cream and wore plastic gloves each night. The *C. diversus,* but not the *K. pneumoniae,* disappeared from her hands when she stopped wearing gloves. In the next 3 months no other infants were identified with *C. diversus* colonization of the umbilicus, nor were there any cases of neonatal *C. diversus* meningitis or sepsis.

Florida: Florida's 3 cases were also all in infants born at 1 hospital. The first, a full-term infant boy weighing 3,060 grams, was born December 11, 1977. His mother had a normal pregnancy, labor, and vaginal delivery. Three days after birth, he was discharged. On December 22, however, he was admitted *to another hospital* with jaundice and lethargy. Spinal fluid cultures yielded *C. diversus.*   After a long hospitalization, in which drainage of brain abscesses was required, he recovered fully.

Another infant boy, a 2,185-gram male, was delivered vaginally to a mother with endometritis on October 10, 1978. Eleven days later, while still in the hospital, he became lethargic and was found to have meningitis and ventriculitis due to *C. diversus.* In January 1979, he had residual parietal encephalomalacia and right hemiparesis. Maternal endometrial cultures at delivery yielded only alpha-hemolytic *Streptococcus* and *Lactobacillus.*

The third Florida case was in a 2,780-gram, full-term infant girl, delivered on December 29, 1978, and discharged 3 days later. On January 5, she was readmitted for meningitis due to *C. diversus;* she died that day.

No isolates of *C. diversus* had been identified among nursery inpatients at this hospital until July and August 1978, when it was recovered from 2 infants with mild omphalitis. On January 24, 1979, 45 of 57 (79%) infants in the nursery were found to have asymptomatic stool colonization by *C. diversus.* Environmental cultures were negative for the organism. Cultures of the next 27 infants born at the hospital revealed that all 27 had negative nasal cultures at the time of delivery, although 3 eventually became colonized in their stools. Four of 110 nurses (none with dermatitis) carried the organism on their hands, even when cultured 2 days after leaving the hospital, and 2 other nurses carried *C. diversus* in their stools.

Several corrective measures were begun: all patients who were carriers were separated from other patients; persons were instructed to wear gloves when feeding and diapering these patients; and the 2 adult intestinal carriers were treated with trimethoprim-sulfamethoxazole. By April 16, the prevalence of *C. diversus* had fallen from 79% to 0.

Reported by MF Parry, MD, J Hutchinson, RN, Stamford Hospital, Stamford, Connecticut; RM Gofstein, MD, MPH, R Murray, Stamford Health Dept; PJ Checko, SM, A Bruce, MS, JN Lewis, MD, MPH, State Epidemiologist, Connecticut State Dept of Health; H Boer, MD, HR, MPH, FE Ariel, RN, Broward General Medical Center, Fort Lauderdale, Florida; RM Yeller, MD, Acting State Epidemiologist, Florida State Dept of Health and Rehabilitative Services; Field Services Div, Epidemiologic Investigations Laboratory Br, Hospital Infections Br, and Special Pathogens Br, Bacterial Diseases Div, Bur of Epidemiology, CDC.

Editorial Note: *Citrobacter* is an uncommon cause of nosocomial neonatal meningitis (*1*). However, the association of personnel with dermatitis and epidemic nosocomial infections has been documented frequently. Dermatitic lesions on the hands of medical personnel may be heavily colonized with gram-positive or gram-negative bacteria; virus transmission has also been implicated. These organisms may be transmitted to patients during routine patient-care activities and may result in colonization of the patients or in sporadic or epidemic disease (*2-5*).

In neither hospital were nurse carriers proven to be primary sources of the organism for all patients with meningitis. However, in Connecticut, 2 observations suggest that the nurse may have been the carrier: (1) she was associated with the second patient as well as with the colonized neonates, and (2) once she was removed from the hospital, there were no more cases or colonizations. How the carrier's hands initially became colonized with *C. diversus* could not be determined. Colonization could have occurred during her exposure to the first patient, or the first patient may have acquired the organism from the carrier. It is also not clear how the 6 Florida nurses became colonized, though they may have acquired the organism changing the diapers of colonized infants.

References
1. Vogel LC, Ferguson L, Gotoff SP: *Citrobacter* infections of the central nervous system in early infancy. J Pediatr 93:86-88, 1978

2. Buxton AE, Anderson RL, Werdegar D, Atlas E: Nosocomial respiratory tract infection and colonization with *Acinetobacter calcoaceticus*. Am J Med 65:507-513, 1978

3. Snydman DR, Hindman SH, Wineland MD, Bryan JA, Maynard JE: Nosocomial viral hepatitis B: A cluster among staff with subsequent transmission to patients. Ann Intern Med 85:573-577, 1976

4. Salzman TC, Clark JJ, Klemm L: Hand contamination of personnel as a mechanism of cross-infection in nosocomial infections with antibiotic-resistant *Escherichia coli* and *Klebsiella aerobacter*, in Hobby GL (ed): Antimicrobial Agents and Chemotherapy. Detroit, Michigan, American Society for Microbiology, 1967, pp 97-100

5. Mortimer EA Jr, Wolinsky E, Gonzaga AJ, Rammelkamp CH Jr: Transmission of staphylococci between newborns: Importance of the hands of personnel. Am J Dis Child 104:289-295, 1962

MMWR 27:358 (9/22/78)

Nosocomial Meningococcemia — Wisconsin

In February 1978, a nurse developed meningococcemia 3 days after assisting in the emergency room evaluation of a patient with meningococcemia and meningitis.

The index patient was a 25-year-old man who was seen in the emergency room with fever, malaise, myalgia, and headache of 24 hours' duration. A diagnostic lumber puncture in the emergency room was unsuccessful because of the patient's lack of cooperation. He was taken to the postoperative recovery room, where he was given inhalation anesthesia and intubated; a lumbar puncture was then performed. The patient vomited several times in the emergency room and during intubation. Hospital personnel assisting with the anesthesia and lumbar puncture did not wear masks or follow other isolation precautions.

The cerebrospinal fluid (CSF) had a protein of 767 mg/dl, a glucose of 6 mg/dl, and a white blood cell count (WBC) of 20,700/mm^3 with 98% neutrophils. Gram stain of the smear showed multiple gram-negative diplococci that were both extracellular and intracellular. No pneumonia was seen on chest X ray. Cultures of the blood and spinal fluid grew *Neisseria meningitidis*, subsequently identified as a sulfonamide-susceptible group B strain. Following diagnosis of the patient's disease, approximately 6 hours after his admission to the emergency room, he was placed in isolation.

Twenty-four medical personnel (physicians, nurses, orderlies, and others) had contact with the patient before he was placed in isolation. These persons were informed of their possible exposure to meningococcal disease. Those with intimate contact with the patient were advised to take rifampin prophylactically for 2 days; 3 nurses and 2 orderlies received prophylaxis.

Three days after the index patient was admitted to the hospital, a 39-year-old nurse developed headache, fever, and malaise. She had assisted with the intubation and suctioning of nasopharyngeal secretions from the index case at the time of his diagnostic lumbar puncture. Two days after onset of her symptoms she presented for examination and was noted to have scattered petechial lesions on her arms and legs. Her WBC was 17,400/mm^3 with 2% bands and 87% neutrophils; her platelet count was normal. Lumbar puncture showed normal CSF; blood cultures were not obtained. Over the next several days she developed a more severe headache, more petechiae, and joint pains. Six days after her initial symptoms she was admitted to the hospital and isolated with a presumptive diagnosis of meningococcemia. A repeat lumbar puncture was performed which revealed a WBC of 25/mm^3, mostly neutrophils, normal glucose and protein concentrations, and negative Gram stain and culture. A blood culture, however, grew group B *N. meningitidis* susceptible to sulfonamides.

The isolates of *N. meningitidis* from both the index patient and the nurse were not typable with available antisera to protein subtype antigens (*1*). However, protein extracts of the 2 strains had similar migration patterns on SDS polyacrilamide gel.

On careful questioning the nurse recalled that she had exposure to the nasopharyngeal secretions from the index patient, but following this exposure she had not received antibiotic prophylaxis. She had no other known contacts with persons with meningococcal disease or colonization, and at the time of these 2 cases no other cases of meningococcal disease were occurring in the community.

Reported by Bur of Biologics, Food and Drug Administration; Hospital Infections Br and Special Pathogens Br, Bacterial Diseases Div, Bur of Epidemiology, CDC.

Editorial Note: Nosocomial transmission of *N. meningitidis* to hospital personnel caring for a patient with meningococcemia or meningitis is rare and has been reported to occur only with extensive contact with the infected individual (*2*). The risk of transmission of infection by patients with meningococcal pneumonia might be greater, however (*3*). In this outbreak, the epidemiologic evidence suggests that the disease was nosocomially transmitted to a person who had intimate contact with respiratory secretions from the index patient; this is supported by the laboratory finding of a common migration pattern of protein extracts of strains of *N. meningitidis* isolated from both patients.

To minimize the risk of nosocomial transmission of meningococcal infection to hospital personnel, a patient who has disease compatible with meningococcal infection should be placed in respiratory isolation when the diagnosis is first suspected. Personnel who have had intimate contact with the patient's respiratory tract secretions should be provided rifampin as chemoprophylaxis or a sulfonamide if the strain of *N. meningitidis* is known to be sensitive to sulfonamides (*4*).

References
1. Frasch CE, Chapman SS: Classification of *Neisseria meningitidis* group B into distinct serotypes. III. Application of a new bacteriocidal-inhibition technique to distribution of serotypes among cases and carriers. J Infect Dis 127:149-154, 1973
2. Artenstein MS, Ellis RE: The risk of exposure to a patient with meningococcal meningitis. Milit Med 133:474-477, 1968
3. MMWR 27:147, 1978
4. Jacobson JA, Fraser DW: A simplified approach to meningococcal disease prophylaxis. JAMA 236:1053-1054, 1976

MMWR 28:277 (6/22/79)

Bacterial Meningitis and Meningococcemia — United States, 1978

A provisional total of 4,081 cases of bacterial meningitis (excluding cases caused by *Mycobacterium*) and 289 cases of meningococcemia were reported to CDC from 38 participating states* in the national bacterial meningitis and meningococcemia surveillance system in 1978. This represents a national rate of reported bacterial meningitis and meningococcemia of 2.69 cases and 0.19 cases per 100,000 population, respectively.

Table 1 shows the reported incidence and case-fatality ratio (CFR) associated with each pathogen responsible for bacterial meningitis, as well as the reported incidence and CFR of meningococcemia. *Hemophilus influenzae, Neisseria meningitidis,* and *Streptococcus pneumoniae* accounted for 84% of all reported cases of bacterial meningitis.

*Represents 69.8% of the U.S. population. Areas not participating include Rhode Island, Michigan, Delaware, Georgia, New Jersey, Tennessee, Texas, Wyoming, Nevada, Alaska, Hawaii, California, and Washington, DC.

TABLE 1. Incidence rate and case-fatality ratio (CFR) of reported bacterial meningitis (by pathogen) and meningococcemia, United States, 1978

Disease	Number of cases	Percent	Incidence*	CFR
Bacterial meningitis				
Hemophilus influenzae	1,885	46	1.24	7.1%
Neisseria meningitidis **	1,095	27	0.72	13.5%
Streptococcus pneumoniae	456	11	0.30	28.2%
Group B Streptococcus	130	3	0.09	22.4%
Listeria monocytogenes	68	2	0.04	29.5%
Other	235	6	0.15	36.6%
Unknown	212	5	0.14	16.7%
Total bacterial meningitis	4,081	100	2.69	13.6%
Meningococcemia	289		0.19	25.1%

*Cases per 10^5 population, estimated July 1978 for the 38 reporting states
**Excludes cases of meningococcemia alone

In 5% of the cases, the organism responsible for disease was unknown. The highest CFR (37%) was observed with the less common pathogens (predominantly gram-negative bacilli); the lowest CFR (7%) was associated with the most common pathogen, *H. influenzae*. The CFR was 14% for persons with meningococcal meningitis and 25% for persons with meningococcemia.

Age-specific incidence rates show that the peak incidence of reported disease occurred in neonates, with the secondary peak in infants 6 to 8 months of age (Table 2); rates were then successively lower in young children, the elderly, and persons between 10 and 59 years of age. Nearly 70% of all reported cases of bacterial meningitis and 55% of all reported cases of meningococcemia occurred in children less than 5 years of age. However, slightly over 20% of cases of bacterial meningitis and 25% of cases of meningococcemia occurred in adults (>20 years).

The distribution of pathogens varied considerably in the different age groups. Neonates were more frequently infected with Group B *Streptococcus, Escherchia coli*, and *Listeria monocytogenes*. Meningitis in individuals in the age group 1 month to 10 years most commonly was caused by *H. influenzae, N. meningitidis,* and *S. pneumoniae*; in persons between 10 and 59 years of age, *N. meningitidis, S. pneumoniae,* and other less common organisms predominated. Individuals over 60 years of age frequently were affected by *S. pneumoniae, N. meningitidis*, and less common organisms. A higher attack rate was observed in males (1.25:1) and also in blacks and in American Indians or Alaskan natives.

Marked seasonal trends were observed. Reported cases of meningitis due to *N. meningitidis* and *S. pneumoniae* peaked in the winter months; cases due to *H. influenzae* peaked in the fall and spring months; and cases due to *L. monocytogenes* peaked in late fall-early winter and in the summer months. No seasonality was demonstrated for *Group B Streptococcus*.

The distribution of meningococcal serogroups reported are as follows: serogroup A, 3.9% (range by state, 1%-12%, with the highest percentage in the Mountain and Pacific States); serogroup B, 49.1% (range 30%-65%, highest in the Central States); serogroup C, 20.2% (range 11%-41%, highest in the New England and Mid-Atlantic States); serogroup Y, 8.6% (range 2%-16%, highest in the South Central States); and other serogroups (predominantly W135), 7.7% (range 0-27%, highest in the South Atlantic and East South Central States). Ten percent of isolates were reported to be ungroupable.

TABLE 2. Age-specific incidence* of bacterial meningitis and meningococcemia, United States, 1978

AGE	ORGANISM								
	Neisseria meningitidis	Hemophilus influenzae	Streptococcus pneumoniae	Group B Streptococcus	Listeria monocytogenes	Other	Unknown	Total bacterial meningitis	Meningococcemia
In months									
<1	4.0	6.0	3.0	42.0	12.0	23.0	6.0	96.0	2.0
1-2	8.0	17.0	5.0	2.0	0.3	5.0	3.0	45.0	1.4
3-5	13.0	46.0	8.0	2.0	0.4	2.0	3.0	73.0	3.6
6-8	13.0	59.0	4.0	0.4	0	0.5	0.9	79.0	5.0
9-11	12.0	41.0	3.0	0	0	0.5	0.9	58.0	2.4
In years									
1-2	5.0	16.0	1.0	0.1	0	0.1	0.5	23.0	1.3
3-4	2.0	3.0	0.3	0	0	0.1	0.4	6.0	0.6
5-9	0.7	0.6	0.2	0	0	0.1	0.3	2.0	0.2
10-19	0.6	0.1	0.1	0	<0.1	0.1	0.1	0.9	0.1
20-29	0.3	<0.1	0.1	<0.1	<0.1	0.1	0.1	0.6	<0.1
30-59	0.2	<0.1	0.2	<0.1	<0.1	0.1	<0.1	0.6	<0.1
>60	0.2	0.1	0.4	0	0.1	0.2	0.1	1.2	0.1

*Per 10^5 population; July 1978 estimate for 38 participating states.

Eighteen percent of *H. influenzae* isolates were reported to be resistant to ampicillin. Little geographical variation in resistance was observed.

Reported by State Epidemiologists from participating states; Special Pathogens Br, Bacterial Diseases Div, Bur of Epidemiology, CDC.

Editorial Note: Surveillance of bacterial meningitis was recommended by the Conference of State and Territorial Epidemiologists to provide baseline information against which the impact of vaccines against *H. influenzae, N. meningitidis,* and *S. pneumoniae* (should these be deployed on a large scale) could be measured and to provide information that would help control bacterial meningitis through chemoprophylaxis and treatment. The national incidence of reported bacterial meningitis observed in this surveillance program in 1978 represents about 30% of the national incidence of culture-proven bacterial meningitis estimated from data collected several years ago (1). The degree of reporting for 1978, the second year of this system, is encouraging and represents an increase of 176% over the reports submitted in 1977. To date, vaccines against *H. influenzae, N. meningitidis,* and *S. pneumoniae* have not been used on a large scale in the highest-risk age groups because of their limited immunogenicity in the young, but attempts continue to develop more immunogenic vaccines.

The wide variation of meningococcal serogroups observed in the different geographic regions may have important implications from the standpoint of sulfonamide chemoprophylaxis. Most serogroup B, Y, and W135 isolates are sensitive to sulfonamides, while a considerable proportion of serogroup C isolates are resistant (2). CDC is currently in the process of reviewing antibiotic susceptibility information for all isolates submitted for serogrouping.

The percentage of *H. influenzae* isolates resistant to ampicillin observed in this survey is considerably higher than that in most other reports. In 1976-1977, a survey of 45 of the largest pediatric medical centers in the United States found that 5% of *H. influenzae* strains causing meningitis or bacteremia were resistant to ampicillin (3). The 18% rate of resistance in reported cases in 1978, an unexpectedly high figure, may be inflated by preferential reporting of cases caused by ampicillin-resistant strains.

Through states participating in the national surveillance program, CDC has recently prospectively examined the risk of acquiring severe *H. influenzae* illness in household contacts of a patient with *H. influenzae* meningitis (4). It was found that the risk for this group (0.2%) in the month after exposure was similar to the risk of acquiring secondary meningococcal disease and was especially high in contacts under 6 years of age (0.5%). These results have prompted a nationwide prospective study to examine the efficacy of chemoprophylaxis in preventing secondary cases of *H. influenzae* disease.

References

1. Fraser DW, Geil CC, Feldman RA: Bacterial meningitis in Bernalillo County, New Mexico: A comparison with three other American populations. Am J Epidemiol 100:297, 1974
2. Jacobson JA, Weaver RE, Thornsberry C: Trends in meningococcal disease, 1974. J Infect Dis 132:480, 1975
3. Ward JI, Tsai TF, Filice GA, Fraser DW: Prevalence of ampicillin and chloramphenicol-resistant strains of *Haemophilus influenzae* causing meningitis and bacteremia: National survey of hospital laboratories. J Infect Dis 138:421, 1978
4. Ward JI, Fraser DW, Plikaytis BD, Baraff L: *H. influenzae* meningitis: A prospective national study of secondary spread in household contacts. Pediatr Res 13:470, 1979

MMWR 27 (A.S., 1978): 42

MENINGOCOCCAL INFECTIONS (Total) — Reported Case Rates by Year, United States, 1920—1978

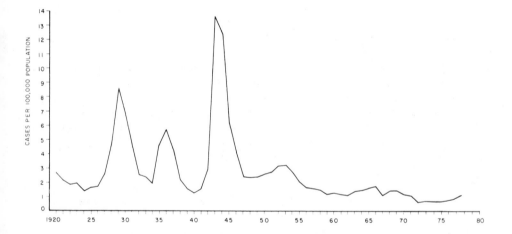

CHAPTER 20

Various Nosocomial Infections

MMWR 27:307 (8/25/78)

An Outbreak of Bacteremia
and Pyrogenic Reactions in a Dialysis Unit — Pennsylvania

On March 18, 1978, 3 patients undergoing hemodialysis at a university hospital in Pennsylvania became ill. All 3, who had previously been well, developed fever and chills during dialysis. One patient became hypotensive. Dialysis was discontinued, and all 3 were admitted for evaluation. *Pseudomonas aeruginosa* was isolated from blood cultures from 2 patients; *Klebsiella pneumoniae* was also isolated from one of these patients' blood. Blood cultures from the third patient were negative. On March 20, 2 more patients undergoing hemodialysis became ill with fever and chills and required hospitalization. Blood cultures from these patients were negative.

The outpatient hemodialysis facility is located in a separate building and consists of a large room containing 10 units and a separate 2-unit area for patients positive for hepatitis B surface antigen. Each unit contains a single-pass dialysis machine equipped with a disposable coil dialyzer. The dialyzers are not reused. An investigation revealed that a sodium hypochlorite pump attached to the dialysis mixing console had not been functioning for the previous 2 weeks because a replacement part had not arrived. Normally, a solution of sodium hypochlorite was pumped through the entire system between each shift. Alkaline glutaraldehyde solutions were also used on a variable schedule. During the 2 weeks before the outbreak, individual units were disinfected daily with sodium hypochlorite. However, without the pump the distribution system and pipes leading to the dialysis machine could not be disinfected.

Cultures taken in the unit grew *P. aeruginosa* in all samples of water and dialysate; heavy growth was present in the storage tank from which mixed dialysate was distributed to individual units and in the tubing leading to the dialysis machines. *K. pneumoniae* and *Enterobacter agglomerans* were also cultured from additional sites in the system. Bacteria were recovered from the inlet and outlet blood tubing as well as from the blood side of the dialyzer used for one of the ill patients.

Following the repair of the sodium hypochlorite pump and thorough disinfection of the unit, there have been no further cases of febrile illness associated with dialysis.

Reported by Hospital Infections Br, Bacterial Diseases Div, Bur of Epidemiology, CDC.

Editorial Note: Chronic hemodialysis as a treatment for patients suffering from end-stage renal disease has been used increasingly in the United States since the early 1960s. In 1978, the total number of patients undergoing chronic hemodialysis in private or nospital-based centers was 37,000—more than triple the 1973 figure. It is estimated that by 1980 there will be 45,000 such patients. Technological advances in hemodialysis systems have been significant in the past 10-15 years; they have allowed chronic hemo-dialysis to become a common procedure and accounted for a dramatic improvement in the clinical state of the art.

However, a significant number of microbiologic parameters were not taken into con-sideration in the design of many hemodialysis systems, and, as a result, there are many situations in which certain types of bacteria, notably, gram-negative water bacteria, can persist and actively multiply in water associated with hemodialysis equipment. This can result in the production of massive levels of gram-negative bacteria in dialysis fluid—levels which have been associated with outbreaks of pyrogenic (fever-producing) reactions and septicemia among patients undergoing hemodialysis. These bacteria contain lipo-polysaccharide or endotoxin, which can produce a pyrogenic response if introduced into the bloodstream. CDC has investigated a number of outbreaks of pyrogenic reactions in the United States, some of which were complicated by septicemia, among patients in hemodialysis centers.

These outbreaks fell into 2 categories. The most common type involved pyrogenic reactions that could be directly associated with high levels of gram-negative bacteria in dialysis fluid. Inadequate disinfection of water-treatment devices and fluid-distri-bution systems and improper design and operation of these systems were the usual causes of excessive bacterial contamination. In 1 such outbreak, in which 2 patients died from septicemia, it was shown that the same pyocin type of *P. aeruginosa* that occurred in high numbers in dialysate was isolated from the blood of patients who were dialyzing. During the same outbreak, bacteriologic assays of dialysate showed that there was a relationship between the level of bacterial contamination and the attack rate of pyrogenic reactions (1). Once the bacteriologic reservoir was identified and eliminated by proper disinfection, modification, or operation of the systems involved, the outbreaks abruptly ceased (2,3). The second general type of outbreak is exemplified by an investigation which traced the source to a high level of bacterial endotoxin in a community water supply. This outbreak occurred in the absence of a large reservoir of bacteria in the center and could have been controlled only by the use of a water-treat-ment system that removed endotoxin from water such as reverse osmosis or ultrafil-tration (4).

The manner in which microorganisms reach the blood stream to cause bacteremia is not entirely clear. It has been reported that bacteria can pass through the dialyzer mem-brane (5). Another possibility is that the blood compartment of the dialyzer may be con-taminated by nonsterile saline used to prime dialyzers prior to connection of the patient. It is common practice to heparinize sterile saline before use. Several saline containers may be heparinized with the same needle and syringe using heparin from multiple-dose vials that are re-entered several times. This procedure often takes place in the dialysis center enviroment in which hands and surfaces may be heavily contaminated with gram-negative bacteria. Strict application of aseptic technique and other precautions asso-ciated with the use of parenteral fluids can, of course, minimize this hazard.

The most probable explanation of the outbreak reported here is that the gram-negative bacteria were able to grow within the water and dialysate distribution systems because of the cessation of routine sodium hypochlorite disinfection. Sodium hypochlorite is used as a disinfectant for hemodialysis systems by a large number of hemodialysis centers in the United States. However, it is corrosive, and consequently it is usually rinsed from the system after a minimum exposure time. Unfortunately, this practice commonly results in negation of the disinfection procedure because water used to rinse the dis-infectant out of the system is not sterile and usually contains gram-negative bacteria.

In recirculating dialysis machines—the most difficult type to disinfect—gram-negative bacteria present in the rinse water can multiply immediately and, if permitted to stand overnight, can significantly contaminate the system. This level of bacterial contamination will increase by 3-5 logs during dialysis.

The optimum strategy for the disinfection of dialysis systems may be to use aqueous formaldehyde (1.5-2.5%) and to allow it to remain in the system for prolonged periods of time when the system is not operational such as for a night or weekend. Although other high-level disinfectants such as alkaline glutaraldehyde could be used, the volume of these systems is so large that their use would be very expensive. The strategies for disinfecting different types of hemodialysis systems as well as bacteriologic guidelines for hemodialysis systems have been published (2,6) and are available from the Hepatitis Laboratories Division, CDC, Phoenix, Arizona 85021.

References
1. Favero MS, Petersen NJ, Boyer KM, Carson LA, Bond WW: Microbial contamination of renal dialysis systems and associated health risks. Trans Am Soc Artif Intern Organs 20A: 175-183, 1974
2. Favero MS, Petersen NJ, Carson LA, Bond WW, Hindman SH: Gram-negative water bacteria in hemodialysis systems. Health Lab Sci 12:321-334, 1975
3. Petersen NJ, Boyer KM, Carson LA, Favero MS: Pyrogenic reactions from inadequate disinfection of a dialysis fluid distribution system. Dialysis Transplantation 7:52-60, 1978
4. Hindman SH, Favero MS, Carson LA, Petersen NJ, Schonberger LB, Solano JT: Pyrogenic reactions during hemodialysis caused by extramural endotoxin. Lancet ii:1-7, 1975
5. Jans H, Bretlau P, Nielsen B: Bacteriological contamination of dialyzers. Nephron 20:10-17, 1978
6. Favero MS, Petersen NJ: Microbiologic guidelines for hemodialysis systems. Dialysis Transplantation 6:34-36, 1977

MMWR 27:513 (12/22/78)

Mycobacterial Infections Associated with Augmentation Mammoplasty — Florida, North Carolina, Texas

Postoperative wound infections caused by organisms of the *Mycobacterium fortuitum* complex have recently been reported from Florida, North Carolina, and Texas. To date, 17 patients who underwent insertion of silicone mammary prostheses for augmentation mammoplasty and then developed infections at 1 or both periprosthetic sites have been identified. All patients were previously healthy women who ranged in age from 20-51 years.

The onset of infection occurred 1-2 weeks to over 1 year after surgery. All infections were localized to the operative site. Typically, infection was manifested by a painful, swollen breast with little or no erythema or incisional drainage and the absence of fever and systemic signs. However, when the breast was re-incised and drained because of the infection, non-odorous, serosanguineous or purulent fluid was often present in the pocket around the prosthesis. Gram stain of the fluid usually revealed many polymorphonuclear leukocytes with few, if any, organisms; initial cultures were often reported to be sterile (1).

The first case occurred in March 1975; the last in October 1978. Clustering in time has been observed in Texas in 3 practices; in each, 2 cases occurred in patients who had received implants within a span of 1 month. Investigation of cases has revealed that the silicone gel-containing prostheses implanted in the patients were made by several different manufacturers. Some prostheses had been sterilized by the manufacturers; others had been nonsterile when distributed but were sterilized just prior to their use.

Review of charts from the practices of 3 surgeons who each reported more than 1 case has yielded no additional cases and has demonstrated uniformly low postoperative wound infection rates after augmentation mammoplasty. A case-control study in the practice of 1 surgeon has failed to demonstrate exposure factors significantly associated with cases. Investigations are continuing in search of possible sources of contamination.

CDC would like to receive, through state health departments, reports of suspected cases of mycobacterial postoperative infections at sites of augmentation mammoplasties.

Reported by MT Foster, MD, Jacksonville, Florida; WE Sanders, MD, Omaha, Nebraska; JL Baker, MD, Orlando, CB Bass, MD, Miami, MM Shuster, MD, HI Wald, MD, Hollywood, Florida; RM Yeller, MD, Acting State Epidemiologist, Florida State Dept of Health and Rehabilitative Services; TR Kitchens, MD, Greensboro; MP Hines, DVM, North Carolina Dept of Human Resources; WE Barnes, MD, Austin; GW Johnson, MD, RJ Wallace, MD, RW Wood, MD, Houston; IR Toranto, MD, Plano; TS Wilkinson, MD, San Antonio; CR Webb Jr, MD, State Epidemiologist, Texas State Dept of Health; Mycobacteriology Br, Bacteriology Div, Bur of Laboratories, Special Pathogens Br, Hospital Infections Br, Bacterial Diseases Div, Bur of Epidemiology, CDC.

Reference
1. Foster MT, Sanders WE: Atypical mycobacterial infections complicating mammary implants, in Eighteenth Interscience Conference on Antimicrobial Agents and Chemotherapy (Abstract 104), 1-4 Oct 1978. Atlanta, 1978

MMWR 28:25 (1/26/79)

Endotoxic Reactions Associated with the Reuse of Cardiac Catheters — Massachusetts

During a 2-week period in July 1978, 3 cases of suspected endotoxic reactions (fever, chills, and hypotension) occurred in patients undergoing cardiac catheterization at a Massachusetts hospital. An investigation revealed that reusable intravascular catheters, although sterile, were contaminated with 0.3 to 7.4 nanograms of endotoxin and that this contamination was related to procedures employed to clean and disinfect the catheters.

At the time the endotoxic reactions occurred, used catheters were rinsed with hospital distilled water, wiped to remove clotted blood, and then soaked in Detergicide,* a quaternary ammonium compound. Next, the bore of the catheter was flushed continuously for 2 hours with distilled water, followed by a second flush with 1 liter of commercial pyrogen-free, sterile, distilled water. Finally, the catheters were wrapped and gas-sterilized. The administration set for the delivery of the pyrogen-free fluid had not been changed regularly.

The hospital-supplied distilled water contained greater than 0.2 ng of endotoxin per ml even when samples were taken directly from the storage tanks. Cultures of samples taken from the cardiac catheterization laboratory's distilled water tap and from the research laboratories contained up to 310 colonies of *Pseudomonas cepacia* per ml, while storage tank samples were sterile.

Five previously used, but subsequently cleaned and sterilized, catheters contained levels of endotoxin ranging from 0.3 ng to 7.4 ng per catheter, as measured by the Limulus Amebocyte Lysate assay. (A level of 0.05 ng is considered pyrogenic by the laboratory performing the assay.) All catheters were sterile when cultured. New, sterile catheters were free of endotoxin. After only 1 use and cleaning, catheter flushes yielded excessive endotoxin. An aliquot of distilled water, used for the first continuous flush, contained greater than 0.2 ng of endotoxin per ml and, on culture, yielded heavy growth of *P. cepacia*. A 4-ml rinse from the administration set used for the second flushing contained 0.06 ng of endotoxin per ml but was sterile on culture. No samples from patients were available.

---

*Use of trade name is for identification only and does not constitute endorsement by the Public Health Service, U.S. Department of Health, Education and Welfare.

Two previously used catheters (1 had just been used) were cleaned in the usual manner through the Detergicide soaking. Flushing the bore of these catheters with pyrogen-free, distilled water reduced levels of endotoxin from as high as 0.275 ng/ml at the beginning of the wash to less than 0.02 ng/ml at the end of the wash, and reduced bacterial contamination from 30 bacterial colonies/ml to zero. Each catheter was then enclosed in a sterile cylindrical container and shaken with 10 ml of pyrogen-free, distilled water to assess contamination of the outer surface of the catheter. This procedure yielded 0.4 ng and 0.75 ng endotoxin, respectively, from the 2 catheters and greater than 10^3 bacterial colonies/ml of wash from the freshly used catheter. It was, therefore, concluded that most of the contamination came from the external catheter surface.

A similar problem occurred in the catheterization laboratory in 1973. The distilled water supply used for washing the reusable catheters was contaminated with *Pseudomonas* species and contained high levels of endotoxin. At that time, institution of a final rinse using sterile, pyrogen-free, distilled water followed by ethylene oxide sterilization was associated with cessation of the outbreak. Since then, occasional reactions had been observed, but frequently the patients had received contrast material prior to the reactions, making an etiologic diagnosis difficult.

This investigation resulted in the recommendation that disposable catheters be used. When this was not possible, it was recommended that pyrogen-free, sterile, distilled water be used in the cleaning procedure, and that both the outer and inner surfaces of the catheter be flushed. Detergicide was freshly prepared daily, using pyrogen-free, sterile, distilled water. After the catheters were cleaned and packaged, they were stored at 4 C until sterilized. In the 5-month period since this outbreak, there have been no further suspected endotoxic reactions.

Reported by E Bauer, RN, P Densen, MD, D Faxon, MD, C Kloster, RN, C Melidossian, RN, University Hospital, Boston; R Kundsin, ScD, P Ryan, BA, Peter Bent Brigham Hospital, Boston; N Fiumara, MD, State Epidemiologist, Massachusetts Dept of Public Health; Hospital Infections Br, Bacterial Diseases Div, Bur of Epidemiology, CDC.

Editorial Note: The precise mechanism by which catheters used for cardiac catheterization were contaminated with endotoxin was not proven, but this investigation suggests that contamination was introduced during the cleaning procedure. Hospital supplies of distilled water, used in cleaning, were contaminated. Furthermore, the detergent-disinfectant preparation that was used in the preliminary cleaning, an aqueous quaternary ammonium formulation, has been shown to be ineffective against *P. cepacia* and may even permit the selective growth of this and other microorganisms (1). Presumably, viable microorganisms were introduced during cleaning from the distilled water, the Detergicide failed to kill the contaminants or permitted their growth, and the final sterilization killed the contaminants but allowed high levels of residual endotoxin to persist. Although a variety of detergent-disinfectants may be used safely for environmental sanitation of floors, surfaces, and the like, these agents must be used with utmost caution with critical medical devices that come in contact with any normally sterile body tissue. An effective sterilizing procedure, such as ethylene oxide, will kill microorganisms but will not remove endotoxin.

This report further highlights the hazards that may result from reuse of some medical devices. Ethylene oxide sterilization and reuse of disposable arterial pressure domes, meant to be used once and discarded, have previously been documented to produce defects in the dome membranes that were followed by epidemic bacteremia (2). Some, but not all, medical devices can be cleaned and safely sterilized. If practical and economical, disposable devices are preferable to reusable devices that are difficult to sterilize.

References
1. Dixon RE, Kaslow RA, Mackel DC, Fulkerson CC, Mallison GF: Aqueous quaternary ammonium

antiseptics and disinfectants. Use and misuse. JAMA 236:2415-2417, 1976
2. MMWR 26:266, 1977

MMWR 28:82 (2/23/79)

Pseudobacteremia due to *Staphylococcus aureus* — New York

In the period June 15-19, 1978, 11 patients in a New York community hospital had blood cultures positive for *Staphylococcus aureus*. Four of the 11 patients had more than 1 positive culture for *S. aureus*. All patients, except 1 premature infant, were febrile at the time cultures were obtained but had been admitted for a variety of reasons, including orthopedic injuries, cardiovascular diseases, and cerebrovascular disease. The patients were hospitalized on 4 different services, and none had *S. aureus* isolated from any site other than blood. Five of the 11 patients were placed on antimicrobial therapy for *S. aureus* infection.

Blood cultures in this hospital are initially inoculated into Brucella Broth.* At the time of the outbreak, specimens were subcultured routinely with a sterile applicator after a 24-hour incubation period to inoculate blood and chocolate agar plates. Investigation revealed that only subculture specimens were positive for *S. aureus*, while the original culture bottles remained sterile.

One of 7 technicians had subcultured all 31 blood-culture specimens on the 4 days involved. Nasopharyngeal cultures of this technician, who remained asymptomatic, revealed *S. aureus*, phage type 94/96, the same type as 8 of the 9 blood-culture isolates that were phage typed. Cultures from other laboratory personnel, the original blood-culture broth media, and subsequent blood cultures from involved patients were all negative for *S. aureus*. The implicated technician had nasopharyngeal cultures negative for *S. aureus* at the 1-week follow-up culture, and further cultures were not performed. Laboratory procedures were changed to avoid opening the original blood-culture bottles to the air during the subculturing, and no further cases of *S. aureus* pseudobacteremia have occurred.

Reported by J Dolan, MT, GR Joachim, MD, A Khapra, MD, Oceanside, New York; P Greenwald, MD, Acting State Epidemiologist, New York State Dept of Health; Hospital Infections Br, Bacterial Diseases Div, Bur of Epidemiology, CDC.

Editorial Note: Outbreaks of pseudobacteremia due to contamination of blood cultures have been reported occasionally, but the contamination has usually been traced to a source in the inanimate environment such as contaminated media, disinfecting agents, and mist tents (1-4). The probable source of contamination in this outbreak was a laboratory technician transiently colonized with *S. aureus* in the nasopharynx. No further cases were noted after laboratory procedures were changed, but since the implicated technician no longer carried *S. aureus* in the nasopharynx on repeat culture, the efficacy of the improved procedures could not be evaluated.

That 5 of 11 patients received unnecessary antistaphylococcal therapy highlights the importance of conducting the necessary epidemiologic studies so that outbreaks of pseudobacteremia can be identified. Transient, asymptomatic nasal colonization with *S. aureus* is common, and other sources of contamination in laboratories are prevalent. Although outbreaks such as this one are rarely reported, 20% or more of positive blood cultures in hospitals may be due to organisms recognized as common skin contaminants (5). Thus, laboratory procedures for collecting and culturing patient specimens should

---

*Use of trade names is for identification only and does not constitute endorsement by the Public Health Service, U.S. Department of Health, Education, and Welfare.

be such as to prevent inadvertent contamination of patient cultures.

References
1. Noble R, Reeves S: *Bacillus* species pseudosepsis caused by contaminated commercial blood culture media. JAMA 230:1002, 1974
2. Kaslow RA, Mackel DC, Mallison GF: Nosocomial pseudobacteremia. Positive blood cultures due to contaminated benzalkonium antiseptic. JAMA 236:2407-2409, 1976
3. Snydman DR, Maloy MF, Brock SM, Lyons RW, Rubin SJ: Pseudobacteremia: False-positive blood cultures from mist tent contamination. Am J Epidemiol 106:154-159, 1977
4. Hoffman PC, Arnow PM, Goldmann DA, Parrott PL, Stamm WE, McGowan JE: False-positive blood cultures associated with nonsterile blood collection tubes. JAMA 236:2073-2075, 1976
5. Scheckler WE: Septicemia in a community hospital 1970 through 1973. JAMA 237:1938-1941, 1977

MMWR 28:177 (4/20/79)

Nosocomial Infections Caused
by *Acinetobacter calcoaceticus* — United States, 1978

Acinetobacter calcoaceticus was reported as causing 474 nosocomial infections by the 82 hospitals participating in the National Nosocomial Infections Study (NNIS) during 1978 for a rate of infection of 3.54 per 10,000 patients discharged. This rate is 14% higher than that reported during the years 1974-1977 (*1*). Of the 2 subspecies of *A. calcoaceticus*, 41.6% of the isolates were var. *anitratus* (formerly *Herellea vaginicola*), and 6.1% were var. *lwoffi* (formerly *Mima polymorpha*); 52.3% of the isolates were not subspeciated. As has been observed previously (*1*), the rate of infection with this pathogen demonstrated a marked seasonal variation with a maximum rate during the summer months (6.52/10,000 in August) and a minimum rate during the winter months (2.29 in February) (Figure 2). Although this trend is clear for var. *anitratus* and unspeciated isolates, the number of isolates of var. *lwoffi* is too small to determine whether a similar seasonal variation exists with this subspecies.

The most frequent site of infection with *Acinetobacter* was the lower respiratory tract, primarily in cases of pneumonia (infection rate 1.3/10,000); almost 38% of isolates of *A. calcoaceticus* were from this site. This is a higher percentage of isolates from this site than for any other pathogen reported to NNIS except *Streptococcus pneumoniae* and *Haemophilus influenzae*, in which over 80% of the nosocomial isolates were from the lower respiratory tract. Per 10,000 patients discharged, the rate of *Acinetobacter* infection was 0.8 for the urinary tract, 0.7 for surgical wounds, 0.3 for blood, 0.2 for skin, and 0.1 for cardiovascular sites. Eight percent of nosocomial *Acinetobacter* infections with a defined site were associated with secondary bacteremia. Overall, 14.8% of infections with this pathogen were bacteremic.

The reported rates of infection varied widely with the service and category of hospital. Patients on the medical service developed nosocomial infection with *A. calcoaceticus* at a rate of 3.3/10,000 patients discharged, whereas patients on the surgical service had a rate of 6.6. The rate of infection on all other services ranged from 0.3 to 0.9. University hospitals reported *Acinetobacter* infections at a rate of 7.2/10,000—almost 5 times the rate reported by community hospitals (*1,5*). Community-teaching, federal, and municipal-county hospitals reported intermediate rates of infection with this pathogen (3.1, 3.2, and 3.8/10,000, respectively).

Reported by Hospital Infections Br, Bacterial Diseases Div, Bur of Epidemiology, CDC.

Editorial Note: *A. calcoaceticus* is one of the less frequently reported nosocomial pathogens, accounting for 1% of the bacterial isolates associated with nosocomial infection reported by the NNIS hospitals. *Acinetobacter* organisms are gram-negative, nonfer-

FIGURE 2. Nosocomial *Acinetobacter calcoaceticus* infection rate, NNIS* hospitals, 1978

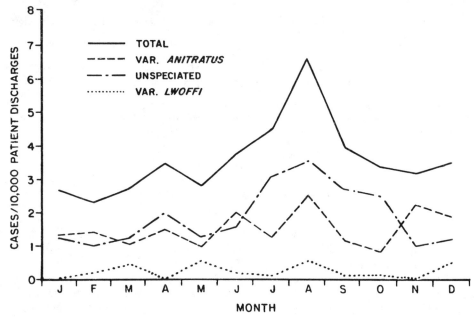

*National Nosocomial Infections Study

mentative, aerobic bacteria. They are widely distributed in nature and frequently form part of the normal flora of humans, particularly of the skin but occasionally also of the oral cavity, upper respiratory tract, and lower gastrointestinal tract. Because of this distribution in humans, evaluation of the clinical significance of isolates from surgical wound and sputum specimens may be difficult. However, reports in the medical literature document the increasing frequency with which this organism is recognized as a nosocomial pathogen associated with both endemic and epidemic disease (1-5). A. calcoaceticus is frequently an opportunistic pathogen, causing disease in severely compromised hosts. This fact may partially explain the markedly higher rate of reported infection with this organism from university hospitals compared with community hospitals.

An unusual feature of nosocomial infections caused by A. calcoaceticus reported by NNIS hospitals is the marked and consistent seasonal fluctuation in rates of infection that peaks in the summer each year (1). This pattern is in contrast to the overall relatively stable trend of reported nosocomial infections from this group of hospitals. This seasonal fluctuation was consistent for all categories of hospitals, for medical and surgical services, and for all major sites of infection. It was consistent for hospitals in the northern and southern United States and for those with and without training programs for house staff. The higher rate was not a reflection of seasonal epidemics at a small number of the NNIS hospitals but rather a general increase in reporting of infections with this pathogen from most hospitals. Information about community-acquired infections is not collected from NNIS hospitals, and it is not known whether the seasonal pattern of infections with this pathogen reflects community-acquired disease or colonization within the hospital.

References
1. Retailliau HF, Hightower AW, Dixon RE, Allen JR: *Acinetobacter calcoaceticus:* A nosocomial pathogen with an unusual seasonal pattern. J infect Dis 139:371, 1979

2. Glew RH, Moellering RC, Kuny LJ: Infections with *Acinetobacter calcoaceticus (Herellea vagini-cola)*: Clinical and laboratory studies. Medicine 56:79, 1977

3. Buxton AE, Anderson RL, Werdegar D, Atlas E: Nosocomial respiratory tract infection and colonization with *Acinetobacter calcoaceticus.* Epidemiologic characteristics. Am J Med 65:507, 1973

4. Castle M, Tenney JH, Weinstein MP, Eickhoff TC: Outbreak of a multiply-resistant *Acinetobacter* in a surgical intensive care unit: Epidemiology and control. Heart Lung 7:641, 1978

5. Abrutyn E, Goodhart GL, Roos K, Anderson R, Buxton AE: *Acinetobacter calcoaceticus* outbreak associated with peritoneal dialysis. Am J Epidemiol 107:328, 1978

MMWR 28:289 (6/29/79)

Nosocomial *Pseudomonas cepacia* Infection

In January and February 1979, 3 patients in a large university hospital acquired serious nosocomial infection with *Pseudomonas cepacia* attributed to the receipt of cryoprecipitate, possibly contaminated when separate units of this substance were combined for administration to patients.

P. cepacia organisms were isolated from blood cultures from 2 patients with septicemia and from 1 mediastinal wound infection of the other patient. The patient with the wound infection and 1 of the septicemic patients had undergone elective cardiac surgery procedures, received cryoprecipitate during their operations, and developed evidence of infection on the fifth and tenth postoperative days, respectively. The other patient, who had liver failure attributed to cytomegalovirus hepatitis, was given cryoprecipitate because of acquired blood-coagulation abnormalities.

An epidemiologic investigation revealed that the 3 cases of infection had few common exposures. Receipt of cryoprecipitate intravenously before onset of infection was significantly associated with disease, however, when cases were compared with 76 procedure-matched controls ($p = 0.007$).

About 100 courses of cryoprecipitate are given each month in the hospital. Single units of cryoprecipitate are supplied in Fenwall Transfer Packs* at −20 C by a central blood bank. For administration to patients up to 20 units of cryoprecipitate are combined in the hospital's blood bank. To prepare the combined pools, the frozen packs are placed in a 37 C water bath to be gently thawed. They are blotted dry, and the protective tabs covering the administration ports are dried with a clean gauze. Cryoprecipitate pools are generally administered within 2 hours after they have been prepared.

A sample of the cryoprecipitate pool received by the last patient was obtained and cultured, and it grew *P. cepacia*. Moreover, cultures of water in the warming bath used to thaw the frozen packs were found to contain 1.8×10^8 *P. cepacia* per ml, although each day these water baths were cleaned with povodine-iodine, and fresh water was added. The *Pseudomonas* isolates from the 3 patients, the cryoprecipitate pool, and the water bath had the same antimicrobial susceptibility patterns. Studies are underway to attempt to determine the exact mechanism of contamination.

Reported by FS Rhame, MD, J McCullough, MD, and the Hospital Infections Br, Bacterial Diseases Div, Bur of Epidemiology, CDC.

Editorial Note: Infections due to *P. cepacia* are almost exclusively limited to drug addicts (*1*), patients with cystic fibrosis, and hospitalized patients. In the last context, they arise

---

*Use of trade names is for identification only and does not constitute endorsement by the Public Health Service, U.S. Department of Health, Education, and Welfare.

because of the organism's ability to proliferate in relatively pure water (2) and in certain dilute aqueous quaternary ammonium disinfectants (3-5). This outbreak and others emphasize the importance of thorough investigation of all nosocomial P. cepacia infections for the possibility of a contaminated common source.

These 3 cases of P. cepacia infection were traced to contaminated pooled cryoprecipitate. The contamination probably occurred during the pooling process after removal of the packs from the contaminated water bath. Even though the packs had been blotted dry, they and the hands of the technician performing the pooling were presumably heavily contaminated with P. cepacia.

Thawing frozen blood products in water baths is widely practiced in blood banks. Preventing further infections of this sort should involve adopting procedures for cleaning water baths to reduce contamination levels and exercising great care to avoid contamination by touch during pooling procedures. A plastic overwrap may be used to protect the packs while in the water bath. Microwave technology is being developed which may allow heating of such items and, in the future, make use of water baths unnecessary.

References
1. Noriega ER, Rubinstein E, Simberkoff MS, Rahal JJ: Subacute and acute endocarditis due to *Pseudomonas cepacia* in heroin addicts. Am J Med 59:29-36, 1975
2. Carson LA, Favero MS, Bond WW, Petersen NJ: Morphological, biochemical, and growth characteristics of *Pseudomonas cepacia* from distilled water. Appl Microbiol 25:475-483, 1973
3. Dixon RE, Kaslow RA, Mackel DC, Fulkerson CC, Mallison GF: Aqueous quaternary ammonium antiseptics and disinfectants. Use and misuse. JAMA 236:2415-2417, 1976
4. Frank MJ, Schaffner W: Contaminated aqueous benzalkonium chloride: An unnecessary hospital infection hazard. JAMA 236:2418-2419, 1976
5. Weinstein RA, Emori TG, Anderson RL, Stamm WE: Pressure transducers as a source of bacteremia after open heart surgery: Report of an outbreak and guidelines for prevention. Chest 69:338-344, 1976

MMWR 28:409 (8/31/79)

Follow-up on Nosocomial *Pseudomonas cepacia* Infection

In a previous article (1), an outbreak of serious nosocomial infection with *Pseudomonas cepacia* was significantly associated with the receipt of cryoprecipitate intravenously. The cryoprecipitate, contained in frozen units, had been thawed in a water bath. P. cepacia organisms were isolated from the bath, but the exact means by which they had contaminated the cryoprecipitate was unclear. Further investigation has now identified a possible mechanism of contamination.

Studies have shown that as little as 0.025 ml of water, when placed between the unopened tabs of Fenwal Transfer Packs,* may contaminate the outlet port of the pack when the tabs are pulled apart (Figure 2). It is important, therefore, that the tabs be dried before they are separated to expose the port. The surfaces of the transfer packs can be kept dry if they are enclosed in an impermeable overwrap, such as a self-sealing plastic bag, while being thawed in the water bath. If an overwrap is not used, the outer surface of the transfer pack must be dried, with special attention being paid to the areas around the tabs.

Reported by FS Rhame, MD, J McCullough, MD, and the Hospital Infections Br, Bacterial Diseases Div, Bur of Epidemiology, CDC.
Reference
1. MMWR 28:289-290, 1979

FIGURE 2. Fenwal transfer pack*

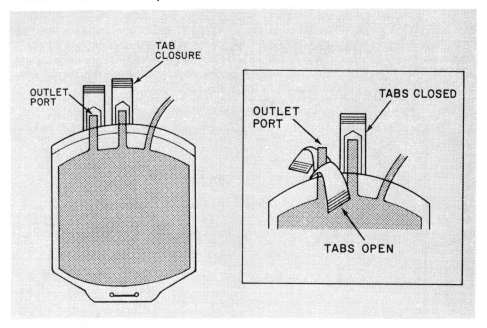

---

*Use of trade names is for identification only and does not constitute endorsement by the Public Health Service, U.S. Department of Health, Education, and Welfare.

CHAPTER 21

Various Bacterial Diseases

MMWR 27 (A.S., 1978): 17

ANTHRAX — Reported Cases in Humans by 5-Year Period, United States, 1920–1978

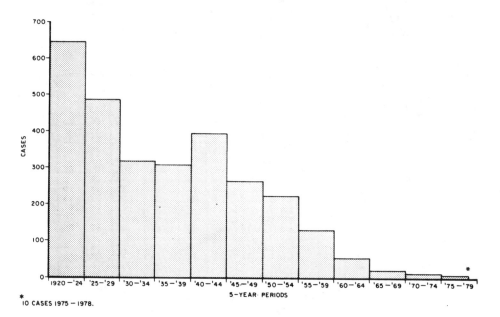

* 10 CASES 1975 – 1978.

MMWR 28:160 (4/13/79)

Anthrax in Humans — United States, 1978

Six cases of anthrax in humans were reported to CDC in 1978. All 6 cases were occupationally acquired: 4 in industrial settings, 2 in agricultural ones. In each case the patient had cutaneous anthrax. All 6 have recovered.

Of the 4 industrial anthrax cases, 2 were associated with a North Carolina textile mill and 2 with a New Hampshire felt mill. The 2 North Carolina cases occurred in January and February 1978 in unvaccinated employees of a textile mill, where imported goat hair is processed into fabrics. The first case was in a 67-year-old man whose duties involved general maintenance of the carding machines. After working in the mill for 7 days, he noticed a painless, nonpruritic postule on the right side of his chin, associated with slight swelling. Two days later he was seen by a physician, who placed him on tetracycline therapy. A 1-cm ulcer with a black eschar at its base subsequently developed at the postule site. Cultures taken after antibiotic therapy was initiated were negative for *Bacillus anthracis*; a blood specimen obtained 58 days after onset and 37 days after he received 1 dose of anthrax vaccine revealed a microscopic indirect hemagglutination titer of 1:640 for *B. anthracis*. The second patient was a 59-year-old man who had hauled waste material from the mill for the past year. He noticed a small pruritic pimple on the left side of his chin. He was seen by his physician and placed on penicillin and ampicillin therapy. Cultures of the lesion yielded *B. anthracis*. Ninety-four (62%) of 151 environmental swab samples and 29 (76%) of 38 bulk waste samples collected during an environmental culture survey of the mill also yielded *B. anthracis*.

The 2 cases of anthrax in the New Hampshire felt mill also occurred in unvaccinated employees who were exposed to imported goat hair. Both had onset in May and had worked in the carding area during the week before their onset. In the first instance a 20-year-old man, who had worked at the mill for 1 year, lanced a small postule on the right lower quadrant of his abdomen at the belt line on May 1. On May 5, he sought medical attention, complaining of a painful, swollen skin lesion on his abdomen, fever, headache, sore neck, anorexia, and malaise. On physical examination, his physician noted a well-developed eschar surrounded by edema and erythema, right inguinal adenopathy, and fever of 100.9 F (38.3 C). A wound culture obtained at the time of the initial diagnostic workup on May 5 yielded *B. anthracis*. The second case was in a 19-year-old man; an eschar developed on the biceps area of his left arm. Anthrax in this patient was also culture confirmed.

The 2 agricultureal anthrax cases occurred in North Dakota and Idaho in August and September and were associated with anthrax in cattle. The North Dakota patient was a 45-year-old veterinarian, who performed a postmortem examination on 1 of 5 cattle that had died suddenly on a ranch in the southeastern part of the state. On August 20, 6 days after the postmortem examination, a 1- to 2-mm vesicle developed on the dorsum of the middle finger of his left hand near the knuckle. At the time of his admission to the local hospital on August 24, he had a purple, pruritic, moderately painful, pustular lesion 10-15 mm in diameter on his finger, axillary adenopathy, and a temperature of 99.8 F (37.6 C). He was treated with tetracycline and penicillin and was discharged on August 27. *B. anthracis* was cultured from specimens from 1 of the cows and from a blood culture obtained from the patient when he was admitted to the hospital. The Idaho patient was a ranchhand, who noted a lesion on his hand a few days after he had assisted the ranch owner and a veterinarian in the postmortem examination of cattle that had died suddenly. *B. anthracis* was positively identified by culture of clinical specimens from the ranchhand and 2 of the dead steers.

Reported by JA Mather, MD, State Epidemiologist, J Westervelt, Southeastern District, Idaho State Dept of Health and Welfare; JI Freeman, State Public Health Veterinarian, MP Hines, DVM, State Epidemiologist, North Carolina State Dept of Human Resources; G Eash, MD, Fargo, North Dakota; K Mosser, State Epidemiologist, HD Neugebauer, North Dakota State Dept of Health; M Hilgameier, MH Mires, MD, New Hampshire State Dept of Health and Welfare; and Bacterial Zoonoses Br, Bacterial Diseases Div, Bur of Epidemiology, CDC, in CDC's Veterinary Public Health Notes, *January 1979.*

Editorial Note: Before anthrax vaccination programs were initiated for persons exposed to industrial anthrax, textile and felt mills were frequent sources of anthrax morbidity in the United States. The widespread use of the vaccine has markedly reduced morbidity in mill employees; however, there is no method of completely eliminating potential exposure except not using imported goat hair and other infective animal materials or instituting expensive decontamination procedures.

An effective vaccine for anthrax in cattle is available; however, the sporadic occurrence of bovine anthrax fails to provide ranchers with incentive to vaccinate their livestock routinely.

The number of cases (6) reported in 1978 is more than double the average annual number (2.4) of cases reported to CDC in the preceding 10 years and is the largest number of cases reported in any 1 year since 7 cases were reported in 1965.

MMWR 28:327 (7/20/79)

Penicillin-Resistant Viridans Streptococcal Endocarditis — North Carolina

A case of endocarditis due to relatively penicillin-resistant viridans streptococci, probably secondary to a minor dental procedure, has occurred in a North Carolina woman receiving oral penicillin both as long-term prophylaxis for rheumatic fever and as short-term prophylaxis for endocarditis.

In December 1978, the patient, a 24-year-old woman, was admitted to a hospital in Winston-Salem, with a 10-day history of daily fever, rigors, malaise, and anorexia. In addition to having a congenital ventricular septal defect, she had developed mitral stenosis thought to be caused by rheumatic fever. She had been taking long-term oral phenoxymethyl penicillin (250 mg twice daily) for rheumatic fever prophylaxis. One month before admission, her teeth had been cleaned; for the 2 days before, the day of, and the 2 days after the dental work, she had increased her penicillin dosage to 250 mg 4 times daily.

All 6 blood cultures, obtained at different times from the patient, were positive for viridans streptococci, and an echocardiogram demonstrated vegetations on the posterior leaflet of the mitral valve. At CDC, the streptococci were identified as *Streptococcus salivarius* and were shown to have a minimal inhibitory concentration (MIC) to penicillin of 2 μg/ml. Other MICs were erythromycin, $\leqslant$0.06 μg/ml; vancomycin, 0.25 μg/ml; gentamicin, 8 μg/ml; and ampicillin, 1 μg/ml.

Treatment for bacterial endocarditis was begun with intravenous aqueous penicillin (24 million units/day) and intramuscular streptomycin (1 g/day) until both peak and trough serum bactericidal levels were reported as less than 1:2. Vancomycin was substituted with good response clinically and *in vitro* (trough serum bactericidal level was 1:112); however, an allergic reaction necessitated changing to ampicillin for the completion of 4 weeks of therapy. The patient has had no recurrence of endocarditis in the 6 months since discharge.

Reported by R Marx, MD, S Pegram, MD, Div of Infectious Diseases and Immunology, Dept of Medicine, B Wasilauskas, PhD, Dept of Pathology, Bowman Gray School of Medicine, Winston-Salem; Antimicrobics Investigation Sect, Staphylococcus and Streptococcus Sect, Clinical Bacteriology Br, Bacteriology Div, Bur of Laboratories, CDC.

Editorial Note: Patients continuously receiving oral penicillin as secondary prophylaxis for rheumatic fever often carry, in the oral cavity, viridans streptococci that are relatively resistant to penicillin (1). Because a few cases of endocarditis caused by relatively penicillin-resistant viridans streptococci have been reported in persons taking long-term penicillin prophylaxis (2-4), the American Heart Association (AHA) has indicated that physicians may choose oral erythromycin or a combination of penicillin and streptomycin as endocarditis prophylaxis before dental procedures for persons taking long-term oral penicillin (5).

To evaluate the efficacy of regimens intended to prevent endocarditis, the AHA has set up a registry of persons who contract endocarditis despite attempts at prophylaxis. Reports of such events, including the name and birth date of the patient and the name, address, and telephone number of the physician, may be telephoned or mailed to the AHA, Endocarditis Prophylaxis Failure Registry, 7320 Greenville Avenue, Dallas, Texas 75231 (Telephone 214-750-5432). The reporting physician will be contacted for clinical details, which will be kept confidential.

References
1. Spencer WH III, Thornsberry C, Moody MD, Wenger NK: Rheumatic fever chemoprophylaxis and penicillin-resistant gingival organisms. Ann Intern Med 73:683-687, 1970
2. Doyle EF, Spagnuolo M, Taranta A, Kuttner AG, Markowitz M: The risk of bacterial endocarditis during antirheumatic prophylaxis. JAMA 201:807-812, 1967
3. Garrod LP, Waterworth PM: The risks of dental extraction during penicillin treatment. Br Heart J 24:39-46, 1962
4. Parillo JE, Borst GC, Mazur MH, et al: Endocarditis due to resistant viridans streptococci during oral penicillin chemoprophylaxis. N Engl J Med 300:296-300, 1979
5. Kaplan EL, Anthony BF, Bisno A, et al: Prevention of bacterial endocarditis: A statement prepared by the Committee on Rheumatic Fever and Bacterial Endocarditis of the Council on Cardiovascular Disease in the Young of the American Heart Association. Circulation 56:139A-143A, 1977

MMWR 28:215 (5/11/79)

Leprosy — Worldwide, 1975

The World Health Organization (WHO) recently reported on the worldwide distribution of leprosy in 1975. Some details of that report follow.

According to information received through questionnaires and other sources, the total number of registered cases in 154 countries was 3,599,949, an increase of about 710,000 over the figure obtained in the previous evaluation in 1968. This is a 25% increase; however, the countries reporting were not identical in the 2 evaluation years, and the populations from which figures were derived had increased by 19% over the 7-year period. Even when this population increase was taken into account, it is clear that the rate of registration has increased since 1968: a true comparison for the period 1968-1975, possible with 110 countries, revealed a 7% increase in registered cases. In Asia there were significant increases in registration, especially in Burma (25%), India (56%), and Indonesia (85%).

In tropical African countries the proportion of lepromatous cases tended to be low (10%—15%), whereas in Asia it was greater (34% in Indonesia, 40% in Thailand). In the Americas it was frequently above 50%, as in Brazil (55%). The proportion was extremely variable in Oceania.

The lack of uniformity in the classification of cases and the varying efficiency in case finding are 2 factors that partially explain the variation in the proportion of each form of leprosy in different countries. In recent years, indefinitely retaining patients with lepromatous leprosy on treatment or surveillance beyond the accepted period of inactivity has led to a rise in the proportion of this form. In other countries tardiness in dropping from the registry fully treated tuberculoid cases also has affected the proportion of the forms of leprosy reported.

Many countries gave data on the number of registered patients receiving treatment. These were presented as a percentage of total under treatment to total registered, by area: Africa, 69%; America, 67%; Eastern Mediterranean, 73%; Southeast Asia, 86%; and Western Pacific, 78%. When an analysis was made of patients receiving regular treatment (at least 75% of the prescribed doses), the percentages fell to much lower levels: Africa, 41%; Eastern Mediterranean, 53%; Southeast Asia, 47%; and Western Pacific, 74%. An estimated 120,000 to 150,000 patients were released from control annually, worldwide. *Reported by WHO in the Weekly Epidemiological Record 54:17-19, 1979*

MMWR 27 (A.S., 1978): 36

LEPROSY — Reported Cases by Year, United States, 1942—1978

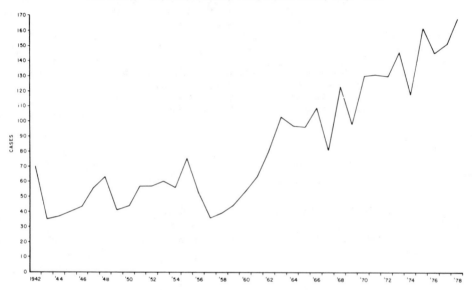

The increase in leprosy cases is most likely due to an increase in imported cases of disease.

MMWR 27 (A.S., 1978): 37

LEPTOSPIROSIS — Reported Cases by Year, United States, 1950—1978

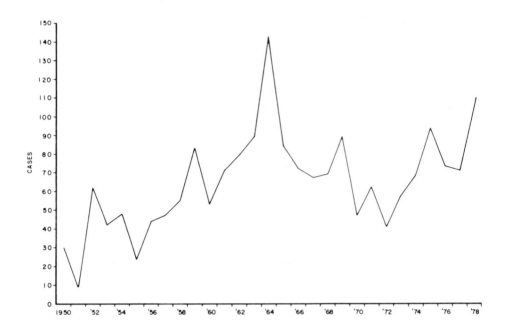

MMWR 27:526 (1/5/79)

Relapsing Fever — California

Tick-borne relapsing fever in the United States is uncommon and may resemble, partic-ularly initially, other febrile illnesses. Although low, the precise incidence of relapsing fever is unknown, in part because reporting is optional. The following case report illus-trates some of the characteristic clinical and epidemiologic features of the disease.

On August 21, 1978, a 29-year-old man was seen in a hospital emergency room with fever of 39.4 C, shaking chills, myalgia, diaphoresis, and headache. Six days previously he had returned from a hiking and camping trip in Yosemite National Park, California. He could not recall tick bites or contact with wild rodents. Physical examination was unre-markable, and laboratory studies revealed a normal urinalysis, hematocrit, and white blood cell count (WBC). A chest X ray was normal. He was diagnosed as having a viral illness and improved spontaneously without specific treatment.

On August 29, the patient had recurrence of fever, chills, myalgia, and headache. He was admitted to the hospital, where physical examination was unremarkable except for a temperature of 38.3 C. There was no skin rash, jaundice, organomegaly, or stiff neck.

Laboratory studies revealed a hematocrit of 42% and WBC of 10,600/mm^3 with 65% neutrophils (9% bands), 24% lymphocytes, and 11% monocytes. The urinalysis showed trace protein. An erythrocyte sedimentation rate (ESR) was 68 mm/hour. Serum creatinine, serum glutamic oxalacetic transaminase, alkaline phosphatase, and bilirubin were normal. A lumbar puncture revealed a normal opening pressure, and normal protein and glucose, but 3 red blood cells and 6 WBC/mm^3 (5 lymphocytes and 1 neutrophil). Serologic tests for brucellosis, tularemia, and leptospirosis were negative. The Weil-Felix reaction revealed a negative *Proteus* OX-19 and OX-2, but the *Proteus* OX-K was positive at 1:80 dilution.

The patient was given symptomatic treatment. His temperature spontaneously resolved by August 30, and he was discharged on September 1.

On September 8, the patient returned with a fever of 40.6 C. Repeat physical examination was again unremarkable. The hematocrit was 37% and the WBC 9,900/mm^3 with 76% neutrophils (3% bands), 20% lymphocytes, and 4% monocytes. *Borrelia* organisms were seen on Wright-stained blood smears. The ESR remained elevated at 65 mm/hour. Repeat *Proteus* OX-19, OX-2, and OX-K were negative, as were tests for brucellosis and tularemia.

The patient was begun on a course of oral tetracycline, 500 mg every 6 hours for 10 days, for treatment of relapsing fever. His fever defervesced within 12 hours of the initial dose of tetracycline, and he has remained well since.

Reported by RM Wilkes, MD, SC Vandervoort, MD, South San Francisco; JM Bodie, MD, San Mateo County Health Dept; J Chin, MD, State Epidemiologist, California Dept of Health Services; Bacterial Zoonoses Br, Bacterial Diseases Div, Bur of Epidemiology, CDC.

Editorial Note: Relapsing fever in the United States is due to the bite of soft ticks that have become infected with *Borrelia* organisms. *Orthnithodoros hermsi, O. turicata,* and *O. parkeri* are of primary importance as vectors of the etiologic agent. Disease usually occurs in the summer months, primarily in the western states. Although the majority of occurrences are sporadic, several recent outbreaks of tick-borne relapsing fever have been reported (*1,2*). Louse-borne relapsing fever is not presently a problem in this country.

O. hermsi is probably responsible for most reported human infections. It is prevalent in forested mountainous regions and inhabits unoccupied cabins or rodent nests in dead trees. Human contact with *O. hermsi* frequently goes unrecognized because the tick feeds briefly at night and has a painless bite.

Visitors exposed in *Borrelia*-endemic areas may return home before showing signs of illness since the disease has an average incubation period of about 7 days. Diagnosis is best made by demonstrating the causative organism in the blood during the febrile phase of the illness. *Borrelia* are readily stained with aniline and acid dyes, and can be recognized on Wright-stained blood films (*3*).

Serologic tests for relapsing fever have been developed; however, they are difficult to perform and are of limited utility. With the exception of certain strains using special media, the organism cannot be cultured. Animal inoculation with patient blood and subsequent demonstration of the spirochete in the animal may be used for cases difficult to diagnose (*3*).

References
1. Thompson RS, Burgdorfer W, Russell R, Francis BJ: Outbreak of tick-borne relapsing fever in Spokane County, Washington. JAMA 210:1045-1050, 1969
2. Boyer KM, Munford RS, Maupin GO, Pattison CP, Fox MD, Barnes AM, Jones WL, Maynard JE: Tick-borne relapsing fever: An interstate outbreak originating at Grand Canyon National Park. Am J Epidemiol 105:469-479, 1977
3. Southern PM, Sanford JP: Relapsing fever. A clinical and microbiological review. Medicine 48:129-149, 1969

MMWR 27 (A.S., 1978): 66

TETANUS — Reported Cases by Year, United States, 1950—1978

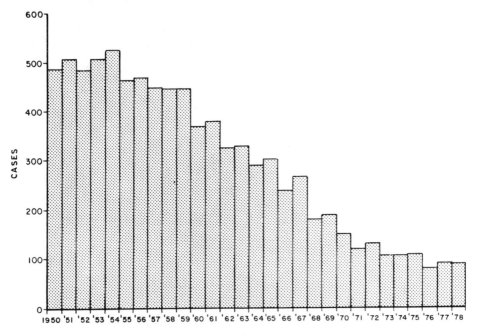

TETANUS — Reported Case Rates by Age Group, United States, 1978

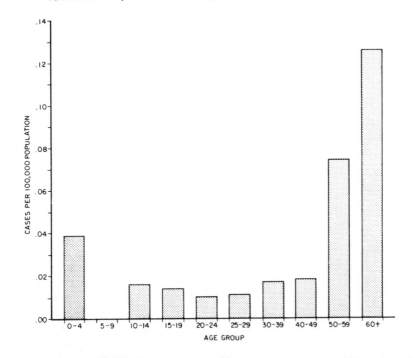

Part II

Diseases Caused by Viruses

CHAPTER 22

Poliomyelitis

MMWR 27:381 (10/6/78)

Follow-up on Poliomyelitis — Netherlands

As of September 29, 1978, there have been a total of 108 cases of poliomyelitis reported to the Ministry of Health, Netherlands. The most recent case, in a person from the province of Gelderland, had onset of illness on September 20. There have been 4 cases reported for the month of September in contrast to 57 cases in June.

All cases to date continue to be among members of religious groups that have refused vaccination. The cases have been geographically confined to a belt that parallels the main population concentrations of these religious communities and runs from the province of Zeeland in the Southwest to the province of Overijssel in the Northeast.

Sixty-six of the cases occurred in males, 42 in females (Table 1) (1). Seventy-eight of the reported cases had paralysis; the remaining 30 had aseptic meningitis. The paralytic cases included 65 cases with spinal paralysis, 8 with bulbar paralysis, and 5 with both spinal and bulbar involvement. There was 1 death in a female infant 3 months of age.

TABLE 1. Poliomyelitis cases, by sex and age group, Netherlands, April 15-September 29, 1978**

Age group (years)	Number of cases			Confirmed virologically
	Male	Female	Total	
<1	2	1	3	3
1 - 4	5	5	10	10
5 - 9	21	7	28	27
10 - 14	12	12	24	23
15 - 19	12	6	18	18
20 - 24	6	6	12	12
25 - 34	7	3	10	10
35 - 44	1	2	3	3
45 - 54	-	-	-	-
≥55	-	-	-	-
Total	66	42	108	106

**provisional data (1)

The present epidemic, caused by type 1 virus, was first detected on May 3, when 2 cases were reported from neighboring villages in the center of the country. These patients had become ill on April 23 and April 24, respectively. Through a retrospective study in the involved regions, a 14-year-old girl from a village near Utrecht—presumably the index case—was discovered to have become ill on April 15. She attended a large, regional, secondary school attended by more than 1,000 pupils from over 100 municipalities. A large number of the pupils came from the few religious groups that refuse vaccination. Schools such as this are felt to have been the major means by which the poliovirus spread throughout the Netherlands.

Canada has reported 6 cases of paralytic poliomyelitis related to this outbreak. In the United States there have been no cases of polio that can be related to this ongoing outbreak.

Reported by H Bijkerk, MD, Office of the Chief Medical Officer, Netherlands; Viral Diseases Div, Bur of Epidemiology, CDC.

Editorial Note: This situation is unique because a major outbreak of poliomyelitis has occurred in a country which exclusively uses the inactivated polio vaccine (IPV) and has an overall vaccine acceptance rate of 95%. In the past, outbreaks in the Netherlands were confined to areas of the country where relatively large numbers of persons were inadequately vaccinated. In well-vaccinated areas only sporadic cases, not outbreaks, were seen. In this outbreak no cases have occurred in fully vaccinated persons.

Reference
1. Bijkerk H: Poliomyelitis epidemic in some Protestant communities in the Netherlands. Paper given at the Fourth International Congress for Virology, The Hague, August 31, 1978. Updated and corrected through September 29, 1978.

MMWR 28:49 (2/9/79)

Poliomyelitis — Pennsylvania, Maryland

The first paralytic poliomyelitis case in the United States with onset in 1979 has been reported in a 22-year-old unvaccinated, female resident of a small Amish community in Franklin County, Pennsylvania. The patient, who has been hospitalized in Maryland, became ill on January 5 with headache, fever, and generalized myalgias. On January 6 and 7, she developed right and then left lower-extremity weakness and decreased deep tendon reflexes. She had no sensory abnormalities. On January 17, the Maryland State Department of Health and Mental Hygiene reported that type 1 poliovirus had been isolated from a stool specimen collected from the patient on January 10.

An epidemiologic investigation revealed that the patient had no known exposure to other individuals with clinical poliomyelitis or to recent recipients of the live virus vaccine. In addition, there was no history of recent travel to known polio-endemic areas. At least 3 weddings of Amish couples had taken place during the period of November through January, resulting in extensive interactions among the Amish communities in Franklin and 8 other Pennsylvania counties and other Amish communities in Maryland, Ohio, Vermont, New York, and Ontario, Canada. The patient's most recent out-of-state travel had been to an Amish community in St. Mary's and Charles Counties, Maryland, in late November. Stool specimens were collected on January 18 and 19 from 17 asymptomatic members of this community; 12 were positive for type 1 poliovirus. In the patient's own community, stool specimens collected on January 18 through 20 from 32 individuals revealed that 16 were positive for poliovirus.

Surveys by the Pennsylvania and Maryland state health departments revealed that very few individuals had been completely immunized in the 2 affected Amish communities. It is being strongly recommended that all members of the affected Amish communities and all non-Amish persons who have had close association with these communities be vaccinated with the trivalent oral poliovirus vaccine. Vaccination clinics have been set up in Pennsylvania and Maryland. Approximately 67% of the target population in Maryland was vaccinated by January 31.

Surveillance for paralytic illness and aseptic meningitis possibly due to poliovirus infection has been intensified in Pennsylvania and Maryland, as well as in Amish communities in other states.

Reported by R Gens, MD, B Kleger, DrPH, E Moore, RN, WE Parkin, DVM, DrPH, State Epidemiologist, Pennsylvania Dept of Health; V Dettor, MD, MPH, Charles County Health Dept; W Marek, MD, MPH, St. Mary's County Health Dept; JM Joseph, PhD, D Sorley, MD, State Epidemiologist, Maryland Dept of Health and Mental Hygiene; Field Services Div, Enteric and Neurotropic Viral Diseases Br, Viral Diseases Div, Bur of Epidemiology, CDC.

Editorial Note: The most common wild-type poliovirus found in the Americas in recent years has been type 1. In this instance the isolation of type 1 virus from many individuals in the communities involved suggests that this virus is a wild strain. Preliminary laboratory tests on the isolate support this conclusion. Sporadic cases of wild poliovirus infection do occasionally occur during the winter months in the United States, but wild-virus activity is generally more frequent in warmer months. Since 1969, there have only been 2 epidemics of poliomyelitis in the United States; both occurred in the period of April through October.

MMWR 28:229 (5/25/79)

Poliomyelitis — United States, Canada

As of May 22, an additional case of polio caused by type 1 poliovirus has been reported in Pennsylvania, bringing to 4 the total number of such cases this year. Two other states have reported suspected cases. Three of the confirmed and both suspected cases are in Amish residents (1,2). In addition, Ontario, Canada, has confirmed a case of paralytic poliomyelitis (type 1 virus) in an Amish woman.

United States: The Pennsylvania Department of Health's most recent report is of a case of non-paralytic polio (aseptic meningitis) in a 36-year-old, non-Amish woman whose vaccination history is unclear. The woman became ill on April 30. She was hospitalized with apparent aseptic meningitis on May 8. The State Laboratory confirmed a poliovirus type 1 isolate from her stool on May 14. The patient is from Mifflin County, where 2 cases of paralytic polio were recently identified in an Amish community (2). Although this woman's husband has had regular contact with Amish farmers in the county, the patient, herself, has had no direct contact with this community. She is the first non-Amish ill person identified in 1979 with confirmed poliovirus type 1.

In addition, Iowa and Wisconsin are each currently evaluating a case of acute paralytic illness in a previously unvaccinated Amish person. These 2 patients became ill on April 30 and May 5, respectively. In Wisconsin at least 8 of 20 stool specimens from the patient's unvaccinated family members showed early growth of probable enterovirus.

Canada: Ontario has reported a case of paralytic poliomyelitis in a previously unvaccinated, 25-year-old Amish woman, hospitalized on May 13 with right lower extremity weakness. Her brother was hospitalized the same day with a similar acute paralytic disorder. Poliovirus type 1 has been confirmed from stool specimens of the woman and from her asymptomatic mother and sister. The female patient had attended an Amish wedding in the United States on April 5; Amish persons from various areas, including Pennsylvania, attended the wedding.

Reported by S Acres, MD, Dept of National Health and Welfare, Ottawa; J Joshua, MD, Ontario Ministry of Health, Toronto; R Gens, MD, WE Parkin, DVM, DrPH, State Epidemiologist, Pennsyl-

vania Dept of Health; LA Wintermeyer, MD, State Epidemiologist, Iowa State Dept of Health; JP Davis, MD, State Epidemiologist, Wisconsin State Dept of Health and Social Services; Bur of State Services, Viral Diseases Div, Bur of Epidemiology, CDC.

Editorial Note: There have now been 5 confirmed and 3 suspected cases of type 1 polio reported in the United States and Canada in 1979. These cases, from geographically distinct areas, are further evidence of the spread of the type 1—presumably wild-type— poliovirus. The virus appears to have spread from 1 unvaccinated Amish group to another, with transmission enhanced by the extensive travel and large social gatherings character- istic of this population. It is unlikely that the wild poliovirus will spread significantly among the general population, even to areas adjacent to Amish groups, because routine immunization practices have led to a high level of community protection.

Because dissemination of poliovirus is occurring among unvaccinated Amish popula- tions, and because of the possibility for increased (often inapparent) transmission through- out the upcoming summer months, CDC considers the entire American Amish popula- tion at risk of infection and recommends vaccination of all unvaccinated Amish persons (including adults) with a full series of trivalent oral poliovirus vaccine (TOPV). TOPV is also recommended for unimmunized persons who are in daily contact with an unvac- cinated community from which a wild-type poliovirus is isolated. Immunization levels of children in areas near Amish communities should be reviewed to assure that routine immunizations are up-to-date.

CDC has notified all 21 states known to have Amish residents of the new cases and of current recommendations. These states include Delaware, Florida, Georgia, Illinois, Indiana, Iowa, Kansas, Kentucky, Maryland, Michigan, Minnesota, Missouri, Montana, New Jersey, New York, Ohio, Oklahoma, Pennsylvania, Tennessee, Virginia, and Wiscon- sin. Particularly in these states, physicians should include polio in the differential diag- nosis of aseptic meningitis and acute paralytic disease.

References
1. MMWR 28:49, 1979
2. MMWR 28:207, 1979

MMWR 28:250 (6/1/79)

Follow-up on Poliomyelitis — United States, Canada

Since the last report (*1*), the United States and Canada have reported 3 more cases of poliomyelitis caused by the type 1 virus; 3 more suspected cases have also been reported. Five of these new patients are Amish, and the other belongs to an old-order Mennonite sect. To date, 8 cases (6 U.S., 2 Canadian) of type 1 polio and 4 suspected cases (all U.S.) have been identified.

United States: Since May 22, Wisconsin has reported a case of polio in a 20-year-old, unvaccinated Amish man from Vernon County. He became ill on May 5 and developed paralysis of both legs on May 11. Although no virus was isolated from this patient, poliovirus type 1 was cultured from a stool specimen of 1 of 20 unvaccinated family members. The second U.S. patient is a 34-year-old, unvaccinated Mennonite man from Lancaster County, Pennsylvania. He developed aseptic meningitis on approximately April 26; poliovirus type 1 was isolated from a stool specimen.

Pennsylvania, Wisconsin, and Iowa have each reported a new suspected case of para- lytic poliomyelitis since May 22. All 3 are in Amish persons, with dates of onset April 5, May 16, and May 23, respectively. The Pennsylvania and Iowa patients are from areas where suspected or confirmed polio cases have been previously reported. The Wisconsin patient is from Taylor County.

Canada: Polio has now been confirmed in the 20-year-old brother of the Amish patient reported last week from Ontario, Canada (1). The patient had a 4-fold rise in polio type 1 antibody. Although poliovirus type 1 has now been isolated from additional family members and unvaccinated neighbors, no new cases have been reported from Canada.

Reported by R Gens, MD, WE Parkin, DVM, DrPH, State Epidemiologist, Pennsylvania Dept of Health; LA Wintermeyer, MD, State Epidemiologist, Iowa State Dept of Health; JP Davis, MD, State Epidemiologist, Wisconsin State Dept of Health and Social Services; Bur of State Services, Viral Diseases Div, Bur of Epidemiology, CDC.

Editorial Note: Transmission of poliovirus is continuing among unvaccinated populations, but apparently not to any significant degree among the surrounding communities with their presumably high levels of immunization. In order to interrupt the ongoing transmission among Amish groups, all states with known Amish populations are now planning or beginning immunization campaigns for these unvaccinated communities. Trivalent oral poliovirus vaccine (TOPV) is recommended for all U.S. Amish residents, regardless of age, and for all who are in regular close contact with these persons. TOPV may also be offered to any unimmunized person living in a community from which a wild-type poliovirus is isolated.

Before traveling to affected Amish areas, children should complete their routine polio vaccination. Routine polio immunization for adults in the United States is not currently recommended, and adult travelers to affected Amish areas who anticipate short stays and little close personal contact with the Amish are probably at minimal increased risk. However, unimmunized adults who anticipate prolonged stays or close contact should ensure that they are protected. This can be accomplished by receipt of at least 2 doses of inactivated poliovirus vaccine (IPV) a month apart before travel or, if IPV is not readily available, at least 2 doses of TOPV, 6-8 weeks apart. If there is time for only 1 dose of vaccine before travel, a single dose of TOPV should be given.

Reference
1. MMWR 28:229, 1979

MMWR 28:275 (6/15/79)

Poliomyelitis Surveillance — United States, Canada

One additional case of suspected paralytic poliomyelitis due to the type 1 virus has now been confirmed in an unvaccinated Amish patient, bringing the overall total of epidemic-associated cases in 1979 to 13 (Pennsylvania 7; Wisconsin 2; Iowa 2; Canada 2). The latest patient is from Lancaster County, Pennsylvania, where 2 previously reported patients reside. In addition, 3 states (Wisconsin, Iowa, and—for the first time—Missouri) have each reported single suspected cases of paralytic polio in unvaccinated Amish individuals.

Immunization Programs: The recently reported cases of polio among Amish persons in Pennsylvania, Iowa, and Wisconsin have led health authorities to consider the entire U.S. Amish population to be at risk of poliomyelitis infection. Consequently, state health departments in the 25 states where Amish persons reside plan to contact and immunize all Amish persons. Some of the immunization programs in the Amish communities are now in progress and will continue. For example, in Lancaster County—the heart of the Amish community in Pennsylvania—over 6,000 of the 12,000 Amish population have recently received at least 1 dose of vaccine.

In response to the initial case of poliomyelitis in Pennsylvania last January, Wisconsin began to offer poliovirus vaccine to Amish in that state. In the 3 communities where cases have been reported, approximately two-thirds of the Amish have subsequently received vaccine.

In Buchanan County, Iowa, where 2 cases of polio have occurred among Amish persons, approximately 50% of the Amish have received at least 1 dose of vaccine.

Immunization clinics for the Amish in Missouri had already been planned before the suspected case from that state was reported on June 5. A clinic in the affected area, Audrain County, was held on June 1, the same day paralysis developed in the suspected case.

In some areas where poliovirus has been found, large-scale immunization programs have been held for both Amish and non-Amish persons. In Mifflin County, Pennsylvania (where 2 paralytic cases occurred in Amish persons and 1 nonparalytic case occurred in a non-Amish person), a 4-day communitywide immunization program for the general population was conducted May 17-20. More than 20,000 of 45,000 residents received polio vaccine. Another special 3-day immunization program for the general population was conducted June 2-4 in Lancaster County, where 2 paralytic cases occurred in Amish persons and 1 nonparalytic case occurred in a Mennonite person. More than 147,000 of approximately 348,000 residents received polio vaccine during this program.

Reported by R Gens, MD, WE Parkin, DVM, DrPH, State Epidemiologist, Pennsylvania Dept of Health; LA Wintermeyer, MD, State Epidemiologist, Iowa State Dept of Health; HD Donnell Jr, MD, State Epidemiologist, Missouri State Dept of Social Services; JP Davis, MD, State Epidemiologist, Wisconsin State Dept of Health and Social Services; Immunization Div, Bur of State Services, Viral Diseases Div, Bur of Epidemiology, CDC.

MMWR 28:309 (7/6/79)

Follow-up on Poliomyelitis — United States, Canada

Since the last report *(1)*, 2 additional epidemic-associated cases of paralytic poliomyelitis have been confirmed. One is in a 16-year-old, unvaccinated Amish male from Buchanan County, Iowa, where 2 other paralytic cases were previously reported *(2)*; type 1 virus was isolated from this boy's stool. The other new case is in a 9-month-old boy from Chester County, Pennsylvania (from a town adjacent to the Lancaster County residence of the most recently reported Pennsylvania case *[1]*). The infant became ill on June 3, 5 days after receiving his first dose of trivalent oral poliovirus vaccine (TOPV). Poliovirus type 2 was isolated from this patient's stool; results of serologic tests are pending.

These additional cases bring the 1979 total, as of July 3, to 15 confirmed, epidemic-associated cases in Canada (2 cases) and the United States (Pennsylvania, 8; Iowa, 3; Wisconsin, 2). The total number of suspected paralytic cases is 2—1 each from Wisconsin and Missouri.

In addition, poliovirus type 1 has been isolated from asymptomatic Amish persons from 6 different areas where paralytic poliomyelitis has not yet appeared. These are Charles and St. Mary's counties, Maryland (January; 37 of 102 positive); Jefferson County, Pennsylvania (May 21; 14 of 25 positive); St. Joseph County, Michigan (June 1; 3 of 6 positive); Branch County, Michigan (June 4; 1 of 5 positive); Pike County, Missouri (June 7; 9 of 30 positive); and Eaton County, Michigan (June 15; 1 of 5 positive).

Reported by LE Wintermeyer, MD, State Epidemiologist, Iowa State Dept of Health; JP Maher, MD, MPH, Chester County Health Dept, Pennsylvania; WE Parkin, DVM, DrPH, State Epidemiologist, Pennsylvania State Dept of Health; NS Hayner, MD, State Epidemiologist, Michigan State Dept of Public Health; D Sorley, MD, Acting State Epidemiologist, Maryland State Dept of Health and Mental Hygiene; HD Donnell Jr, MD, State Epidemiologist, Missouri State Dept of Social Services; Immuniza-

tion Div, Bur of State Services, Viral Diseases Div, Bur of Epidemiology, CDC.

Editorial Note: The origin of disease in the Amish infant from Pennsylvania has not yet been determined. The isolation of poliovirus type 2 from a recent TOPV recipient is not unusual and does not necessarily implicate that virus as the cause of disease. In a situation such as described here, when a person living in an epidemic area—and potentially exposed to wild poliovirus (type 1)—receives TOPV, more than 1 poliovirus type may be isolated from the stool. To explore this possibility, specimens are being retested in Pennsylvania and at CDC. Results of serologic tests may be useful in establishing the poliovirus type responsible for disease in this patient.

The circulation of wild poliovirus in areas without a paralytic case is not unusual, as the inapparent-to-apparent infection rate for poliovirus, though variable, can be quite high. For every 100 persons with poliovirus cultured from their stool, 90-95 will be asymptomatic; 4-8 will have "minor illness" (gastroenteritis, upper-respiratory-tract symptoms, or an influenza-like illness); 1 or 2 will have aseptic meningitis; and 0.1 to 1 will have paralytic disease (*3*).

Immunization campaigns for the Amish (who have a total U.S. population of approximately 75,000) are continuing. Of the 23 states now known to have Amish residents, 18 have achieved immunization levels of ≥50% and 5 of these have achieved levels ≥90%. In the 3 states with the largest Amish populations (Ohio, Pennsylvania, and Indiana; total of 56,000 Amish), 46%-60% immunization levels have been achieved, and campaigns are continuing. Most states are trying to achieve immunization of at least 80% of their total Amish populations.

References
1. MMWR 28:275, 1979
2. MMWR 28:255, 1979
3. Horstmann DM: Clinical epidemiology of poliomyelitis. Ann Intern Med 43.526-533, 1955

MMWR 28:345 (7/27/79)

Follow-Up on Poliomyelitis — United States, Canada, Netherlands

No new cases of epidemic-associated poliomyelitis have been reported to CDC during the past month. Two cases previously reported as suspected have now been confirmed, bringing the 1979 total of confirmed cases in the United States and Canada to 17. Fourteen of these cases (all paralytic) occurred in unvaccinated Amish persons; 2 (both nonparalytic) were in unvaccinated non-Amish persons, who lived in or near an Amish area; and 1 case (paralytic) occurred in an Amish infant, who received oral poliovirus vaccine 5 days before becoming ill. In the latter case, the patient had laboratory evidence of recent infection with both type 1 and type 2 poliovirus; the other 16 cases were clearly due to a wild (type 1) poliovirus. These 17 cases have been reported from 4 different states (Pennsylvania, 8 cases; Iowa, 3; Wisconsin, 3; Missouri, 1) and Canada (2). Immunization campaigns for the Amish are continuing; at least half of the nation's Amish have now received 1 or more doses of oral poliovirus vaccine.

Antigenic marker tests, consisting of (a) the van Wezel Method, using cross-absorbed rabbit antisera against vaccine and nonvaccine (wild) poliovirus strains and (b) the modified Wecker method, using guinea pig antisera against vaccine strains, have been performed on the poliovirus type 1 strains isolated from 5 U.S. cases and from a household contact of a sixth case. All isolates were nonvaccine-like in their antigenic characteristics.

The type 1 poliovirus isolated from the first 1979 poliomyelitis patient (an Amish female from Pennsylvania) shows a resemblance to a wild type 1 strain isolated in Kuwait in 1977 (1). Type 1 strains from cases occurring in the 1978 epidemic in the Netherlands and Canada also showed a resemblance to the Kuwait poliovirus strain (1).

Epidemiologic information also links last year's poliomyelitis epidemic in the Netherlands and Canada with this year's outbreak in the United States and Canada. During the 1978 outbreak, members of the affected religious group traveled from the Netherlands to Canada, where cases subsequently appeared. An Amish family from an Ontario town 15 miles from the affected area moved in late summer 1978 to the Pennsylvania town where the first U.S. Amish case subsequently occurred, in January 1979. There were also other, less well-defined contacts between Amish persons in Ontario and Pennsylvania.

Reported by Dr. A. van Wezel and Dr. van Zermarel, Rijks Institute voor der Volksgezondheit, the Netherlands; S Acres, MD, Dept of National Health and Welfare, Ottawa; State Epidemiologists from Iowa, Missouri, Pennsylvania, and Wisconsin; Virology Div, Bur of Laboratories, and Viral Diseases Div, Bur of Epidemiology, CDC.

Editorial Note: Both laboratory and epidemiologic information have suggested a link between the poliovirus type 1 strain from the 1979 outbreak in the United States and Canada with the type 1 strain responsible for last year's outbreak in the Netherlands and Canada. The onset of illness in the last case occurring in Canada in 1978 was in August, more than 4 months before the onset of illness in the first 1979 case, which occurred in Pennsylvania. Nearly 3 months elapsed before the next 1979 cases occurred, and these were also in Pennsylvania. These data suggest that the wild poliovirus circulated inapparently through several generations without causing paralytic disease. The absence of new cases of paralytic poliomyelitis reflects, in part, the success of the multi-state immunization campaigns for the Amish; the possibility of new cases remains, because the wild type 1 poliovirus may continue to be excreted by some infected persons throughout the summer months. However, the risk of additional cases is diminishing as more of the susceptible Amish persons receive vaccine.

Reference
1. van Wezel A: Personal communication.

MMWR 28:483 (10/12/79)

Poliomyelitis — United States, 1978-1979

1979—In 1979, the United States experienced the first epidemic of poliomyelitis since 1972. Through September 21, there were 15 epidemic-associated cases (13 paralytic; 2 nonparalytic) in the United States and 2 additional epidemic cases (both paralytic) in Canada. All paralytic cases occurred in unvaccinated Amish persons.

In addition, there have been 8 reported endemic cases—i.e., non-epidemic-associated cases that were indigenous to the United States. All 8 were paralytic and have been epidemiologically classified as vaccine associated. Five occurred in recent recipients of trivalent oral poliovirus vaccine (OPV) and 3 in contacts of such recipients.

1978—In 1978, there were 9 cases of paralytic poliomyelitis, including 1 death, reported in the United States. None were epidemic associated: 1 was imported, and 8 were endemic. The imported case was in an unimmunized woman who had traveled to Mexico before onset of illness. Six of the 8 endemic cases met the standard epidemiologic criteria for vaccine association. Four were in vaccine recipients, 2 in contacts. In 1 of the other 2 endemic cases, OPV was also implicated, as the patient's child had received OPV 3 days and 70 days before onset of disease, and there was no known exposure to wild poliovirus.

The last endemic case occurred in an 11-year-old boy who had received 4 doses of

OPV as an infant. Following a 2-week catarrhal illness in late July, he developed difficulty with swallowing and speaking on August 5 and suffered a respiratory arrest (presumably from choking) that same day. He died 18 days later of neurologic sequelae of the
arrest. Poliovirus type 1 was isolated from a throat swab obtained on August 7. Using the
Wecker serologic test and a new method developed in the Netherlands by Dr. A. van
Wezel (1), CDC characterized the virus as nonvaccine-like. A monotypic rise in neutralizing antibody titer in serum was demonstrated to type 1 poliovirus. The clinical and
laboratory data in this case suggest that the patient died of bulbar poliomyelitis due to
a wild type 1 poliovirus. This case is the first known OPV failure in an otherwise normal
patient who had received, in the United States, ≥3 vaccine doses.

*Reported by T Halpin, MD, MPH, State Epidemiologist, Ohio State Dept of Health; Enteric Virology
Br, Virology Div, Bur of Laboratories, Enteric and Neurotropic Viral Diseases Br, Viral Diseases Div,
Bur of Epidemiology, CDC.*

Editorial Note: From January 1, 1969 through September 21, 1979, there were a total
of 185 cases of paralytic poliomyelitis reported to CDC through the National Poliomyelitis Surveillance System. Of these, 43 were epidemic associated; 73 endemic, vaccine
associated (23 in recipients; 50 in contacts); 39 endemic, nonvaccine associated; 19
imported; and 11 in immunodeficient persons. The number of paralytic cases per year
from 1969 through 1978 ranged from 5 to 32. There have been 21 paralytic cases reported to date in 1979.

   Vaccines against poliomyelitis (injectable [inactivated poliomyelitis vaccine] and oral
[OPV]) have been largely responsible for the dramatic decline in the incidence of the
disease in this country over the past 25 years. Since 1964, there have been less than 100
paralytic cases reported per year, except in 1966, when 102 cases occurred. With the widespread use of oral poliovirus vaccines since the early 1960s, naturally occurring polioviruses have been virtually replaced in the United States by attenuated vaccine viruses.
Thus, in the 1970s, epidemics caused by wild polioviruses have become rare and have
been almost completely confined to communities of inadequately vaccinated persons.
Most of the few cases that have continued to occur each year can be attributed either to
the vaccine viruses themselves or, occasionally, to sporadic imported wild viruses.

Reference
1. MMWR 28:345, 1979

MMWR 28:510 (11/2/79)

Poliomyelitis Prevention

   *This revised ACIP recommendation on poliomyelitis prevention addresses issues impor-
tant in poliomyelitis control in the United States today. Specifically, situations that
constitute increased risk are defined, and alternatives for protection are outlined. Recommendations for immunization of adults are presented, clarifying the role of Inactivated
Polio Vaccine in immunizing adults. These recommendations also address the problems
of interrupted immunization schedules and completion of primary immunization. Oral
Polio Vaccine remains th e vaccine of choice for primary immunization of children.*

INTRODUCTION
   Poliovirus vaccines, used widely since 1955, have dramatically reduced the incidence
of poliomyelitis in the United States. The annual number of reported cases of paralytic
disease declined from more than 18,000 in 1954 to less than 20 in 1973-1978. The risk
of poliomyelitis is generally very small in the United States today, but epidemics are

certain to occur if the immunity of the population is not maintained by immunizing children beginning in the first year of life.

The proportion of the U.S. population fully immunized against poliomyelitis appears to have declined in recent years. The United States Immunization Survey in 1978 indicated that only 60% of 1- to 4-year-old children had completed primary vaccination against poliomyelitis. Rates for infants and young children in disadvantaged urban and rural areas were even lower. Recent intensive immunization efforts have reversed this downward trend, but clearly there remain many unimmunized (or incompletely immunized) children.

Laboratory surveillance of enteroviruses shows that the circulation of wild polioviruses has diminished markedly. Inapparent infection with wild strains no longer contributes significantly to establishing or maintaining immunity, making universal vaccination of infants and children even more important.

POLIOVIRUS VACCINES

Two types of poliovirus vaccines are currently licensed in the United States: Oral Polio Vaccine (OPV)* and Inactivated Polio Vaccine (IPV).†

Oral Polio Vaccine (OPV)

Since it was licensed in the United States in 1963, trivalent OPV, the live attenuated vaccine combining all 3 strains of poliovirus, has almost totally supplanted the individual monovalent OPV antigens used in the early 1960s. Full primary vaccination with OPV will produce long-lasting immunity to all 3 poliovirus types in more than 95% of recipients. Most recipients are protected after a single dose.

OPV consistently induces intestinal immunity that provides resistance to reinfection with polioviruses. Administration of OPV may interfere with simultaneous infection by wild polioviruses, a property which is of special value in epidemic-control campaigns. In rare instances (once in approximately 3 million doses distributed) OPV has been associated with paralytic disease in vaccine recipients or their close contacts. In the 10-year period 1969-1978, approximately 242 million doses of OPV were distributed, and 76 cases of paralysis associated with vaccine were reported. Eighteen cases of paralysis occurred in otherwise healthy vaccine recipients, 47 cases in healthy close contacts of vaccine recipients, and 11 cases in persons (recipients or contacts) with immune deficiency conditions.

Inactivated Polio Vaccine (IPV)

Licensed in 1955, IPV has been extensively used in this country and many other parts of the world. It is given by subcutaneous injection. Where extensively used, IPV has brought about a great reduction in paralytic poliomyelitis cases. Approximately 428 million doses have been administered in the United States, mostly before 1962. Although IPV has not been widely used in this country for more than a decade, a Canadian product licensed for use in the United States is now available.

It is generally accepted that primary vaccination with 4 doses of IPV produces immunity to all 3 poliovirus types in more than 95% of recipients. Additional experience with the currently available, more potent, IPV product is necessary to establish whether the duration of immunity is comparable to that induced by OPV. Experience in other countries forms the basis for the present recommendations on booster doses.

---

*Official name: Poliovirus Vaccine, Live, Oral, Trivalent.
†Official name: Poliomyelitis Vaccine.

There is considerable evidence from epidemiologic studies that immunizing with IPV diminishes circulation of wild poliovirus in the community, although it is known that persons vaccinated with IPV can subsequently be infected with, and become intestinal carriers of, either wild strains or attenuated vaccine virus strains. No paralytic reactions to IPV are known to have occurred since the 1955 cluster of poliomyelitis cases caused by vaccine that contained live polioviruses that had escaped inactivation. Serious adverse reactions are not anticipated with the current IPV product.

ROUTINE IMMUNIZATION

Rationale for Choice of Vaccine

Although IPV and OPV are both effective in preventing poliomyelitis, OPV is the vaccine of choice for primary immunization of children in the United States when the benefits and risks for the entire population are considered. OPV is preferred because it induces intestinal immunity, is simple to administer, is well accepted by patients, results in immunization of some contacts of vaccinated persons, and has a record of having essentially eliminated disease associated with wild polioviruses in this country. The choice of OPV as the preferred polio vaccine in the United States has also been made by the Committee on Infectious Diseases of the American Academy of Pediatrics (1) and a special expert committee of the Institute of Medicine, National Academy of Sciences (2).

Some poliomyelitis experts contend that greater use of IPV in the United States for routine vaccination would provide continued control of naturally occurring poliovirus infections and simultaneously reduce the problem of OPV-associated disease. They argue that there is no substantial evidence that OPV and currently available IPV differ in their ability to protect individuals from disease. They question the public health significance of higher levels of gastrointestinal immunity achieved with OPV. Finally, they question whether the transmission of vaccine virus to close contacts contributes substantially to the level of immunity achieved in the community.

Some countries prevent poliomyelitis successfully with IPV. However, because of many differences between these countries and the United States, particularly with respect to risks of exposure to wild polioviruses and the ability to achieve and maintain very high vaccination rates in the population, their experiences with IPV may not be directly applicable here. Based on current achievements in the United States with other vaccines, it is doubtful that a sufficient number of persons would regularly receive vaccination with IPV to sustain the present level of poliomyelitis protection in the community and to prevent recurrence of outbreaks.

Prospective vaccinees or their parents should be made aware of the polio vaccines available and the reasons why recommendations are made for giving specific vaccines at particular ages and under certain circumstances. Furthermore, the benefits and risks of the vaccines for individuals and the community should be stated so that vaccination is carried out among persons who are fully informed.

RECOMMENDATIONS FOR INFANTS, CHILDREN, AND ADOLESCENTS

Primary Immunization

OPV: For infants, children, and adolescents (up to the 18th birthday) the primary series of OPV consists of 3 doses. In infancy the primary series is integrated with DTP vaccination, and the first dose is commonly given at 6-12 weeks of age. At all ages the first 2 doses should be separated by at least 6, and preferably 8, weeks. The third dose is given at least 6 weeks, and preferably 8-12 months, after the second dose.

IPV: The primary series consists of 4 doses of vaccine; volume and route of injection are specified by the manufacturer. In infancy, the primary schedule is usually integrated with DTP vaccination, as with OPV. Three doses can be given at 4- to 8-week intervals; the fourth dose should follow 6-12 months after the third.

All children should complete primary immunization with OPV or IPV before entering school.

Supplementary Immunization

OPV: Before school entry, all children who previously received primary immunization with OPV (3 doses) in early childhood should be given a fourth dose. This additional dose will increase the likelihood of complete immunity in the small percentage of children who have not previously developed serum antibodies to all 3 types of polioviruses. The need for supplementary doses after the 4 basic doses of OPV has not been established, but children considered to be at increased risk of exposure to poliovirus (as noted below under RECOMMENDATIONS FOR ADULTS) may be given a single additional dose of OPV.

IPV: Before entering school, all children who previously received primary immunization with IPV (4 doses) in early childhood should be given at least 1 dose of OPV or 1 additional dose of IPV. Use of a primary series of OPV would eliminate the need for subsequent booster doses of IPV. Children who received primary immunization with IPV should obtain a booster dose of IPV every 5 years until the age of 18 years, unless a primary series of OPV is given. The need for supplementary doses after the 5 basic doses of the currently available IPV product has not been firmly established. Further experience may lead to alteration of this recommendation.

Children Incompletely Immunized

The preadolescent years are a good time to re-evaluate polio vaccination status and to complete the immunization of those who are inadequately protected.

OPV: To help assure seroconversion to all 3 serotypes of poliovirus, completion of the primary series of 3 doses of OPV is recommended. Time intervals between doses longer than those recommended for routine primary immunization do not necessitate additional doses of vaccine. Individuals who received only 1 dose of each of the monovalent OPVs in the past should receive 2 doses of trivalent OPV at least 6 weeks apart. One dose of each monovalent OPV (poliovirus types 1, 2, and 3) is at least equivalent to 1 dose of trivalent OPV.

IPV: Regulations for vaccine licensure adopted since 1968 require a higher potency IPV than was previously manufactured. Four doses of IPV administered after 1968 are considered a complete primary series. As with OPV, time intervals between doses longer than those recommended for routine primary immunization do not necessitate additional doses.

Incompletely immunized children who are at increased risk of exposure to poliovirus (as noted below under RECOMMENDATIONS FOR ADULTS) should be given the remaining required doses or, if time is a limiting factor, at least a single dose of OPV.

RECOMMENDATIONS FOR ADULTS

Routine primary polio vaccination of adults (those past the 18th birthday) residing in the United States is not necessary. Most adults are already immune and have a very small risk of exposure to poliomyelitis. Immunization is recommended for certain adults

who are at greater risk of exposure to poliovirus than the general population, including:
1. travelers to areas or countries where poliomyelitis is epidemic or endemic;
2. members of communities or specific population groups with disease caused by wild poliovirus;
3. laboratory workers handling specimens which may contain polioviruses;
4. health care workers in close contact with patients who may be excreting polioviruses.

For individuals in the above categories, polio vaccination is recommended, as detailed below.

Unvaccinated Adults

For adults at increased risk of exposure to poliomyelitis, primary immunization with IPV is recommended whenever this is feasible. IPV is preferred because the risk of vaccine-associated paralysis following OPV is slightly higher in adults than in children. Three doses should be given at intervals of 1-2 months; a fourth dose should follow 6-12 months after the third.

In circumstances where time will not allow at least 3 doses of IPV to be given before protection is required, the following alternatives are recommended:
1. If less than 8, but more than 4, weeks are available before protection is needed, 2 doses of IPV should be given at least 4 weeks apart.
2. If less than 4 weeks are available before protection is needed, a single dose of OPV is recommended.

In both instances the remaining doses of vaccine should be given later, at the recommended intervals, if the person remains at increased risk.

Incompletely Immunized Adults

Adults who are at increased risk of exposure to poliomyelitis and who have previously received less than a full primary course of OPV or IPV should be given the remaining required doses of either vaccine, regardless of the interval since the last dose.

Adults Previously Given a Complete Primary Course of OPV or iPV

Adults who are at increased risk of exposure to poliomyelitis and who have previously completed a primary course of OPV may be given another dose of OPV. The need for further supplementary doses has not been established. Those adults who previously completed a primary course of IPV may be given a dose of either IPV or OPV. If IPV is used exclusively, additional doses may be given every 5 years, but their need also has not been established.

Recommendations for Unvaccinated Parents of Children to be Given OPV

Unvaccinated parents of infants who are to be given OPV are at a very small risk of developing OPV-associated paralysis. Therefore, when OPV strains are to be introduced into a household with adults who have never received any polio vaccine, some health care personnel may elect to give these adults at least 2 doses of IPV a month apart—if not the full primary series—before the children receive OPV. Vaccination of the children must be assured and not unduly delayed by this process—the primary concern is immunization of the child.

PRECAUTIONS AND CONTRAINDICATIONS

Pregnancy

Although there is no convincing evidence documenting adverse effects of either OPV or IPV on the developing fetus or pregnant woman, it is prudent on theoretical grounds to avoid vaccinating pregnant women. However, if immediate protection against polio-myelitis is needed, OPV is recommended.

Immunodeficiency

Patients with immune deficiency diseases, such as combined immunodeficiency, hypogammaglobulinemia and agammaglobulinemia, should not be given OPV because of their substantially increased risk of vaccine-associated disease. Furthermore, patients with altered immune states due to diseases such as leukemia, lymphoma, or generalized malignancy, or with immune systems compromised by therapy with corticosteroids, alkylating drugs, antimetabolites, or radiation should not receive OPV because of the theoretical risk of paralytic disease. OPV should not be used for immunizing immuno-deficient patients and their household contacts; IPV is recommended. Although a pro-tective immune response to IPV in the immunodeficient patient cannot be assured, the vaccine is safe and some protection may result from its administration. If OPV is inad-vertently administered to a household-type contact of an immunodeficient patient, close contact between the patient and the recipients of OPV should be avoided for at least 2-3 weeks after vaccination. Because of the possibility of immunodeficiency in other children born to a family in which there has been 1 such case, OPV should not be given to a member of a household in which there is a family history of immunodeficiency until the immune status of the recipient and other children in the family is documented.

ADVERSE REACTIONS

OPV

In rare instances, administration of OPV has been associated with paralysis in healthy recipients and their contacts. Other than efforts to identify persons with immune defi-ciency conditions, no procedures are currently available for identifying persons likely to experience such adverse reactions. Although the risk of vaccine-associated paralysis is extremely small for vaccinees and their susceptible close personal contacts, they should be informed of this risk.

IPV

No serious side effects of currently available IPV have been documented. Since IPV contains trace amounts of streptomycin and neomycin, there is a possibility of hyper-sensitivity reactions in individuals sensitive to these antibiotics.

CASE INVESTIGATION AND EPIDEMIC CONTROL

The occurrence of a single case of poliomyelitis should prompt an immediate epidemi-ologic investigation, including an active search for other cases. If evidence implicates wild poliovirus and there is a possibility of transmission, a vaccination plan designed to contain spread should be developed. If evidence implicates vaccine-derived poliovirus, no vac-cination plan need be developed, as no outbreaks associated with vaccine virus have been documented to date. Within an epidemic area, OPV should be provided for all persons over 6 weeks of age who have not been completely immunized or whose immunization status is unknown, with the exceptions noted above under **Immunodeficiency.**

References
1. American Academy of Pediatrics: Report of the Committee on Infectious Diseases. 18th ed. Evanston, Illinois, AAP, 1977
2. Nightingale E: Recommendations for a national policy on poliomyelitis vaccination. N Engl J Med 297:249-253, 1977

SELECTED BIBLIOGRAPHY

CDC: Neurotropic Diseases Surveillance: Poliomyelitis Summary 1974-1976. Issued October 1977

CDC: Poliomyelitis — United States, 1978-1979. MMWR 28:483-484, 1979

Hardy GE, Hopkins CC, Linneman CC Jr, et al: Trivalent oral poliovirus vaccine: A comparison of two infant immunization schedules. Pediatrics 45:444-448, 1970

Krugman S, Katz SL: Childhood immunization procedures. JAMA 237:2228-2230, 1977

Nightingale E: Recommendations for a national policy on poliomyelitis vaccination. N Engl J Med 297:249-253, 1977

Salk J, Salk D: Control of influenza and poliomyelitis with killed virus vaccines. Science 195: 834-847, 1977

Sanders DY, Cramblett HG: Antibody titers to polioviruses in patients ten years after immunization with Sabin vaccine. J Pediatr 84:406-408, 1974

Schonberger LB, McGowan JE, Gregg MB: Vaccine-associated poliomyelitis in the United States, 1961-1972. Am J Epidemiol 104:202-211, 1976

The relation between acute persisting spinal paralysis and poliomyelitis vaccine (oral): Results of a WHO enquiry. Bull WHO 53:319-331, 1976

Replaces previous recommendation on poliomyelitis, published in MMWR 26:329-330, 335-336, 1977.

CHAPTER 23

Encephalitis

MMWR 27:164 (5/12/78)

Imported Tick-borne Encephalitis — Ohio

On July 15, 1977, a 4-year-old girl from Cleveland was noted to have a swollen right hand and pale appearance and to refuse solid foods. By July 17, she complained of headache and had a temperature of 38 C (100 F). Between July 19-21 she had 4 episodes of vomiting fluids and periods of increased irritability alternating with lethargy. When she was admitted to a hospital in Cleveland on July 21, she was ataxic and complained of neck pain. Her vital signs on admission were temperature, 38 C (100 F); blood pressure, 104/56; pulse, 120, and respiration, 30. Other than an elevated leukocyte level and slightly depressed hemoglobin level, laboratory results were within normal ranges. However, 381 leukocytes were found in cerebrospinal fluid, and there was a total absence of normal waking rhythms by EEG.

Three serum samples, collected July 22, July 26, and August 12, were sent to CDC for determination of antibody to arboviruses. Hemagglutination inhibition (HI) tests were performed with a battery of antigens including those of St. Louis encephalitis, yellow fever, Powassan (POW), Langat (LGT) and California encephalitis subtype LaCrosse (LAC) viruses. The results revealed antibody to all 4 flaviviruses but not to LAC virus (Table 1). Serologic conversion to LGT and stable titers to the other flaviviruses suggested a recent infection with a member of the tick-borne encephalitis (TBE) complex of that group. CF test results confirmed this, demonstrating an 8-fold rise to LGT and detection of antibody to POW. Because of the potential hazards to laboratory workers inherent in further testing with flaviviruses of the TBE complex, neutralization tests were not performed.

Patient history revealed that the child recently had visited her native Hungary with her adoptive parents. On

TABLE 1. Results of hemagglutination-inhibition (HI) and comple-ment-fixiation (CF) tests with serum from a 4-year-old girl, Ohio, July-August, 1977

Serum No.	Date	Test	Antibody titer* to antigen shown				
			St. Louis encephalitis	Powassan virus	Langat virus	Yellow fever	LaCrosse virus
1	7-22-77	HI	20	—**	20	20	—
		CF	—	—	32	—	—
2	7-26-77	HI	20	—	20	20	—
		CF	—	—	32	—	—
3	8-12-77	HI	40	10	80	20	—
		CF	—	16	256	—	—

*Given as reciprocals
**Blank signifies <10 (HI) or <8 (CF)

June 22, she had hiked in an open area near the city of Nastori, about 25 kilometers from the Bakony Forest. The latter is an enzootic focus of TBE virus approximately 100 kilometers southwest of Budapest. Three days later she had a temperature of 39 C (102 F), and a tick of undetermined species and gender was removed from her scalp. She was started on a course of antibiotics. Within 5 days after this treatment began, the fever resolved. Afterward, however, she became more hostile, negativistic, and irritable. She returned to Cleveland, and no additional problems were noted until July 15. Follow-up EEG readings, performed at approximately 1-month intervals, indicated improved but continued aberrant rhythms simultaneous with a return to good physical health and psychosocial normality.

Reported by SM Bannister, MD, RP Cruse, DO, AD Rothner, MD, Cleveland Clinic, Cleveland; T Halpin, MD, State Epidemiologist, Ohio Dept of Health; Arbovirus Reference Br, Vector-borne Diseases Div, Bur of Laboratories, CDC.

Editorial Note: Of the 58 known flaviviruses, 15 are considered to be principally tick-borne, and a number have been isolated in eastern Europe, including Hungary. In such areas TBE is considered an important, if not wide-spread, problem. TBE virus in east central Europe is mainly transmitted by ixodid ticks, often of the species *Ixodes ricinus*. The remission and recurrence of symptoms and the serologic responses described in this case are characteristic of biphasic meningoencephalitis caused by the tick-borne viral encephalitides.

These findings emphasize the need for a complete case history, including recent travel and insect exposure, in this day of rapid and direct long-distance travel.

MMWR 27:279 (8/4/78)

California Encephalitis — Wisconsin, Minnesota

On July 14, 1978, a 3-year-old girl from DeSoto, Wisconsin, was hospitalized in near-by LaCrosse with a diagnosis of acute encephalitis. The girl's condition worsened, and she died on July 18. Virus was isolated from brain tissue collected at autopsy. It was subsequently identified at the University of Wisconsin on July 24 as LaCrosse or a close-ly related strain of California encephalitis (CE) group virus by specific fluorescent anti-body staining of original brain tissues and passaged virus.

The child had lived on a wooded farm 1 mile east of the Mississippi River. Her parents recalled that she had been bitten so frequently by mosquitoes that, when hospitalized, she had a rash of the exposed parts of her body. When the cause of her death was estab-lished, Wisconsin health officials, with the assistance of family and relatives, searched the area for breeding sites of *Aedes triseriatus*, the vector mosquito. Mosquito larvae were collected from tree holes, rubber tires, discarded containers, and a disused and partially water-filled boat. The larvae were removed for viral study, and the breeding sites were drained or destroyed.

A survey of hospitals in those areas of southwestern Wisconsin and adjacent southeast Minnesota known to be endemic for CE revealed that 16 children had been admitted with signs of encephalitis in July. The fatal case, when tested by the counterimmune electro-phoresis technique at the hospital where she was admitted, was found to be one of 4 children with encephalitis who had evidence of antibodies to CE virus. Laboratory studies are pending at the Wisconsin and Minnesota state laboratories to determine the etiologies of the illnesses of the 16 children with encephalitis.

State and local health officials in the affected areas have issued news releases to inform the public of the situation. *A. triseriatus* breeds in water collected in naturally occurring cavities in trees and in artificial containers, such as discarded tires. Prevention of human infection depends on eliminating breeding sites around houses and residential areas and on preventing mosquito bites in persons visiting wooded areas.

Reported by C Gunderson, MD, LaCrosse Lutheran Hospital; W Thompson, DVM, Dept of Preventive Medicine, University of Wisconsin; E Fifer, MD, State Epidemiologist, R Wade, PhD, J Washburn, MS, Minnesota Dept of Health; IE Imm, MA, State Epidemioloigst, M LaVenture, MPH, Wisconsin State Dept of Health and Social Services; Vector-Borne Diseases Div, Bur of Laboratories, Vector Biology and Control Div, Bur of Tropical Diseases, and Viral Diseases Div, Bur of Epidemiology, CDC.

Editorial Note: Typical reports of CE involve children with acute encephalitis or meningi-tis in midwestern states. Fatal cases of documented CE are rare: Only 3 have been re-ported. Isolation of the LaCrosse virus has been reported only from 1 other case, also fatal.

Elimination of infected breeding sites is important because CE virus is perpetuated by transovarial transmission to successive generations of mosquitoes.

MMWR 27:449 (11/10/78)

Encephalitis Outbreak — India

According to releases from Air India Radio, an outbreak of viral encephalitis has resulted in 448 deaths in Uttar Pradesh, India's most populous state. Most of the cases have been reported from the eastern districts of that state, although some have also been reported from New Delhi, the nation's capital, and 27 deaths have been reported from

Bihar State, east of Uttar Pradesh.

Japanese B encephalitis infection has been shown to be the cause of the outbreak by serologic testing and viral isolation performed at the Calcutta School of Tropical Medicine and the Indian National Institute of Virology on serum and tissue specimens from a small number of cases.

Reported by Viral Diseases Div, Bur of Epidemiology, CDC.

Editorial Note: Japanese B encephalitis is a mosquito-borne disease that is endemic in much of Asia. Studies have shown that hundreds of inapparent or mild infections may occur for each case of clinical encephalitis, but that the fatality rate for encephalitic patients may exceed 20% (1). It is typically a rural disease, and the vector mosquitoes, such as those of the *Culex vishnui* group, breed abundantly in rice paddies found in agricultural areas. Inactivated vaccine is commercially produced in Japan, but it is not licensed for use in the United States.

Because of the paucity of accurate, official information regarding the outbreak, it is difficult to assess the severity or the geographic extent of the Japanese B virus activity. Nevertheless, based on the prevalence of the mosquito vector and pattern of past outbreaks, travelers to urban areas, even in northeastern India, are probably at very low risk of infection.

Reference
1. Horsfall FL, Tamm I (eds): Viral and Rickettsial Infections of Man. 4th ed. Philadelphia, Lippincott, 1965, pp 626-631

MMWR 27:464 (11/24/78)

Follow-up on Japanese B Encephalitis — India

As of November 9, a total of 5,459 confirmed and clinically suspected cases of Japanese B encephalitis have been reported this year in India. There have been 1,869 deaths. The outbreaks have been occurring in at least 7 states, but they have been particularly severe in Uttar Pradesh, which has over 2,000 reported cases with 768 deaths, and West Bengal (1,600 reported cases; 532 deaths). The attack rate is estimated to be about 4 per hundred thousand population.

The high mortality rate reported in children has declined, particularly in Uttar Pradesh. Intensive and massive spray operations have been carried out to rid the areas, many of them flood-ridden, of the mosquito vector, and people have been asked to use mosquito nets, appropriate clothing, and mosquito repellants. The Director General of Health Services has secured 40,000 doses of Japanese encephalitis vaccine from Japan, and expects 87,000 more doses by January. An intensive collaborative epidemiologic study has been started in Uttar Pradesh and Bihar to identify possible asymptomatic infections.

Reported by B Sankaran, Director General of Health Services, India.

MMWR 28:310 (7/6/79)

St. Louis Encephalitis — Ohio, 1978

Five serologically documented cases of St. Louis encephalitis (SLE), 1 fatal, were reported from Ohio in 1978. All of the patients had onset of symptoms between September 16 and November 11. Two cases occurred in Urbana, in Champaign County, and 1 case occurred in each of the following areas: Rocky River, Cuyahoga County;

Columbus, Franklin County; and Chillicothe, Ross County. Cases of SLE have been diagnosed in Columbus each year since the 1975 epidemic, which involved much of the Mississippi and Ohio River valleys; however, human cases had not been detected in the other 3 counties since that time.

In a statewide arbovirus surveillance program conducted from June through mid-September 1978, 6,081 avian blood samples were tested for SLE antibody by the hemagglutination-inhibition (HI) test. The resulting rate of seropositivity was 0.25%. A total of 39,204 *Culex* mosquitoes, tested on duck-embryo-cell culture, yielded a single isolate of of SLE virus. The virus isolation was made from a pool of 50 *C. pipiens* collected at Cedar Bog, approximately 6.4 km south of Urbana, on July 20.

SLE Case-Cuyahoga County: The Cuyahoga County Health Department initiated a surveillance program (41 hospitals in the 6-county Cleveland metropolitan area) during the summer and fall of 1978 to monitor encephalitis-like illnesses. On September 19, a 23-year-old woman with a 1-day history of severe frontal headache and temperature of 39 C was examined and admitted to a hospital participating in the surveillance program. She reported minimal pain when flexing her neck, but otherwise her physical examination was unremarkable. Except for a brief visit, 3 weeks earlier, to a camping area in southern Ohio, she had no history of recent travel.

Laboratory results included a white blood cell (WBC) count of 9,800/mm³ with normal differential, a hemoglobin of 13.4 g/dl, and a normal chest X ray. Cerebrospinal fluid (CSF) contained 799 WBC/mm³ (99% polymorphonuclear leukocytes, 1% lymphocytes), a protein level of 50 mg/dl, and a glucose level of 55 mg/dl. The blood sugar level was 37 mg/dl. On examination of Gram-stained spinal fluid, numerous polymorphonuclear cells and 2 or 3 questionable gram-negative diplococci were seen, but blood and CSF cultures yielded no bacterial growth.

The patient was started on intravenous penicillin. On the night of admission she had a transient macular rash covering her extremities and experienced a left-sided, focal seizure. A repeat lumbar puncture after 48 hours revealed 160 WBC/mm³ (80% lymphocytes, 20% polymorphonuclear leukocytes) and a red blood cell count of 2,000/mm³. The protein level was 71 mg/dl, and the glucose, 67 mg/dl. Her blood sugar level was 110 mg/dl. No organisms were seen in the Gram-stained smear. On the fourth hospital day the patient became confused and rapidly deteriorated into a comatose state. At this stage, chloramphenicol was added. She remained febrile and developed a decerebrate posture and early signs of papilledema. On the seventh hospital day, she became hypotensive, had a cardiorespiratory arrest, and died.

At autopsy, the brain appeared grossly normal. Serum from the acute phase of illness had an HI antibody titer to SLE of <1:10 and a complement-fixing (CF) antibody titer of <1:8; serum collected on the seventh day had an HI titer of 1:20 and a CF titer of 1:32. Testing of 351 *C. pipiens* and serum specimens from 26 house sparrows from the areas frequented by the patient did not demonstrate SLE virus or other evidence of recent SLE activity.

SLE Field Studies, Champaign and Ross Counties: After the first reports of human SLE cases, which had occurred in the area in mid- to late September, field investigations were initiated to determine the extent of SLE infection in the mosquito and avian populations in Champaign and Ross counties. Resting mosquitoes were aspirated from culverts and storm sewers in Urbana and Chillicothe from October 23 through November 7, 1978. *C. pipiens* accounted for over 90% of collections in both cities. A single isolation of SLE virus was made from 7,381 mosquitoes collected from Urbana, and another, from 1,718 mosquitoes collected in Chillicothe. In both instances, virus was detected in a pool of 50 *C. pipiens.*

During the period October 24-December 1, 1978, avian serum samples were collected in Urbana and Chillicothe and at sites within an 18-km radius of both cities. Immature house sparrows accounted for over 97% of all specimens obtained. HI-testing revealed SLE seropositivity rates of 8.2% (33/401) in Urbana and 5.6% (11/196) in Chillicothe. Over one-third (34.1%) of all seropositive birds from Urbana and Chillicothe were found to have antibody titers of $\geqslant$1:120, strongly suggesting recent infection with SLE virus. Seropositivity rates were substantially lower (0-0.5%) in birds collected 6-18 km from both cities, indicating that SLE activity was concentrated in the urban areas. The highest rate of seropositivity outside either city (2.5%) was detected at a farm located 7.1 km from Urbana and 1.6 km from Cedar Bog, the site from which the mosquitoes that originally yielded SLE virus were collected on July 20.

Reported by J Berner, MD, K V Gopalakrishna, MD, K Kapoor, MD, L Maim, MD, W Wilder, MD, Lutheran Medical Center, Cleveland, Ohio; OG Glasser, MD, J Jackson, RS, Cuyahoga County Board of Health; SW Gordon, ED Peterson, RL Berry, PhD, RA Restifo, JA Kertesz, MA Parsons, Vector-Borne Disease Unit, GT Bear, DVM, Veterinary Unit, TJ Halpin, MD, State Epidemiologist, Bur of Preventive Medicine, D Keiper, K Elliot, Bur of Laboratories, Ohio Dept of Health; Enteric and Neurotropic Viral Diseases Br, Viral Diseases Div, CDC.

Editorial Note: These observations suggest that SLE activity was concentrated in the locations associated with the human cases. The seropositivity rates of avian samples collected at points surrounding the Urbana and Chillicothe cases declined from greater than 5% to less than 1% within a 15-km radius. Similarly, geographically limited activity may be the reason mosquito and bird specimens collected in Cuyahoga County were negative.

Close, active surveillance was an important factor in establishing the cause of encephalitis in the Cuyahoga County patient. Most clinical cases of SLE are described in association with outbreaks, and fatalities in patients less than 40 years old are infrequently observed.

MMWR 28:462 (10/5/79)

St. Louis Encephalitis — South Florida

Late in August 1979, sentinel chickens from 5 locations in Collier County, Florida, and separate locations in Charlotte and Hendry counties developed antibodies to the St. Louis encephalitis (SLE) virus, indicating recent infection. When these serologic results were confirmed, the public was warned to avoid mosquitoes, and local medical communities were alerted. Hospital surveillance for SLE cases was increased, and ecological studies for SLE were initiated in south Florida. Control activities for *Culex nigripalpus*, the mosquito vector of human SLE in Florida, were also intensified.

In mid-September the Florida state laboratories confirmed the first human case of SLE and made the first isolation of SLE virus from mosquitoes in Florida since 1977. The case occurred in a 65-year-old woman from Palm Beach County who developed acute encephalitis on August 27. She had traveled widely in peninsular Florida in the weeks before the onset of her illness but not in the counties with evidence of SLE activity. She is recovering. The isolation of SLE virus was from mosquitoes collected in Highlands County, located in south-central Florida.

Surveillance and control activities are continuing in south Florida. Further SLE activity through mid-September has been indicated by additional serologic conversions in sentinel chickens from Charlotte, Collier, and Hendry counties. As a result of recent heavy rains in south Florida, *C. nigripalpus* populations are increasing sharply.

Reported by county health units and mosquito control districts from Charlotte, Collier, Hendry, Highlands, and Palm Beach counties, Florida; E Buff, MS, RA Gunn, MD, State Epidemiologist, HT Janowski, MPH, JA Mulrennan, Jr, PhD, NJ Schneider, PhD, FM Wellings, ScD, Florida State Dept of Health and Rehabilitative Services; Enteric and Neurotropic Viral Diseases Br, Viral Diseases Div, Bur of Epidemiology, CDC.

Editorial Note: In the fall of 1977, an outbreak of SLE occurred in central Florida. A total of 77 confirmed cases, including 8 deaths, were reported from 20 Florida counties. Following the outbreak, a program of integrated surveillance to monitor possible SLE activity in birds, mosquitoes, and humans throughout the state was developed by the Florida Department of Health and Rehabilitative Services. The surveillance program began operation early in the arbovirus season of 1978, but no evidence of recent SLE activity in sentinel chickens, in mosquito collections, or in human patients was found until the activity reported here.

This represents one of the first times that an animal surveillance system has detected epizootic SLE activity before human cases have been recognized.

MMWR 28:485 (10/19/79)

Arboviral Activity — United States, 1979

As of October 12, little epidemic activity had been observed in the 1979 arboviral season. With the exception of a cluster of St. Louis encephalitis (SLE) cases in the residents of the Delta area of Mississippi, arboviral cases have been scattered. A total of 78 California encephalitis cases have been confirmed in 9 states. Only 12 cases of SLE, 2 of Eastern equine encephalomyelitis, and 1 of Western equine encephalomyelitis have been confirmed. There is evidence of ongoing SLE activity in birds and mosquitoes in south Florida.

California encephalitis: With 3 exceptions, cases have been reported from states where California encephalitis (CE) is recognized as endemic: Minnesota (27), Wisconsin (19), Ohio (15), Illinois (8), Iowa (5), and New York (1). The age of patients and clinical severity of most cases have followed the usual pattern—i.e. children with relatively mild encephalitis.

The geographic exceptions occurred in 3 southern states. One of these cases—and also the first reported U.S. case of the season—was in a 13-year-old boy from Stateline, Mississippi, who had onset of febrile headache on May 21. He became confused, clinical encephalitis developed, and he was hospitalized in Mobile, Alabama. He improved rapidly, and the diagnosis of CE was subsequently confirmed by the Alabama state laboratories. CE infection was also confirmed in a 7-year-old girl hospitalized early in July with fever and seizures at the Public Health Service Hospital in Cherokee, North Carolina. (In 1976 and 1977, 6 confirmed cases of CE were diagnosed in children from Cherokee and surrounding areas of western North Carolina.) The Georgia state laboratories have also confirmed CE infection in a 7-year-old boy from Macon, Georgia, who was hospitalized with clinical encephalitis in July. This is the first case of CE ever reported from Georgia.

St. Louis encephalitis: An outbreak of SLE in the Delta area of Mississippi, near Greenville, occurred in August and September *(1)*. A total of 5 laboratory-confirmed and 4 laboratory-presumptive cases (2 fatal) have been identified, and other cases of clinical encephalitis from the area are currently under laboratory investigation. Cases of confirmed SLE have also been reported from Florida (2), Tennessee (2), Texas (2), and Indiana (1). SLE activity in southern Florida, as detailed in a previous report *(2)*, now involves a band of 14 counties across south central Florida which show evidence of SLE infection in humans, birds, and/or mosquitoes. Human cases have been identified in Hillsborough County (1 confirmed and 1 presumptive) and in Palm Beach County (1 confirmed and 1 presumptive).

Eastern equine encephalomyelitis: Only 2 cases of Eastern equine encephalomyelitis (EEE) in humans have been identified this year. The first involved a resident of Newcastle, Delaware, who developed encephalitis in early July. Delaware laboratories subsequently confirmed the case to be EEE. The second case involved a woman who was hospitalized September 11 in Bryn Mawr, Pennsylvania, with acute encephalitis, later laboratory confirmed as EEE. She was most likely infected while vacationing near Somers Point, New Jersey.

Western equine encephalomyelitis: The only confirmed human case of Western equine encephalomyelitis (WEE) this year was reported from South Dakota. The patient, a 32-year-old resident of Sioux Falls, developed acute encephalitis on August 21.

Reported by participating State Epidemiologists; Vector-Borne Diseases Div, Bur of Laboratories, Vector Biology and Control Div, Bur of Tropical Diseases, and Enteric and Neurotropic Viral Diseases Br, Viral Diseases Div, Bur of Epidemiology, CDC.

References
1. MMWR 28:474-475, 1979
2. MMWR 28:462-463, 1979

MMWR 27 (A.S., 1978): 24

ENCEPHALITIS — Reported Cases by Month of Onset, United States, 1970–1977

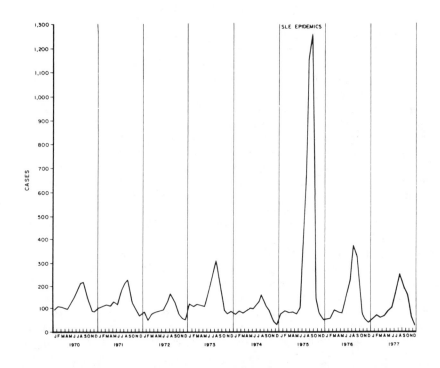

ENCEPHALITIS — Reported Cases by Etiology and Month, United States, 1977

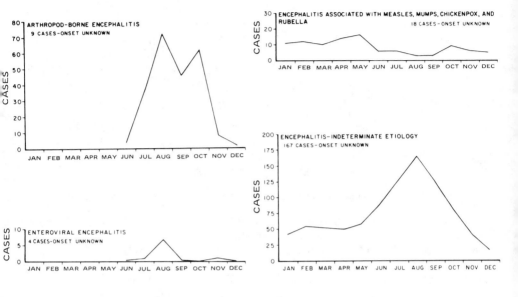

CHAPTER 24

Rabies

MMWR 28:109 (3/16/79)

Human-to-Human Transmission of Rabies by a Corneal Transplant — Idaho

On October 10, 1978, a 37-year-old Boise, Idaho, woman died of rabies. She had received a corneal transplant 7 weeks earlier (August 21) from a 39-year-old man from Baker, Oregon, who had died of presumed Guillain-Barré syndrome (GBS). The temporal relationship between the recipient's illness and the corneal transplant prompted her physician to send serum, cerebrospinal fluid (CSF), and fresh brain tissue from the woman and fixed brain tissue and the frozen eyes from the donor to the Infectious Diseases Branch, National Institute of Neurological and Communicative Diseases and Strokes, National Institutes of Health (NIH), Bethesda, Maryland, for further diagnostic studies. The possibility of rabies was first raised when investigators found inclusion bodies in brain tissue from both patients. Fresh brain tissue then was sent to CDC, where fluorescent antibody (FA) studies confirmed the diagnosis in the recipient on October 23. Subsequently, the diagnosis was confirmed in the donor by identifying rabies virus in the donor's frozen eye by FA studies and virus isolation (1).

The donor had been healthy until July 28, when he developed lumbar and thoracic back pain. Over the next few days he developed weakness (first in his legs and then in his arms), diplopia, and ataxia; on August 4 he was hospitalized in Baker, Oregon. The next day, because of difficulty swallowing and breathing, he was transferred to a hospital in Boise, with the diagnosis of GBS. While in the hospital he developed progressive weakness, suffered a cardiopulmonary arrest, became comatose, and died on August 20 from complications presumed to be secondary to GBS. CSF studies on August 5 revealed 8 white blood cells (WBCs)/mm^3 with 7 lymphocytes and 1 neutrophil and a protein of 63 mg/dl. Within 90 minutes of the donor's death, his eyes were removed and refrigerated. The following day a cornea from 1 eye was transplanted into the right eye of the woman for treatment of keratoconus. The recipient's postoperative course was uneventful until 30 days after the transplant, when she developed right retroorbital headache. Over the next few days her headache worsened, and she developed hypesthesia on the right side of her face, dysphagia, dysarthria, and difficulty walking. She was hospitalized on September 27; thereafter she developed a flaccid paralysis, became progressively obtunded, and died on October 10. CSF studies on September 29 revealed 14 WBCs/mm^3 (13 lymphocytes and 1 neutrophil) and a protein of 53 mg/dl. Serum collected on October 2 was negative for rabies antibody, but serum collected on October 5 was positive at a titer of 1:23.

The donor's family members, friends, and fellow workers were questioned in an attempt to identify a source of exposure to rabies. No history of an animal bite was found. However, the donor had risk of exposure from his job as a professional lumberman, from his work with livestock, and from trapping, shooting, and skinning coyotes. It is unlikely that a source of rabies for him will be identified. The woman had no history of an animal bite or risk of rabies exposure. The only rabid animals identified in eastern Oregon or Idaho since 1968 have been bats.

Because the 2 patients were not isolated for 23 of their combined 31 hospital days, many persons were potentially exposed. Individuals who had had contact with the donor or recipient were identified by interviewing family, friends, hospital personnel, and others and by a review of hospital records. Contacts were interviewed to determine their risk of exposure to rabies. It was recommended that those contacts who potentially had open cuts or wounds or mucous membranes that could have been exposed to saliva or other infectious body fluids receive rabies postexposure treatment. Wyeth Laboratories provides experimental human diploid cell strain rabies vaccine (W-HDCS) on an emergency basis; thus, persons were given the choice of receiving the experimental vaccine or duck embryo vaccine (DEV). In addition, all those treated were given human rabies immune globulin (HRIG). Ninety-three persons elected to take W-HDCS and 1, DEV. For those receiving W-HDCS, informed consent was obtained, and each person was given 1 dose of W-HDCS plus 1 dose of HRIG (20 I.U./kg) on the first day of treatment. Then single doses of W-HDCS were given 3, 7, 14, and 28 days later. Serum samples will be drawn on the first day of treatment and 7, 14, 28, 42, 90, and 365 days later. No person has become ill, to date.

Reported by RC Burton, Boise, Idaho; I Johnson, RN, L Lemon, RN, St. Alphonsus Hospital, Boise; R McKim, MD, Baker, Oregon; YM Johnson, RN, St. Elizabeth Hospital, Baker; B Baggerly, RN, G Ward, MD, Baker County Health Dept, Oregon; W Lechtenberg, FR Dixon, MD, Idaho Central District Health Dept, Boise; JA Mather, MD, State Epidemiologist, Idaho State Dept of Health and Welfare; JA Googins, MD, State Epidemiologist, LP Williams, DVM, State Public Health Veterinarian, Oregon Dept of Human Resources; Infectious Diseases Br, National Institute of Neurological and Communicative Diseases and Strokes, NIH; Viral Zoonoses Br, Virology Div, Bur of Laboratories, Respiratory and Special Pathogens Br, Viral Diseases Div, Bur of Epidemiology, CDC.

Editorial Note: This is the first case of rabies acquired from a tissue transplant of any kind. The lack of a history of other possible exposure to rabies, the rarity of human rabies in the United States, the temporal relationship to the transplant, and the onset of symptoms with right retroorbital headache (pain, paresthesia, or hypesthesia at the site of virus inoculation is a classic symptom of rabies) implicate the transplanted cornea as the source of rabies in the recipient. This case highlights concern about the transmission of infectious agents by corneal transplants first raised by the report of transmission of Creutzfeldt-Jakob disease by a corneal transplant (2), and suggests that the criteria for accepting donors should be reevaluated.

These 2 cases demonstrate how hard it is to diagnose rabies if an animal bite is not noted and the patient presents with an ascending paralysis without the excitement and agitation classically associated with rabies. When the patient is alive, the diagnosis, if suspected, can sometimes be confirmed by immunofluorescent studies showing rabies antigen in corneal impressions (3), by neck skin biopsy (4), by isolation of virus from saliva or body fluids, or by demonstration of rabies antibody in serum or CSF (5). After death, the diagnosis can be made by identifying Negri bodies and then showing rhabdovirus by electron microscopy in fixed brain tissue, by immunofluorescent studies of fresh brain tissue, or by virus isolation. As occurred in connection with a recent rabies case in Pennsylvania (6), the difficulty persons had in remembering the circumstances of their contact with the patients—a contact that occurred 14-100 days earlier—and the many days the patients were not on isolation precautions, resulted in the recommendation that many persons receive rabies post-exposure treatment.

References
1. Hough SA, Burton RC, Wilson RW, Henson TE, London WT, Baer GM, *et al*: Human-to-human transmission of rabies virus by a corneal transplant. N Engl J Med 300:603-604, 1979
2. Duffy P, Wolf J, Collins G, *et al*: Possible person-to-person transmission of Creutzfeldt-Jakob disease. N Engl J Med 290:692-693, 1974
3. Koch FJ, Sagartz JW, Davidson DE, *et al*: Diagnosis of human rabies by the cornea test. Am J Clin Pathol 63:509-515, 1975
4. Smith WB, Blenden DC, Fuh TH, *et al*: Diagnosis of rabies by immunofluorescent staining of frozen sections of skin. J Am Vet Med Assoc 161:1495-1501, 1972
5. Hattwick MAW, Gregg MB: The disease in man, in Baer GM (ed): The Natural History of Rabies. New York, Academic Press, 1975, pp 281-304
6. MMWR 28:75, 1979

MMWR 28:256 (6/8/79)

Follow-up on Animal Rabies — U.S.-Mexican Border

From January 1 through May 25, 1979, a total of 49 cases of animal rabies have been reported from 12 of the 26 U.S. Border counties (28 dogs, 15 skunks, 4 bats, 1 fox, and 1 bovine). Seventy-two cases have been reported from 3 of the 12 border cities in Mexico (71 dogs and 1 cat). Outbreaks of canine rabies are occurring in 3 areas along the Border: 1. Cd. Juarez, Chihuahua (55 dogs); El Paso County, Texas (18 dogs, 1 bat); Dona Ana County, New Mexico (3 dogs, 2 skunks); 2. Maverick County, Texas (9 dogs); Piedras Negras, Coahuila (3 dogs); and 3. Mexicali, Baja California (13 dogs, 1 cat).

Intensive immunization and programs to capture stray animals are continuing in the affected areas. In Cd. Juarez, for example, since January 1, 1979, approximately 2,000 dogs have been captured, and over 32,000 dogs have been immunized.

Reported by B Velimirovic, MD, El Paso Field Office, Pan American Health Organization; L R Hutchinson, VMD, BF Rosenblum, MD, El Paso City-County Health Unit; WR Bilderback, DVM, Texas State Dept of Health; JM Mann, MD, State Epidemiologist, Health Services Div, New Mexico State Health and Environment Dept; GL Humphrey, DVM, Veterinary Public Health Unit, California Dept of Health Services; Respiratory and Special Pathogens Br, Viral Diseases Div, Bur of Epidemiology, CDC.

MMWR 28:315 (7/13/79)

Human Rabies — United States

A second case of human rabies from Texas has been reported to CDC. As with a case reported in June (*1*), this case occurred near the U.S.-Mexican Border, where a rabies epizootic is continuing. Further information is now available on the 2 suspected cases reported previously (*1*).

A 7-year-old girl from Eagle Pass, Texas, was bitten on the left leg on May 31, 1979, by a dog proven rabid by fluorescent antibody (FA) testing. On June 5 she was given human rabies immune globulin (HRIG) and was begun on daily doses of duck embryo vaccine (DEV). On June 24, after she had received 20 doses of DEV, she developed fever, severe headaches, vomiting, stiff neck, and myalgias. On June 26, she was admitted to a hospital in Eagle Pass. Two days later, she was transferred to a hospital in San Antonio, where she was noted to have fever, a stiff neck, and no lower-extremity reflexes. Over the next few days she became less responsive and dysphonic and had 2 generalized seizures; she also had hallucinations and difficulty handling secretions. On the evening of July 2, she had a cardiorespiratory arrest, but was resuscitated; she died the following day. Cerebrospinal fluid (CSF) obtained on June 29 had 45 white blood cells per mm^3 (30 lymphocytes, 15 neutrophils), a protein level of 20 mg/dl, and a glucose level of 69 mg/dl. Corneal impressions taken on June 29 were nondiagnostic. Serum and CSF obtained on June 29 revealed a rabies antibody titer of 1:16 and <1:5, respectively. Postmortem brain specimens were positive for rabies by FA.

Follow-up on previously reported cases

The diagnosis of rabies has been confirmed for the 8-year-old boy from Piedras Negras, Mexico, who was hospitalized in San Antonio, Texas, on June 7. The initial diagnosis was based on a positive FA test of corneal impressions and a rabies antibody titer of 1:145 in serum collected on the 16th day of illness (1). Serum and CSF taken on the 23rd day of illness had rabies antibody titers of 1:1,300 and 1:56, respectively. Viral isolation studies are pending. As of July 9, the patient remains comatose and on a respirator.

An 18-year-old man from Vancouver, Washington, was suspected of having rabies because of a positive FA test of brain biopsy material obtained on the sixth day of his clinical illness and because of positive corneal impressions made on the eighth day. Serum from the 16th day of illness, 5 days after HRIG was given, had a titer of 1:16. Serum from the 29th day and CSF from the 27th day both had titers of <1:5. Viral isolation studies are negative, to date. As of July 9, the patient was confused, quadraplegic, and on a respirator.

Reported by FA Guerra, MD, J Seals, MD, San Antonio, Texas; E Blizard, MD, R Fisher, MD, R Kim, MD, Vancouver, Washington; RF Bell, San Antonio Metropolitan Health District, San Antonio; CR Webb, Jr, MD, State Epidemiologist, Texas State Dept of Health; JW Taylor, MD, State Epidemiologist, Washington State Dept of Social and Health Services; Viral Zoonosis Br, Virology Div, Bur of Laboratories, Respiratory and Special Pathogens Br, Viral Diseases Div, Bur of Epidemiology, CDC.

Editorial Note: The diagnosis of rabies has been confirmed in the 2 cases from Texas: in 1 by the combination of a positive corneal impression and high serum and CSF rabies antibody titers and in the other by a positive FA test of brain material. The case from Washington does not appear to be rabies because of the lack of antibody in the CSF, the decreasing serum antibody titer, and the, to date, negative viral isolation studies. The reason that the FA test of brain material and the corneal impressions were both false-positive is not clear at this time. The corneal impression test is being reviewed for sensitivity and specificity in animal studies, and the conjugated antirabies serum will be tested for specificity against other viruses.

The girl from Texas developed clinical rabies and died in spite of treatment with HRIG and DEV. Although most failures with vaccine and globulin therapy have, as in this case, been associated with delay in onset of therapy, rare cases of rabies have developed after timely, appropriate, postexposure treatment (2-5).

The 2 cases from the Texas-Mexican Border area highlight the importance of controlling canine rabies because of the close contact between humans and dogs and, therefore, the high risk of rabies transmission. Since January 1, approximately 40,000 dogs have been vaccinated in Ciudad Juarez (6). Health officials in Texas have initiated an intensive dog vaccination and stray-animal-control program in the Eagle Pass area. These cases are the first human cases confirmed from Border communities since 2 were reported in Ciudad Juarez in 1967.

References

1. MMWR 28:292, 1979
2. Anderson JA, Daly FT, Kidd JC: Human rabies after antiserum and vaccine postexposure treatment. Ann Intern Med 64:1297-1302, 1966

3. MMWR 15:326, 1966
4. MMWR 19:293, 1970
5. MMWR 25:235, 1976
6. Pan American Health Organization, El Paso Field Office: Rabies follow-up—El Paso/Cd. Juarez/ Doña Ana County. Border Epidemiological Bulletin 7(5), May, 1979

MMWR 28:476 (10/12/79)

Human Rabies — Oklahoma

On September 26, 1979, CDC was notified of a possible case of human rabies occurring in a man from northeastern Oklahoma.

The 24-year-old man was well until September 15, when he had onset of insomnia, headache, nausea, vomiting, malaise, myalgia, and fever (101 F). Two days later, when symptoms persisted and tremulousness, intermittent confusion, and hallucinations began, he was hospitalized. He became hyperactive, hyper-responsive to environmental stimuli, and diaphoretic, and developed a left seventh cranial nerve palsy. Localized and generalized seizures began on the sixth day of his clinical illness. He was intubated and treated with dopamine for hypotension. On September 22, he was transferred to another hospital. Cerebrospinal fluid (CSF) specimens obtained on September 23 contained 34 lymphocytes and 1 monocyte/mm,^{3} a protein level of 176 mg/dl, and a glucose level of 133 mg/dl. The patient became obtunded on September 22 and progressively comatose over the next 4 days. An electroencephalogram revealed diffuse, slow, non-focal dysrhythmia. Serum rabies virus neutralizing antibody titers were 1:12, 1:10, and 1:42 on September 22, September 23, and September 28, respectively. CSF antibody titers were <1:5. The patient's condition continued to deteriorate, despite intensive support, and he died on October 4. A postmortem brain biopsy contained fluorescing rabies antigen.

The patient's occupation as a woodcutter and his activities before his illness provided the potential for exposure to rabid wild or domestic animals. Thus far, however, no such contact has been documented. Friends and family contacts of the patient and employees of the 2 hospitals at which he was treated are being investigated to determine the degree of their exposure to the patient. As of October 5, 18 family/friend contacts and 34 hospital employees have been identified as having a possibly significant exposure. These persons are beginning a course of postexposure prophylaxis.

Reported by L Kerton, RN, S Schwartz, MD, Tulsa, Oklahoma; EM Cleaver, MD, FA Reynolds, MD, Tulsa City County Health Dept; J Grim, RN, MA Roberts, MPH, Acting State Epidemiologist, M Ward, MD, Oklahoma State Dept of Health; Field Services Div, Viral Diseases Div, Bur of Epidemiology, CDC.

Editorial Note: The patient's clinical course, the rising neutralizing antibody titers in the absence of any antirabies therapy, and the presence of rabies virus in the brain, identified by fluorescence, provide strong evidence to support a diagnosis of rabies. Although a corneal impression fluorescently stained for rabies virus antigen was strongly positive, CDC is not currently using this as a diagnostic test because of several false-positive tests in human non-rabies cases. The corneal impression test appears to be a very reliable diagnostic test in animal models (1) and is sometimes positive in man (2,3), but its diagnostic capabilities have not been fully evaluated in human rabies.

If a likely exposure to rabies is not found, this man will be the fourth of 8 cases of human rabies reported to CDC since January 1978 in which no source of rabies was discovered. The most probable explanation for this was the inability of the patients to communicate at the time rabies was entertained as a diagnosis. Thus, rabies should be considered as a possible cause of encephalopathic illness of undetermined etiology, despite a negative contact history.

With the exception of a corneal transplant recipient (4), no human-to-human transmission of rabies has been documented. However, because of the theoretical possibility of human-to-human transmission in limited circumstances, CDC currently recommends treating contacts of human rabies cases who have possible risk exposure. Risk exposure is considered to be the contamination of open wounds or mucous membranes with saliva or other potentially infectious materials such as neural tissue, autopsy tissue, or spinal fluid. Although any risk of acquiring rabies under these circumstances is unlikely, CDC recommends postexposure prophylaxis for contacts with these exposures.

References

1. Larghi CP, Gonzalez L, Held JR: Evaluation of the corneal test as a laboratory method for rabies diagnosis. Appl Microbiol 25:187-189, 1973
2. Cifuentes E, Calderon E, Bijlengn G: Rabies in a child diagnosed by a new intravitam method-the corneal test. J Trop Med Hyg 74:23-25, 1971
3. Koch FJ, Sagartz JW, Davidson DE, Lawhaswasdi K: Diagnosis of human rabies by the cornea test. Am J Clin Pathol 63:509-515, 1975
4. MMWR 28:109-111, 1979

MMWR 28:590 (12/14/79)

Human Rabies — Kentucky

On December 6, 1979, the diagnosis of rabies was made by fluorescent antibody (FA) staining of a brain tissue specimen from a 45-year-old man from Frankfort, who died on November 30. This is the fifth case of human rabies in the United States in 1979—the most cases in any year since 1959.

The man had been in good health until November 20, when dizziness, vomiting, diaphoresis, and an unstable gait developed. Over the next 2 days dysarthria, difficulty swallowing, diplopia, and spasms in his extremities also developed, and he was admitted to a hospital in Frankfort with the presumptive diagnosis of tetanus. There he was noted to be alert, with a temperature of 38.7 C, tremors, and generalized spasms of the muscles of his extremities. The spasms were precipitated by noise, change in lighting, or passive movement of his body. The patient was treated with human immune tetanus globulin and penicillin.

Late on November 23, he was transferred to a hospital in Lexington, where he was intubated and treated with dopamine for hypotension. He then had mild renal failure and was treated for presumed tetanus with a muscle relaxant and a neuromuscular blocking agent. On November 26, then off medication, he was found to be comatose and have a flaccid paralysis. He remained comatose and developed diabetes insipidus, pulmonary infiltrates, and raised intracerebral pressures. He died on November 30.

Cerebral spinal fluid (CSF) obtained on November 22 was normal, and a repeat study 5 days later showed 23 white blood cells/mm^3 (95% lymphocytes) and a protein level of 146 mg/dl. Serum and CSF specimens, a neck skin biopsy, and buccal mucosal, nasal mucosal, and tongue scrapings, all taken on November 28, were negative. A corneal impression test from November 28, however, was positive.

When he was lucid, the patient gave no history of a potential rabies exposure, and his family and friends have similarly been unable to recall any bites by animals. He worked as a mechanic in a distillery near Frankfort, raised tobacco, and hunted deer occasionally. His next-door neighbor had a dog that died of rabies 5 years ago, to which the patient presumably was not exposed, and he killed an ill-appearing groundhog in the spring of 1979. He had not been outside his county of residence (Franklin) in the last 2 years. In that county, no animals have been reported rabid in 1979, although 11 skunks have been reported rabid in the 6 surrounding counties.

Reported by HJ Cowherd, MD, Frankfort; S Reeves, RN, S Riegler, MD, PD Walzen, MD, University of Kentucky Medical Center; C Hernandez, MD, State Epidemiologist, JW Skaggs, DVM, Kentucky State Dept for Human Resources; Viral Zoonoses Br, Virology Div, Bur of Laboratories; Respiratory and Special Pathogens Br, Viral Diseases Div, Bur of Epidemiology, CDC.

Editorial Note: The increase in cases of human rabies in the United States this year parallels an increase in reports of rabies in animals.

The case reported here is the second one this year—and the fourth in 2 years—in which no potential bite exposure could be identified, despite intensive questioning of families and friends. There are 3 possible explanations: these patients knew of, but did not relate to others, an animal bite; the patients were unaware of a bite exposure (e.g., a bat bite while sleeping); or the patients had a nonbite exposure to rabies.

Although this patient's clinical symptoms were not classic for rabies and he had no exposure history, the diagnosis was suspected. The staff, therefore, took extra precautions to avoid contact with his respiratory secretions, and a laboratory confirmation of a diagnosis was sought. Because of the extra precautions, few hospital personnel were exposed or needed postexposure prophylaxis. The diagnostic studies performed while the patient was alive were negative except for the corneal impression test, which has given frequent false-positive and false-negative results in possible human rabies cases investigated by CDC, making the results difficult to interpret. Thus, in this instance the diagnosis of rabies could not be made until after the patient died.

Serum and CSF specimens can be negative as late as 2 weeks after onset of symptoms (1). Laboratory confirmation of clinical rabies may be difficult during the early stages of illness because of the lack of diagnostic changes in body tissues or fluid or the unreliability of diagnostic tests.

Reference
1. Hattwick MAW, Gregg MB: The disease in man, in Baer GM (ed): The Natural History of Rabies. New York, Academic Press, 1975, pp 281-304

MMWR 27:499 (12/15/78)

Rabies — United States, 1977

A total of 3,182 laboratory-confirmed cases of rabies were reported in the United States and areas under U.S. jurisdiction (Guam, Puerto Rico, and Virgin Islands) in 1977—36 more cases than for 1976 but approximately 7% below the annual average for the preceding 5 years. Forty-seven states and Puerto Rico reported infected animals; only the District of Columbia, Hawaii, Rhode Island, Vermont, Guam, and the Virgin Islands reported no rabies cases. States reporting over 100 cases were California (434), Texas (389), Minnesota (342), Oklahoma (243), Georgia (210), South Dakota (139), Iowa (134), North Dakota (122), and Arkansas (118). Sixteen states reported more cases of rabies in 1977 than in 1976, and 32 states and Puerto Rico reported less. Ninety-seven percent of the reported cases occurred in 7 kinds of animals: skunks, 51%; bats, 20%; raccoons, 9%; cattle, 6%; foxes, 4%; dogs, 4%; and cats, 3%. One case of human rabies was reported. A laboratory technician who worked in the rabies laboratory of the New York Department of Health is surviving with sequelae 1 year after infection (1,2).

Of the total 3,182 rabies cases reported, 2,736 occurred in wild animals (approximately 86% of the total cases) (Figure 1), and 445 occurred in domestic animals (14%). The major wildlife hosts were skunks (59.6%), bats (23.3%), raccoons (10.3%), foxes (4.5%), and mongooses (1.4%).

FIGURE 1. Counties reporting wild animal rabies, 1977

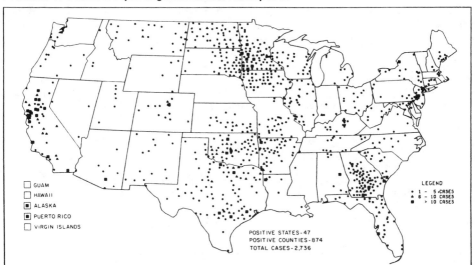

GUAM
HAWAII
ALASKA
PUERTO RICO
VIRGIN ISLANDS

LEGEND
• 1 – 5 CASES
▲ 6 – 10 CASES
■ > 10 CASES

POSITIVE STATES-47
POSITIVE COUNTIES-874
TOTAL CASES-2,736

Skunks: For the 17th consecutive year, infected skunks were the animals most frequently reported. States that reported over 100 cases in skunks were Minnesota (260), Texas (257), California (247), Oklahoma (188), and South Dakota (105).

Bats: Forty-three states reported a total of 637 cases of rabies in bats in 1977, 100 fewer cases than in the previous year but 17% higher than the annual average for the preceding 5-year period. In 12 states the only rabies cases in wildlife that were reported occurred in bats; these states were Colorado, Connecticut, Delaware, Idaho, Maryland, Massachusetts, Mississippi, Nevada, New Hampshire, New Jersey, North Carolina, and Oregon. For the eighth consecutuve year California reported the largest number of cases (166), followed by Colorado (56), and Texas (51). Cases of rabies in bats continued to be more widely distributed than those in any other animal host.

Racoons: Thirteen states reported that 281 cases of rabies had occurred in raccoons, 4 more cases than were reported in the previous year and 97 more than the annual average for the preceding 5 years. This is the highest number of cases ever reported for a year. Georgia (175) and Florida (69) reported 87% of the total cases. Except for an outbreak of 17 cases that occurred in South Carolina, which may have resulted from infected raccoons from Georgia and/or Florida crossing state boundaries, the other cases were scattered and did not appear to be geographically or temporally associated.

Foxes: Eighteen states reported 122 fox rabies cases in 1977, 65 fewer than in 1976 and the lowest total of such cases reported in any year on record. Only 2 states reported foxes as the animals most frequently infected: Alaska and Maine. The states reporting the most cases were Alaska (34), Maine (24), and New York (19).

Other: Various other wildlife species also were reported as positive for rabies in 1977. Thirty-eight cases of mongoose rabies were reported by Puerto Rico, where rabies is enzootic in this species. Other cases occurred in wolves (3), weasels (2), opossums (2), an otter, a mink, a ringtail, and a woodchuck.

Domestic animals: Thirty states and Puerto Rico reported that 445 cases had occurred in domestic animals in 1977, 25 more cases than in 1976 and 31% below the average annual total for the preceding 5 years. Cases occurred in 186 cattle, 120 dogs, 108 cats, 18 horses and mules, 10 sheep and goats, and 3 swine. Generally, cases in domestic animals were reported from areas where rabies is highly endemic in skunks and foxes.

Reported by Respiratory and Special Pathogens Br, Viral Diseases Div, Bur of Epidemiology, CDC.

References
1. MMWR 26:183, 1977
2. MMWR 26:249, 1977
▲ A copy of the report from which these data were derived is available from: CDC, Attn: Chief, Respiratory and Special Pathogens Br, Bur of Epidemiology, Atlanta, Ga. 30333.

MMWR 27 (A.S., 1978): 53

RABIES — Reported Cases in Wild and Domestic Animals by Year, United States, 1953—1978

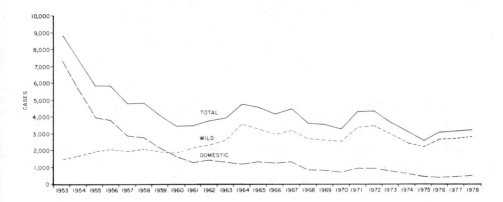

RABIES — Reported Cases in Humans by Year, United States, 1950—1978

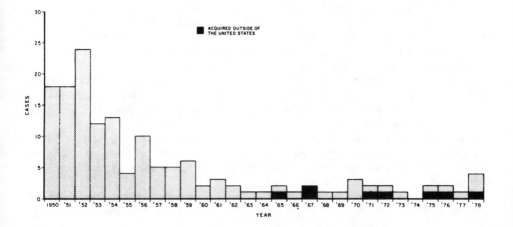

MMWR 27:333 (9/8/78)

Human Diploid Cell Strain Rabies Vaccine

A recently developed vaccine against rabies—human diploid cell strain rabies vaccine—is now available through CDC on a limited, experimental basis. Persons may be eligible to receive the vaccine if: (1) they have a serious allergy to duck embryo vaccine (DEV); (2) they do not show an adequate antibody titer to DEV; or (3) they have been bitten by a proven rabid animal. For pre-exposure, only persons at high risk of being exposed to rabies, primarily laboratory personnel, will be considered for the new vaccine.

The vaccine was developed in the 1960s by inactivating a strain of rabies virus grown in human diploid cell tissue culture. The first human trials were conducted in 1971 (1). It is now being produced by Merieux Institute in France (M-HDCS), Behringwerke in Germany (B-HDCS), and Wyeth Laboratories in the United States (W-HDCS). W-HDCS, the vaccine to be available in the United States, is similar but not identical to its European counterparts: It is inactivated by tri-n-butyl phosphate, instead of B-propiolactone, and it is a subunit vaccine. M-HDCS and B-HDCS have been licensed and used to treat more than 100,000 persons in Europe. W-HDCS is not yet licensed; it is currently being used in human trials in the United States and Israel.

All 3 vaccines have been well studied for pre-exposure rabies prophylaxis and have demonstrated excellent antibody response and a low rate of adverse reactions (1-3). Antibody response is approximately 10 times higher with HDCS vaccine than with DEV (4). Conversion rates are also higher. One study reported an antibody titer to rabies, by the rapid fluorescent focus inhibition technique, in 100% of 775 persons and, by the mouse neutralization technique, in 98.4% of 634 persons receiving 3 doses of W-HDCS. It also showed that 60 to 90% of persons who received 1 to 2 doses developed a detectable antibody titer (5). On the other hand, only 80 to 90% of persons receiving from 16 to 23 doses of DEV develop a rabies antibody titer (6).

Reactions to HDCS vaccines have been minimal. No serious anaphylactic, neuroparalytic, or systemic reactions have been reported. Mild local and systemic reactions, however, have been noted. CDC has accumulated data on 186 persons treated for pre-exposure and post-exposure rabies prophylaxis with W-HDCS by primary-care physicians in the field. The vaccine was well tolerated, and no treatment was discontinued because of an adverse reaction. Of the recipients, 28% reported local reactions, 4.8% fever, 4.8% nausea, and lower percentages a variety of other mild reactions; 61% reported no reactions. With few exceptions the symptoms persisted for less than 48 hours after the vaccine was given.

There have been a number of studies on the efficacy of post-exposure antirabies treatment with HDCS vaccine. In Iran, 45 persons who had been bitten by proven rabid animals were protected from clinical rabies by use of M-HDCS and antirabies serum (7). In Germany, 31 persons who had been bitten by proven rabid animals were treated with M-HDCS or B-HDCS (18 of 31 also received human rabies immune globulin HRIG), and all 31 were protected from clinical rabies (8). Efficacy data for W-HDCS are still being accumulated, but the excellent antibody response and the high antigenic value strongly suggest that it will be comparable with M-HDCS and B-HDCS and more protective against rabies than DEV.

The World Health Organization recommends that post-exposure treatment with M-HDCS or B-HDCS consist of 6 doses of vaccine. On the first day of treatment, 1 dose of vaccine should be given along with anti-rabies serum or globulin. The other 5 doses of vaccine should be administered in single doses 3, 7, 14, 30, and 90 days later.

Since some studies *(8,9)* have shown that antibodies persist for 1 year after a primary series without a booster dose on day 90, CDC is conducting trials of post-exposure treatment with 5 doses of W-HDCS given intramuscularly (single doses given on the first day of treatment and 3, 7, 14, and 28 days later, plus HRIG on the first day of treatment). Antibody response will then be assessed.

Requests for the vaccine should be made to CDC at (404) 633-3311, Ext. 3727.

Reported by Respiratory Special Pathogens Br, Viral Diseases Div, Bur of Epidemiology, CDC.

References
1. Wiktor TJ, Plotkin SA, Koprowski H: Development and clinical trials of the new human rabies vaccine of tissue culture (human diploid cell) origin. Dev Biol Stand 40:3-9, 1977
2. Kuwert EK, Marcus I, Hoher PG: Neutralizing and complement fixing antibody responses to pre- and post-exposure vaccines to a rabies vaccine produced in human diploid cells. J Biol Stand 4:249-262, 1976
3. Plotkin SA, Wiktor TJ, Koprowski H, et al: Immunization schedules for the new human diploid cell vaccine against rabies. Am J Epidemiol 102:75-78, 1976
4. Hafkin B, Hattwick MAW, Smith JS: A comparison of a WI-38 vaccine and duck embryo vaccine for pre-exposure rabies prophylaxis. Am J Epidemiol 107:439-443, 1978
5. Tint H, Rosanoff EI: Clinical response to T(n)BP-disrupted HDCS (WI-38) rabies vaccine. Dev Biol Stand 37:287-289, 1976
6. Hattwick MAW, Rubin RH, Music S, et al: Post-exposure rabies prophylaxis with human rabies immune globulin. JAMA 229:407-410, 1974
7. Bahmanyar M, Fayaz A, Nour-Salehis, et al: Successful protection of humans exposed to rabies infection: Post-exposure treatment with the new human diploid cell rabies vaccine and antirabies serum. JAMA 236:2751-2754, 1976
8. Kuwert EK, Marcus I, Werner J, et al: Post-exposure use of human diploid cell culture rabies vaccine. Dev Biol Stand 37:273-286, 1977
9. Plotkin SA, Wiktor TJ: Rabies vaccination. Annu Rev Med 29:583-591, 1978

MMWR 28:46 (2/2/79)

Use of New Rabies Vaccine Restricted

CDC has had to restrict its distribution of Wyeth Laboratories human diploid cell strain rabies vaccine (W-HDCS) to only those persons needing rabies treatment who have life-threatening reactions to the duck embryo vaccine (DEV) or who have not responded with an adequate antibody titer to DEV.

CDC has been distributing W-HDCS for human treatment on an experimental basis under several protocols for the past 4 years. Last summer *(1,2)*, it extended the use of the vaccine to persons who had been bitten by a proven-rabid animal regardless of that person's sensitivity to DEV.

Unfortunately, licensure of the vaccine has now been delayed. Because the supply of W-HDCS is limited and at its present rate of use it would be exhausted before licensure, treatment with W-HDCS must now be restricted to those persons unable to take DEV or unresponsive to DEV.

Reported by the Respiratory and Special Pathogens Br, Viral Diseases Div, Bur of Epidemiology, CDC.

References
1. MMWR 27:333, 1978
2. MMWR 27:413, 1978

CHAPTER 25

Influenza

MMWR 27:507 (12/15/78)

Influenza — New York, California

New York City: An influenza A(H1N1) isolate has been reported from a *13*-year-old individual in New York City, who was hospitalized on November 7 with mild pneumonia that developed 3 days after the onset of an upper respiratory tract infection.

California: Additional isolates of H1N1 influenza A have been obtained in California. The first of these was from a 13-year-old male in Los Angeles, whose illness began on November 17. Three additional isolates were obtained from siblings aged 9, 11, and 12 living in Santa Barbara County. They became ill November 24 and 25. During late October to mid-November, several outbreaks of influenza-like illness were reported among persons less than 25 years old in Ventura and Santa Barbara Counties. By December 11, outbreaks of influenza-like illness had been reported in schools in many areas of the state, with absenteeism in some places reaching 50%.

An influenza isolate from a 22-year-old patient in Los Angeles, who developed an upper respiratory illness on November 18, has been identified as influenza type C by CDC.

Reported by J Cherry,MD, University of California at Los Angeles; Los Angeles County Health Dept; California Dept of Health Services; I Spigland, MD, Montefiore Hospital, New York City; JS Marr, MD, New York City Epidemiologist, Bur of Preventable Diseases; Immunization Div, Bur of State Services, and WHO Collaborating Center for Influenza, Bur of Laboratories, CDC.

Editorial Note: Influenza C is rarely isolated, possibly because the virus normally grows only in the amniotic cavity of embryonated hens' eggs, it agglutinates a restricted range of indicator red blood cells (e.g., chicken and human "O," but not guinea pig cells), and it elutes from red blood cells rapidly unless maintained at refrigerated temperatures throughout the hemagglutination test (*1,2*). On the basis of serologic surveys, the virus is believed to infect the majority of the population during childhood. Illness is probably less severe than that caused by most influenza A or B viruses, and it has not been recognized as a cause of epidemics in the United States. Little evidence of antigenic drift has been observed in influenza C viruses since the first isolate was obtained in 1947, and no subtypes have been defined. Because expanded surveillance programs in young persons may result in greater frequency of isolation of influenza C than in the past, this virus should be considered when identifying putative influenza-like agents that have been isolated in the amniotic cavity of embryonated eggs and do not appear to be current influenza A or B strains.

References
1. Dowdle WR, Noble GR, Kendal AP: Orthomyxovirus—influenza: Comparative diagnosis unifying concept, in Kurstak E, Kurstak C(eds): Comparative Diagnosis of Viral Diseases, Vol 1. New York, Academic Press, 1977, pp 489-491
2. Taylor RM: Studies on survival of influenza virus between epidemics and antigenic variants of the virus. Am J Public Health 39:171-178, 1949

MMWR 28:22 (1/19/79)

Guillain-Barré Syndrome

Surveillance, January-June 1978: After an association was demonstrated between Guillain-Barré syndrome (GBS) and vaccination with the A/New Jersey influenza vaccine (1), the usefulness of monitoring trends of GBS became apparent. In February-April 1978, with the cooperation of the American Academy of Neurology and the State and Territorial Epidemiologists, CDC asked members of the Academy to report GBS cases to the CDC; 1,990 neurologists agreed to participate in an ongoing surveillance program. Based on the membership roles of the Academy, it was estimated that this included approximately 50%-60% of the neurologists in private practice and academic settings who would be seeing patients with GBS. For the purpose of this surveillance, a case was defined as a patient with objective signs of muscle weakness diagnosed by a neurologist as GBS. The following is a summary of the preliminary findings on GBS for the first 6 months of 1978.*

From January 1 through June 30, 268 neurologists reported to CDC a total of 327 cases of GBS from 42 of the 50 states. Six of the patients (1.8%) had had GBS previously. The attack rate was significantly higher in males, who accounted for 56% of cases (p<.05), than females (Table 1), and a significant correlation was noted between advancing age and attack rate (p<.005).

TABLE 1. Age-adjusted attack rates for Guillain-Barré syndrome, by sex, United States January 1-June 30, 1978

Sex	Cases		Age-adjusted attack rate**
	Number reported	Percent	
Female	145	44	.26
Male	181	56	.35
Total	326*	100	

$\chi^2 = 5.6$, p<.05
*Not specified for 1 case
**Cases per 100,000 population per year, based on 1976 estimates

Ninety-one percent of patients were white, 8% black, and 1% Asian. The age-adjusted semiannual attack rate for whites was 0.15/100,000 population; this compared with 0.11/100,000 population for blacks, a difference which is not statistically significant. Two hundred thirty-two (71%) of the patients had an associated acute illness within 8 weeks before onset on GBS; 70% of these had fever, 82% had respiratory symptoms, and 31% had gastrointestinal symptoms.

Follow-up on Guillain-Barré Syndrome and the 1976 National Influenza Immunization Program (NIIP): In early 1977, each state conducted an inventory of its unused A/New Jersey influenza vaccine. This enabled determination of the proportions of monovalent vaccine (containing only A/New Jersey/76 antigen) and bivalent vaccine (containing both A/New Jersey/76 and A/Victoria/75 antigens), by manufacturer, that were received by each state but not on hand for inventory. These proportions and the monthly reports of vaccine administered, in turn, enabled estimation of GBS attack rates by manufacturer and revealed that no single manufacturer's vaccine had a significantly different rate of GBS than the other manufacturers combined. There was also no significant difference in GBS attack rates between whole-virus and split-virus vaccines.

Based on a lot-specific inventory completed in June 1978 after vaccine was placed in centralized storage facilities, the net national distribution of vaccine was calculated by subtracting inventory data for each lot from the total doses of each lot distributed.

*A copy of the report from which some of these data were derived is available from: CDC, Attention: Bureau of Epidemiology, Viral Diseases Division.

Although these net distributions included numbers of doses lost in shipment, wasted, or otherwise unaccounted for, they provided rough but the best available estimate of the number of doses of each lot of vaccine administered. One hundred seven (76%) of the total 141 lots used during the NIIP Program were known to be associated with at least 1 case of GBS within a 6-week period after vaccination. Of these, 91% were associated with between 1 and 6 cases. The maximum number of cases associated with any single lot within the period was 11. The distribution of the observed number of cases associated with lots grouped by 100,000 dose sizes was not significantly different from what would be expected based on the number of doses in each group and the rate of cases for all lots combined (.10>p>.05). When the rate of each of the 141 lots was compared statistically to the rate of the remaining lots combined, each of 3 lots among those with the highest attack rate differed from all the remaining lots with a relatively high degree of statistical significance ($\chi^2 > 7.92$). The lot with the most significant elevation ($\chi^2 = 9.52$) was associated with cases from Ohio only; there was an unexplained statistically significant lower attack rate associated with this lot's distribution outside Ohio when compared to the attack rate inside Ohio. When information provided by the Bureau of Biologics was used, the lot-specific attack rates did not correlate significantly with thimerosal concentration, protein concentration, formaldehyde concentration, potency, or endotoxin levels.

In June 1978 CDC convened an expert group to review and comment on these data relating to GBS cases and vaccine lots. The group concluded that there was no substantive evidence for any single lot or group of lots having any unusual or significant propensity to produce GBS beyond that which would be expected by normal biological variation. The statistically significant association between GBS and the A/New Jersey influenza vaccine, however, was reaffirmed.

Reported by the Viral Diseases Division, Bureau of Epidemiology, CDC.
Reference
1. MMWR 26:7, 1977

MMWR 28:231 (5/25/79)

Influenza Vaccine

INTRODUCTION

Influenza virus infections occur every year in the United States, but they vary greatly in incidence and geographic distribution. Infections may be asymptomatic, or they may produce a spectrum of manifestations, ranging from mild upper respiratory infection to pneumonia and death. Influenza viruses A and B are responsible for only a portion of all respiratory disease. However, they are unique in their ability to cause periodic widespread outbreaks of febrile respiratory disease in both adults and children. Influenza epidemics are frequently associated with deaths in excess of the number normally expected. During the period from 1968 to 1979, more than 150,000 excess deaths are estimated to have occurred during epidemics of influenza A in the United States.

Efforts to prevent or control influenza in the United States have been aimed at protecting those at greatest risk of serious illness or death. Observations during influenza epidemics have indicated that influenza-related deaths occur primarily among chronically ill adults and children and in older persons, especially those over age 65. Therefore, annual vaccination is recommended for these "high-risk" individuals.

Influenza A viruses can be classified into subtypes on the basis of 2 antigens: hemagglutinin (H) and neuraminidase (N). Four subtypes of hemagglutinin (HO-H3) and 2 subtypes of neuraminidase (N1, N2) are recognized among viruses causing widespread disease among humans. Immunity to these antigens reduces the likelihood of infection and reduces the severity of disease in infected persons. However, there may be sufficient antigenic variation within the same subtype over time (antigenic drift) that infection or immunization with 1 strain may not induce immunity to distantly related strains. As a consequence, the antigenic composition of the most current strains is considered in selecting the virus strain(s) to be included in the vaccine.

The predominant influenza strain in the United States during 1978-79 was A/Brazil/78—a variant of the H1N1 prototype A/USSR/77. This strain caused outbreaks in schools, colleges, and military bases, as had been the case with the prototype strain. People over 25 years of age generally were not affected, presumably because of previous infection with antigenically related strains that had circulated throughout the world in the early 1950s. Strains of the subtype H3N2 were not isolated in the United States, but other countries reported the isolation of both H1N1 and H3N2 strains. Since it is uncertain which strain will predominate in the future, continued circulation of strains related to A/Texas/77 (H3N2) and A/Brazil/78 (H1N1) must be anticipated.

Outbreaks caused by influenza B viruses occur less frequently than influenza A epidemics, but influenza B infection can also cause serious illness or death. Influenza B viruses have shown much more antigenic stability than influenza A viruses. Strains of influenza B that were isolated in 1978 and 1979 in the United States and elsewhere resembled the B/Hong Kong/5/72 virus.

INFLUENZA VIRUS VACCINE FOR 1979-80

Influenza vaccine for 1979-80* will consist of inactivated trivalent preparations of antigens representative of influenza viruses expected to be prevalent: A/Brazil/78 (H1N1), A/Texas/77 (H3N2), and B/Hong Kong/72. The formulation will contain 7 micrograms of hemagglutinin of each antigen in each 0.5 ml dose. Persons 27 years and older will require only 1 dose. Because of lack of previous contact with H1N1 strains, persons less than 27 who did not receive at least 1 dose of the 1978-79 trivalent vaccine will require 2 doses of the 1979-80 vaccine. Those who received the 1978-79 vaccine will require only 1 dose. The vaccine will be available as whole virion (whole-virus) and subviron (split-virus) preparations. Based on past data, split-virus vaccines have been associated with somewhat fewer side effects than whole-virus vaccines in children. Thus, only split-virus vaccines are recommended for persons less than 13 years of age. The vaccines prepared for the 1978-79 respiratory disease season contained A/USSR/77 as the H1N1 component. Because of the antigenic similarities between the A/USSR/77 and the A/Brazil/78 strains, the stocks of vaccine remaining from last year may be used, until the expiration date, according to the instructions on the package insert.

VACCINE USAGE

General Recommendations

Annual vaccination is strongly recommended for all individuals at increased risk of adverse consequences from infections of the lower respiratory tract. Conditions predisposing to such risk include (1) acquired or congential heart disease associated with altered circulatory dynamics, actual or potential (for example, mitral stenosis, congestive heart failure, or pulmonary vascular overload); (2) any chronic disorder with compromised pulmonary function, such as chronic obstructive pulmonary disease, bronchiectasis, tuberculosis, severe asthma, cystic fibrosis, neuromuscular and orthopedic disorders with impaired ventilation, and residual pulmonary dysplasia following the neonatal respiratory

---

*Official name: Influenza Virus Vaccine, Trivalent.

TABLE 1. Influenza vaccine* dosage, by age, 1979-80

Age group	Product	Dosage (ml)	Number of doses
27 years and older	whole virion (whole virus) or subvirion (split virus)	0.5	1
13-26 years	whole virion (whole virus) or subvirion (split virus)	0.5	2**
3-12 years	subvirion (split virus)	0.5	2**
6-35 months***	subvirion (split virus)	0.25	2**

   * Contains 7 µg each of A/Brazil/78, A/Texas/77, B/Hong Kong/72 hemagglutinin antigens in each 0.5 ml.
  ** 4 weeks or more between doses; both doses essential for good protection, unless the individual received at least 1 dose of 1978-79 vaccine.
*** Based on limited data. Since the likelihood of febrile convulsions is greater in this age group, special care should be taken in weighing relative risks and benefits.

distress syndrome; (3) chronic renal disease with azotemia or the nephrotic syndrome; (4) diabetes mellitus and other metabolic diseases with increased susceptibility to infection; (5) chronic, severe anemia, such as sickle cell disease; and (6) conditions which compromise the immune mechanism, including certain malignancies and immunosuppressive therapy.

Vaccination is also recommended for older persons, particularly those over age 65, because excess mortality in influenza outbreaks occurs in this age group.

In considering vaccination of persons who provide essential community services or who may be at increased risk of exposure, such as medical care personnel, the inherent benefits, risks, and cost of vaccination should be taken into account.

Table 1 summarizes vaccine and dosage recommendations by age group for 1979-80.

Use in Pregnancy

Although the issue has been much discussed, only in the pandemics of 1918-19 and 1957-58 has strong evidence appeared relating influenza infections with increased maternal mortality. Although several studies have reported an increased risk of congenital malformations and childhood leukemia among children born to women who had influenza infection during pregnancy, other studies have not shown an increased risk; the issue is not settled.

Physicians prudently limit prescription of drugs and biologics for pregnant women. However, no evidence has been presented to suggest that influenza vaccination of pregnant women poses any special maternal or fetal risk. Furthermore, because influenza vaccine is an inactivated viral preparation, it does not share the theoretical risks that impel caution in the use of live virus vaccines. Taking the above uncertainites into account, physicians should evaluate pregnant women for influenza immunization according to the same criteria applied to other persons. (See VACCINE USAGE—General Recommendations.)

SIDE EFFECTS AND ADVERSE REACTIONS

Recent influenza virus vaccines have been associated with few side effects. Local reactions, consisting of redness and induration at the site of injection lasting 1 or 2 days, have been observed in less than one-third of vaccinees. Three types of systemic reactions to influenza vaccines have been described.

1. Fever, malaise, myalgia, and other systemic symptoms of toxicity, although infrequent, occur more often in children and others who have had no experience with influenza viruses containing the vaccine antigen(s). These reactions, which begin 6-12 hours after vaccination and persist 1-2 days, are usually attributed to the influenza virus itself (even though it is inactivated) and constitute most of the side effects of influenza vaccination.

2. Immediate—presumably allergic—responses, such as flare and wheal or various respiratory expressions of hypersensitivity occur extremely rarely after influenza vaccination. They probably derive from sensitivity to some vaccine component, most likely residual egg protein. Although current influenza vaccines contain only a small quantity of egg protein, on rare occasions they can provoke hypersensitivity reactions. Individuals with anaphylactic hypersensitivity to eggs should not be given influenza vaccine. This would include persons who, upon ingestion of eggs, develop swelling of the lips or tongue or who experience acute respiratory distress or collapse.

3. Guillain-Barré syndrome (GBS) is an uncommon illness characterized by ascending paralysis which is usually self-limited and reversible. Though most persons with GBS recover without residual weakness, approximately 5% of cases are fatal. Before 1976, no association of GBS with influenza vaccination was recognized. That year, however, GBS appeared in excess frequency among persons who had received the A/New Jersey/76 influenza vaccine. For the 10 weeks following vaccination the excess risk was found to be approximately 10 cases of GBS for every million persons vaccinated—an incidence 5-6 times higher than that in unvaccinated persons. Younger persons (under 25 years) had a lower relative risk than others and also had a lower case-fatality rate. Preliminary analysis of data from GBS surveillance during the 1978-79 influenza season suggests that, in contrast to the 1976 situation, the risk of GBS in recipients of the 1978-79 vaccine was not significantly higher than that in non-vaccinees. Nonetheless, persons who receive influenza vaccine should be made aware of this possible risk as compared with the risk of influenza and its complications.

SELECTED BIBLIOGRAPHY

Clinical studies on influenza vaccines—1976. (A conference held at the National Institutes of Health, Bethesda, Maryland, January 20-21, 1977.) J Infect Dis 136 (Suppl): S345-S742, 1977

Dowdle WR, Coleman MT, Gregg MB: Natural history of influenza type A in the United States, 1957-1972. Prog Med Virol 17:91-135, 1974

Eickhoff TC: Immunization against influenza: Rationale and recommendations. J Infect Dis 123: 446-454, 1971

Kilbourne ED (ed): The Influenza Viruses and Influenza. New York, Academic Press, 1975

Leneman F: The Guillain-Barre syndrome. Arch Intern Med 118:139-144, 1966

Parkman PD, Galasso GH, Top FH, Noble GR: Summary of clinical trials of influenza vaccines. J Infect Dis 134:100-107, 1976

Wright PF, Dolin R, LaMontagne JR: Summary of clinical trials of influenza vaccines II. J Infect Dis 134:633-638, 1976

MMWR 27 (A.S., 1978): 89

PNEUMONIA-INFLUENZA — Reported Deaths in 121* Selected Cities by Week, United States, September 1970— June 1979

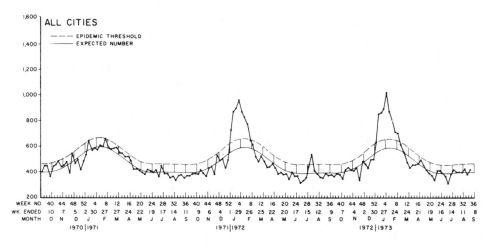

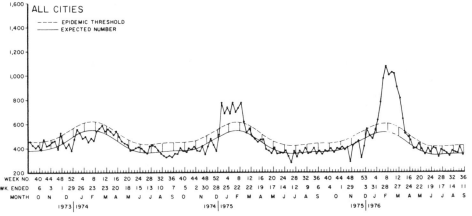

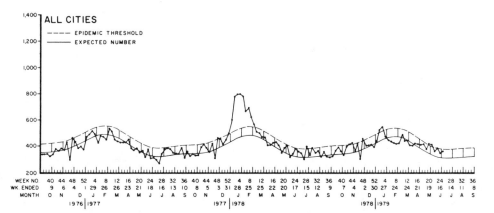

*117 Cities, September 1978— June 1979.

Pneumonia-Influenza

The predominant influenza strain in the United States during 1978-79 was A/Brazil/78, a variant of the H1N1 prototype A/USSR/77. This strain caused outbreaks in schools, colleges, and military bases, as had been the case with the prototype strain. People over 25 years of age generally were not affected, presumably because of previous infection with antigenically related strains that had circulated throughout the world in the early 1950s. Therefore, the elderly were spared and increased influenza-associated mortality was not observed. Influenza B viruses resembling the B/Hong Kong/72 strain were isolated from a small number of outbreaks in this country. Strains of the subtype H3N2 were not isolated in the United States during 1978-79, but other countries reported the isolation of both H1N1 and H3N2 strains.

During the 1978-79 influenza season, epidemics of influenza A (H1N1) that first occurred in California and in several other western states in December were preceded by virus isolations from sporadic cases or localized outbreaks in Texas and Puerto Rico in October. Reported activity decreased during the Christmas holidays, then spread to other parts of the country in early 1979. A few localized outbreaks of influenza B occurred late in the spring.

CHAPTER 26

Parainfluenza and RSV Infections

MMWR 27:475 (12/1/78)

Parainfluenza Outbreaks in Extended-Care Facilities — United States

Since October 1977, 4 outbreaks of respiratory illness caused by parainfluenza (PI) viruses in extended-care facilities have been reported to CDC.

Alabama: In October and November 1977, a 125-bed nursing home reported respiratory illness characterized by fever and cough in 28 residents and 21 employees. Eight residents were hospitalized with pneumonia; 3 of these died, but the role of infections in their deaths could not be ascertained. With fever and respiratory symptoms used as diagnostic criteria, the attack rates for residents and employees were 22.4% and 28.2%, respectively. Employees having direct patient contact had a 35% attack rate while those without patient contact had an 11% attack rate, suggesting person-to-person spread. Elevated titers to PI-type 3 virus were found in 8 out of 9 (89%) of the residents and 2 of 2 employees. No intrinsic host-susceptibility factors were found. The outbreak abated spontaneously.

California: Forty-six cases of a febrile illness occurred in residents of a state mental hospital from May 1 through July 19, 1978. The illness was marked by fever, cough, rhinorrhea, and pharyngitis. Eight cases developed pneumonia, and 1 case died after a complicated clinical course.

The majority of patients resided in 2 of the 34 housing units at the hospital. The median age was 28 (range 15-63 years); 17 were females, 29 males. The attack rate in these 2 units was 56% (36/64). PI-3 virus was isolated from 1 of 8 throat cultures. Paired serum specimens showed a diagnostic rise to PI-3 in 11/30 patients (37%) and to PI-1 in 5/30 (17%). Single high titers were present in 17 (57%) and 21 (70%), respectively. Diagnostic titers to *Mycoplasma pneumoniae* occurred in 7 of 31 patients (23%). Fifteen employees from the 2 housing units reported similar illness without complication. No serology was performed.

New York: In April 1978, a nursing home reported 11 hospitalized cases of a respiratory illness with 1 associated death. The illness was characterized by pneumonia or fever of ⩾101 F. The patients ranged in age from 65 to 102 years; 72.7% were women. There was no increase in respiratory illness identified among the attending staff. Eight of 8 serum specimens had persistently high titers to PI-3 virus.

Oregon: A 240-resident retirement condominium was investigated for respiratory illness in February and March 1978. Twenty-three people reported 1 or more influenza-like symptoms, and 5 had illness marked by fever, cough, sputum production, coryza, and sore throat. PI-3 was isolated from a throat swab from the index patient; he and 4 other patients had elevated convalescent serologic titers to PI-3. In addition, 2 patients had elevated PI-1 titers, and 2 patients had elevated influenza A titers, suggesting multiple causes for the outbreak. All 5 patients knew each other, and nearly all residents ate in common dining rooms.

Reported by M Dale, MD, FS Wolf, MD, State Epidemiologist, Alabama Dept of Public Health; J Chin, MD, State Epidemiologist, California Dept of Health Services; JS Marr, MD, New York City Epidemiologist, Bur of Preventable Diseases, S Millian, PhD, New York City Dept of Health; JA Googins, MD, State Epidemiologist, Oregon Dept of Human Resources; Bacterial Diseases Div, Field Services Div, and Viral Diseases Div, Bur of Epidemiology, CDC.

Editorial Note: Parainfluenza types 1, 2, and 3 are the most frequent causes of upper and lower respiratory disease attributed to the 4 parainfluenza virus types. Serologic surveys have indicated that infection, usually mild, is common in children; 59%-100% have had infection by age 5 (1). However, immunity is not complete, reinfections commonly occur, and the illness has been recognized in adults (2,3). Attack rates are similar regardless of sex, race, and occupation. Disease distribution is worldwide. Transmission is from person to person. PI-1 and PI-2 viruses cause small outbreaks at regular or irregular intervals. PI-3 virus is endemic, causing illness in all seasons of the year, but most frequently during the winter (4,5). Vaccination and other control measures have not clearly shown benefit.

Diagnosis is made by isolation of the organism or by noting a 4-fold rise in the hemagglutination inhibition titer between acute and convalescent serum specimens. Since some cross-reactivity occurs between the antigens of PI types 1, 2, and 3, which can produce heterologous antibody responses, care must be exercised in interpreting serologic data.

Three of these 4 outbreaks are unusual in that they occurred in elderly patients in nursing homes and that pneumonia was prominent. Whether the pneumonia cases were bacterial or viral was not established. Except for several deaths, clinical manifestations were similar to those usually seen in parainfluenza infections. Case-clustering in living units and among contacts in common dining areas, and the illness in employees with patient-care responsibility suggest person-to-person spread. Isolation of individuals from the dining area may have played a role in interrupting one of the outbreaks. These 4 outbreaks suggest that parainfluenza infection should be considered in the differential diagnosis of febrile acute respiratory disease in chronic-care institutions.

References
1. Glezin WP, Loda FA, Denny FW: The parainfluenza viruses, in Evans AS (ed): Viral Infections of Humans. New York, Plenum Medical Book Co., 1976, pp 337-349
2. Monto AS: The Tecumseh study of respiratory illness. V. Patterns of infection with the parainfluenza viruses. Am J Epidemiol 97:338-348, 1973
3. Gross PA, Green RH, McCraeCurnen MG: Persistent infection with parainfluenza type 3 virus in man. Am Rev Respir Dis 108:894-898, 1973
4. Paramyxoviridae, in Fenner FJ, White DO (eds): Medical Virology. 2nd ed. New York, Academic Press, 1976, pp 398-400
5. Cooney MK, Fox JP, Hall CE: The Seattle virus watch. VI. Observations of infections with and illness due to parainfluenza, mumps, respiratory syncitial viruses, and *Mycoplasma pneumoniae*. Am J Epidemiol 101:532-561, 1975

MMWR 28:369 (8/10/79)

Parainfluenza Virus Isolations — Alabama

Investigations of outbreaks of influenza-like illness in Alabama during the first 2 months of 1979 indicated that some of the illnesses were associated with infection by parainfluenza, type 3 virus. The illnesses for the most part were confined to school and university students and resulted in a marked increase in absenteeism.

In the period January 11-February 16, 151 oropharyngeal, nasopharyngeal, or throat gargle specimens from 123 patients with an influenza-like illness were forwarded for virus isolation to the Public Health Laboratory, Virology Section, in Birmingham, Alabama, or to CDC. Viruses were recovered from 36 patients and included parainfluenza, type 3; influenza A/Brazil/78; parainfluenza, type 2; and adenovirus, type 4 (Table 3). Parainfluenza, type 3 isolates were from patients widely distributed throughout the state, whereas the influenza A/Brazil/78 isolations were confined to patients in 2 counties. Six of the isolates—3 influenza A/Brazil/78; 2 parainfluenza, type 3; and 1 adenovirus, type 4—were from a group of 23 students from 1 school that had had approximately 30% absenteeism. Seven other isolates—including 5 parainfluenza, type 3, and 2 influenza A/Brazil/78 viruses—were associated with an influenza-like outbreak among recruits at a U.S. Army training facility in Alabama.

Symptoms of illness associated with parainfluenza, type 3 infections were reported to the laboratory for 27 of the 123 patients for whom specimens were submitted. These symptoms included fever (in 14 cases), upper respiratory infection (8), sore throat (7), neurological symptoms (6), pneumonia (5), and gastrointestinal illness (4). The patients, 10 males and 17 females, ranged in age from 4 days old to 70 years; the majority (56%) were between 10 and 23 years old. In 6 instances, the virus was recovered from infants, ages 3 months or less. The age of 2 patients was not known. One fatality was reported, a female infant, age 2 months.

Convalescent serum was obtained from 1 person from whom parainfluenza, type 3 virus had been isolated, and the neutralization test performed was compatible with the virus isolation (titer of 1:32).

Reported by DE Macquigg, MD, Lexington, Alabama; J Dunkin, RN, HC Woodworth, MD, Northwest Alabama Health District; WJ Alexander, MD, JR Holmes, Jefferson County Health Dept; RJ Atkins, J Bynum, TJ Chester, MD, MPH, State Epidemiologist, B Edwards, MS, C Jennings, JL Holston, DrPH, J McCall, C Sullivan, Alabama Dept of Public Health; Respiratory Virology Br, Virology Div, Bur of Laboratories, Field Services Div, Viral Diseases Div, Bur of Epidemiology, CDC.

Editorial Note: Although parainfluenza infections of young children are usually associated with symptoms of croup, such symptoms were not reported in this outbreak—a finding that demonstrates the value of obtaining viral cultures to establish the etiology of febrile acute respiratory illness. Parainfluenza type 3 is an endemic virus that can produce disease ranging from asymptomatic infection to pneumonia. Types 1 and 2 parainfluenza occur sporadically in sharper outbreaks (*1*).

As would be expected, the majority of isolates in this outbreak came from the population less than 23 years old. Isolates were obtained, however, from young adults and from

TABLE 3. Virus isolation from specimens submitted on 123 patients with influenza-like illness, Alabama, January 11-February 16, 1979

Virus	Patients	Percent
Parainfluenza, type 3	27	22.0
Influenza A/Brazil/78	7	5.7
Parainfluenza, type 2	1	0.8
Adenovirus, type 4	1	0.8
TOTAL	36	29.3

2 elderly persons age 64 and 70. Parainfluenza reinfection with illness in persons over 20 years of age has been recognized (*2,3*), and sharp outbreaks of illness occasionally associated with increased mortality have been described in elderly nursing-home residents (*4-6*). The possible availability in the future of an effective vaccine for parainfluenza

infections underscores the importance of studying the epidemiology of these illnesses, particularly in the elderly, among whom their impact may be unappreciated.

References
1. Jackson GG, Muldoon RL (eds): Virus Causing Common Respiratory Infections in Man. Chicago, University of Chicago Press, 1975, pp 51-93
2. Wenzel RP, McCormick DP, Beam Jr WE: Parainfluenza pneumonia in adults. JAMA 221:294-295, 1972
3. Bloom HH, Johnson KM, Jacobsen R, Chanock RM: Recovery of parainfluenza viruses from adults with upper respiratory illnesses. Am J Hyg 74:50-59, 1961
4. Knight V (ed): Viral and Mycoplasmal Infections of the Respiratory Tract. Philadelphia, Lea and Febriger, 1973, p 128
5. MMWR 27:198, 1978
6. MMWR 27:475, 1978

MMWR 27:260 (7/28/78)

Nosocomial Respiratory Syncytial Virus Infections in an Intensive Care Nursery — California

An outbreak of upper respiratory infection and pneumonia involving 9 infants and caused by respiratory syncytial virus (RSV) occurred in a 16-bed intensive care nursery (ICN) of a hospital and medical center in San Francisco, California, from February 25 through March 19, 1978 (Table 2).

On February 25, an 18-week-old premature infant with hyaline membrane disease and bronchopulmonary dysplasia developed fever with respiratory distress and had a convulsion. A nasopharyngeal viral culture taken then was subsequently positive for RSV. Two days later 2 other premature infants (aged 13 and 35 weeks) developed sneezing, cough, rhonchi, and rales. The 13-week-old was in isolation for a previously documented cytomegalovirus infection. Nasopharyngeal viral cultures from both of these infants were reported positive for RSV on March 2.

At that time the following procedures were instituted: (1) RSV fluorescent antibody (FA) screening and viral cultures were performed on nasopharyngeal swabs from all ICN patients; (2) all positive patients were isolated in a separate room; (3) strict handwashing, gowning, and gloving procedures were required before contact with all ICN patients (masking was not required); (4) certain nursing staff were assigned exclusively to infected infants; and (5) all nursing staff with upper respiratory symptoms were considered infected with RSV. If well enough to work, they were allowed to care only for already-infected infants.

On the basis of direct FA screening, 2 additional infants were found positive for RSV on March 2 and were isolated. One (patient 4, Table 2) had a collapsed right upper lobe; a culture was positive for RSV. The other (patient 5) had no respiratory symptoms; 2 of 3 FA studies were borderline-positive for RSV, and none of 8 viral cultures was positive.

FA screening was repeated March 6 on the remaining 11 patients in the unit, but no new cases were identified. The following day 2 patients, both aged 6 weeks, developed mild upper respiratory symptoms. Repeat FA testing was positive on both; cultures taken at this time subsequently grew RSV.

On March 19, a 6-day-old infant who had been in the ICN since birth developed nasal congestion. FA studies were negative, and he was discharged from the hospital 2 days later. Viral cultures taken before discharge were later positive for RSV.

One additional infant developed RSV infection in association with this outbreak. The child, born on February 28, remained in the newborn nursery, a room adjoining the ICN,

TABLE 2. Clinical data on 9 infants with nosocomial RSV infection, California, Feb. 25-March 19, 1978

Patient	Age (weeks)	Sex	Date of first symptom	FA results	Culture results	Interval between +FA and +culture (days)	Fever	Upper respiratory symptoms	Pneumonia	Severity of illness
1	18	M	2/25	+	+	N/A*	yes	no	yes	severe
2	13	F	2/27	+	+	N/A*	yes	no	yes	severe
3	35	M	2/24	N/D†	+	N/A	yes	yes	yes	moderate
4	3	M	2/28	+	+	8	yes	yes	yes	moderate
5	11	F	unknown	+	−	N/A	no	no	no	unknown
6	6	F	3/2	+	+	5	no	yes	no	mild
7	6	M	3/7	+	+	2	no	yes	no	mild
8	6 days	M	3/19	−	+	N/A	no	yes	no	mild
9**	2	F	3/10	+	+	5	no	yes	no	mild

*N/A = not applicable. Patients 1 and 2 had positive RSV cultures reported before FA screening was begun.
†N/D = not done
**This patient was not in the Intensive Care Nursery.

for 6 days because of neonatal hyperbilirubinemia. She was discharged on March 7 but was readmitted to another hospital ward on March 15 because of rhinorrhea and cough of 5 days' duration. FA studies and viral culture were both positive for RSV at the time of readmission. The child had had no direct contact with ICN babies during her first hospitalization. The nursing staffs of the intensive care and newborn nurseries are separate, but patients in both units are cared for by the same house staff members.

Routine viral screening of nursing and house staff members was not performed. However, from March 7-March 21 FA studies and viral cultures were performed on 2 pediatric house officers, 11 ICN nurses, 1 nursery X-ray technician, and 1 phlebotomist, who regularly bled patients in the ICN. All 15 reported upper respiratory illnesses with onset occurring from 1 to 13 days (mean 4.9 days) before viral testing. The RSV FA test was strongly positive in 1 nurse and weakly positive in 4 additional nurses and the phlebotomist. None of the adults was positive by culture, perhaps owing to the delay in obtaining cultures after onset of symptoms.

Reported by R Ballard, MD, WL Drew, MD, PhD, L Mintz, MD, R Roth, MD, S Sniderman, MD, Mount Zion Hospital and Medical Center, San Francisco; Respiratory Section, Respiratory and Special Pathogens Br, Viral Diseases Div, Bur of Epidemiology, CDC.

Editorial Note: Nosocomial RSV infections have been described in pediatric wards (1) and in newborn (2) and premature infant (3) nurseries. In these settings, transmission appears to occur primarily via the hands and clothing of staff members rather than by direct patient-to-patient contact or aerosol spread (1). Preventive measures such as handwashing, gowning and gloving, and isolation of infected children appear to be effective in reducing nosocomial spread (4).

Identification of RSV-infected patients by viral culture necessarily entails a delay of several days until culture results are known. The speed and sensitivity of viral isolation can be enhanced by direct bedside inoculation of tissue culture cells (5). This technique was utilized in the present outbreak and resulted in viral isolation within 3 to 8 days of culture (mean 4.9 days). The use of direct FA staining of nasopharyngeal smears, on the other hand, permitted identification of infected infants within hours of receipt of the specimen. This technique identified 7 of 8 culture-positive infants (87.5%). Direct fluorescent antibody staining was extremely useful in the rapid detection of RSV infection in infants and permitted prompt institution of specific infection-control measures.

References
1. Wenzel RP, Deal EC, Hendley JO: Hospital-acquired viral respiratory illness on a pediatric ward. Pediatrics 60:367-371, 1977
2. Neligan GA, Steiner H, Gardner PS, McQuillin J: Respiratory syncytial virus infection of the newborn. Br Med J 3:146-147, 1970
3. Berkovich S: Acute respiratory illness in the premature nursery associated with respiratory syncytial virus infections. Pediatrics 34:753-760, 1964
4. Hall CB, Geiman JM, Douglas RG Jr, Meagher MP: Control of nosocomial respiratory syncytial virus (RSV) infections. Pediatr Res 11:436, 1977
5. Hall CB, Douglas RG Jr: Clinically useful method for the isolation of respiratory syncytial virus. J Infect Dis 131:1-5, 1975

CHAPTER 27

Dengue

MMWR 27:304 (8/18/78)

Follow-up on Dengue — Puerto Rico, United States

Puerto Rico: There have been 8,413 suspected cases of dengue reported thus far in 1978 in Puerto Rico. This figure is markedly greater than that for the same time period in 1976 or 1977 (Table 4).

TABLE 4. Reported incidence of dengue-like illness, Puerto Rico, cumulative totals, 1976-1978

Year	Number of cases cumulative, week 31	Yearly
1976	266	412
1977	277	11,824
1978	8,413	--

Several hundred cases in the early months of 1978 were associated with the outbreak that began in 1977, but there was a sharp increase in reported cases beginning in May, indicating a new outbreak (Figure 1). Dengue-like disease has been reported in 1978 from all Puerto Rican municipios.

The largest number of cases was reported in June 1978 (3,883), following a period of heavy rain. During July there was little rain (less than 1 inch/week, average), and the number of reported cases fell to 2,418. The rainy season in Puerto Rico began the week of August 7.

Dengue virus type 1 was first isolated in Puerto Rico in December 1977 toward the end of that year's outbreak. Nearly all (97/103) confirmed dengue isolates in 1978 have been the type 1 strain. Type 3 dengue virus was the major strain isolated during the Puerto Rican outbreak of 1963-64. Type 2 prevailed from 1968 through the peak of the 1977 outbreak.

Although there have been no reported cases of dengue shock syndrome, to date, in the Caribbean, there have been reports of patients with minor hemorrhagic manifestations. In Puerto Rico there are at least 7 patients (age range: 6 weeks-63 years), with findings including one or more of the following hemorrhagic manifestations: positive tourniquet test, petechiae, epistaxis, hematuria, guaiac positive stool, and/or thrombocytopenia ($<$100,000/mm^3). Also, dengue virus has been isolated from at least 5 women during the first trimester of pregnancy. Follow-up on these patients and their offspring is pending.

FIGURE 1. Reported cases of dengue-like illness, by month, Puerto Rico, 1977-1978

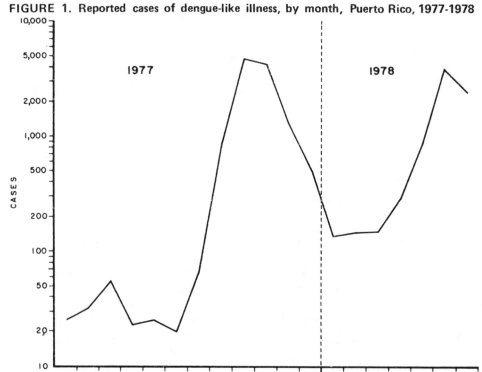

Larval indices for *Aedes aegypti,* the mosquito vector of dengue, are increased over those from previous years, indicating an increased vector population in the areas examined. The Breteau index* reported from the July 1978 larval survey in Ponce was 31, the highest in that area for that month since surveying began in 1973. However, in 2 areas with active programs to clean up the environment the index from January-July 1978 was 3–60% lower than the average of those areas from 1973-1977. By contrast, the index from 2 comparable areas without such programs was 30% higher than the 1973-1977 average. Malathion spraying efforts continue throughout Puerto Rico, particularly in the San Juan metropolitan area and towns reporting large numbers of suspected cases.

United States: Twenty-two cases of serologically confirmed dengue have been reported in 1978 in persons entering the United States from the Caribbean (20 cases) and Tahiti (2). Reports are from 12 different states. A secondary type serologic response (suggesting that the patients had had a previous Group B arboviral infection) was demonstrated in nearly half of the cases; there has been no report of hemorrhagic complications in any of the 22 patients. During 1977 there were a total of 70 confirmed cases of dengue imported into the United States.

Reported by J Chiriboga, MD, Environmental Health, Puerto Rico Dept of Health; San Juan Laboratories, Bur of Laboratories, Vector Biology and Control Div, Bur of Tropical Diseases, and Viral Diseases Div, Bur of Epidemiology, CDC.

Editorial Note: Dengue fever is a disease of interest throughout the Caribbean area, particularly as the peak of the rainy season approaches. Vector populations generally

---

* (The number of positive containers ÷ total number of houses) X 100

increase following heavy rainfall, and increased viral transmission may subsequently occur.

The large number of cases in 1978 may reflect the impact of the appearance of dengue virus type 1 infection upon a susceptible population. Also, other illnesses resembling dengue may be present, as the rate of serologic confirmation has decreased since May from 81% to 70% positive among specimens tested. During the 1977 outbreak many cases of influenza A were identified among specimens negative for dengue. Currently, the CDC San Juan Laboratory is testing negative specimens for measles and influenza antibodies.

U.S. travelers to areas with known dengue activity are encouraged to take measures to prevent mosquito bites and to report to their physicians any illness with fever, headache, myalgias, and rash with onset within 4 weeks of leaving those areas.

MMWR 27:476 (12/1/78)

Dengue Hemorrhagic Fever with Shock in an American Traveler

While visiting in India, a 7-year-old girl from Ohio developed dengue hemorrhagic fever with shock; she recovered. This is the first report to CDC of a case of dengue hemorrhagic fever (DHF) with shock in a U.S. citizen.

The child, who is of Indian descent, became ill with fever to 103 F (39.4 C) on August 7, 1978, while staying with her grandparents in Madras State, India. Two days after the onset of fever, she was seen by a physician who prescribed symptomatic medication. At that time she was noted to be anorectic, but there were no other clinical findings; her hemoglobin was 16.1 g/dl. Because of continuing fever, she was hospitalized on August 14 for observation and care. At that time she was noted to have hepatomegaly, but no jaundice or rash. Blood cultures were obtained, and intravenous fluids were started.

Twelve hours after admission she became restless, and no blood pressure was obtainable. She was noted to have petechiae on her arms and back. A single episode of hematemesis occurred, followed by several tarry stools. Her prothrombin time was 25 seconds (control, 18 seconds), and platelets were markedly reduced on smear. A transfusion of fresh whole blood (450 ml) and intensive supportive care, however, resulted in the gradual return of her blood pressure to normal values over the next 24 hours. The following day her hemoglobin was 17.1 g/dl, and no platelets were seen on smear. Her prothrombin time was 60 seconds (control, 20 seconds). Over the next 48 hours she improved markedly: the hepatomegaly disappeared, her hemoglobin count returned to normal, and platelets reappeared on smear. Her convalescence was uneventful except for 1 episode of hematemesis, which did not require a transfusion or additional supportive care. Serologic tests on the patient are summarized in Table 1.

Pertinent past medical history included a trip to India 3 years earlier during which time she had a 7-day history of febrile illness unaccompanied by rash or other abnormal physical findings.

Reported by M Rammohan, MD, Warren, Ohio; San Juan Laboratories, Bur of Laboratories, and Viral Diseases Div, Bur of Epidemiology, CDC.

Editorial Note: The patient's clinical history is compatible with classic grade IV DHF; grades III and IV DHF are synonymous with dengue shock syndrome (DSS) (Table 2).

CDC's serologic testing for dengue routinely includes measurement of hemagglutination-inhibition (HI) and sometimes complement-fixation (CF) antibodies to 3 or 4 dengue subtypes—D1, D2, D3, and D4—and to other non-dengue flaviviruses (Table 1). Usually, the HI antibodies rise early in the course of illness, and recent dengue infection is generally indicated by a ≥4-fold rise in HI titer. However, in this patient the diagnosis was made on the basis of demonstrated rises of CF antibodies to all 4 dengue serotypes. These results suggest that her illness was due to the dengue virus, but they do not meet CDC laboratory criteria for a secondary-type serologic response (i.e., broadly reactive antibodies to all dengue serotypes and to at least 1 other flavivirus, with a titer of ≥640 to at least 1 dengue type). These results are also not those typically seen with a first dengue infection; there is usually a more type-specific ≥4-fold titer rise with lesser titer rises to the other dengue serotypes and non-dengue flaviviruses. The documented rise is unlikely to be due to transfusion of antibody-containing blood early in the patient's

TABLE 1. Results of arboviral antibody screen in U.S. citizen with DSS, 1978

Serologic test	Agent (antigen)	Reciprocal antibody titers in serum samples		
		Mid-acute (day 15)	Convalescent (day 30)	Late convalescent (day 57)
Hemagglutination inhibition	dengue type 1	160	320	320
	dengue type 2	40	80	40
	dengue type 3	80	160	80
	yellow fever	80	160	80
	St. Louis encephalitis	10	20	20
	eastern equine encephalitis	<10	<10	<10
Complement fixation	dengue type 1	<8	32	64
	dengue type 2	<8	16	32
	dengue type 3	<8	128	256
	dengue type 4	<8	32	32

TABLE 2. The World Health Organization's clinical classification of dengue hemorrhagic fever (DHF) (1)

Grade	Clinical features	Laboratory findings
I	fever constitutional symptoms positive tourniquet test	hemoconcentration thrombocytopenia
II	grade I plus spontaneous bleeding (e.g., skin, gums, gastro-intestinal tract)	hemoconcentration thrombocytopenia
III	grade II plus circulatory failure agitation	hemoconcentration thrombocytopenia
IV	profound shock (blood pressure = 0)	hemoconcentration thrombocytopenia

*DSS = dengue shock syndrome

hospital course; such antibody would be expected to have declined significantly in the late convalescent serum.

Although this is the first case of DSS reported to CDC, 1 other case is known to have occurred in an American citizen—a 16-month-old Caucasian infant who developed fatal DSS while living in Thailand (2). Since 1967 the only cases of DHF documented in the literature that occurred in the Western Hemisphere were in outbreaks in Curacao (3) and Jamaica (4).

DHF is a serious problem in Southeast Asian children. Although classic dengue fever (a milder viral syndrome) has been documented in hundreds of Caucasian Americans and Europeans in Thailand (2), DHF is notably rare among these groups. There is no substantial evidence to support a genetic or nutritional explanation for this difference. Current theories explaining the cause of DHF/DSS include the following: 1) in a second dengue infection, the heterotypic antibody response predisposes one to have more severe disease; 2) with a first or second dengue infection, activation of complement is responsible for subsequent severe disease; and 3) virulence among dengue virus strains differs (a theory not currently well-accepted).

This patient is of Indian descent and had DSS without evidence of a prior infection. This may be a case of DSS with primary dengue infection, or it may represent a serologically unrecognizable secondary infection with primary exposure 3 years before in India.

References
1. World Health Organization: Technical Guides for Diagnosis, Treatment, Surveillance, Prevention and Control of Dengue Hemorrhagic Fever. Geneva, 1975
2. Russell PK, Chumdermpadetsuk S, Piyaratn P: A fatal case of dengue hemorrhagic fever in an American child. Pediatrics 40:804-807, 1967
3. van Der Sar A: An outbreak of dengue hemorrhagic fever on Curacao. Trop Geogr Med 25:119-129, 1973
4. Fraser HS, Wilson WA, Thomas EJ, et al: Dengue shock syndrome in Jamaica. Br Med J 1:893-894, 1978

MMWR 28:194 (5/4/79)

Dengue Type 4 — French Polynesia

During the first 3 months of 1979, an outbreak of dengue type 4 began in French Polynesia, the first recognized appearance of the type 4 virus outside Southeast Asia.

In January 1979, local physicians on Tahiti and Moorea reported an increased incidence of dengue and influenza. The same month, dengue virus type 4 was isolated, and influenza was identified serologically, thus confirming the presence of 2 concurrent outbreaks. Throughout February and March, surveillance was conducted; it consisted of daily telephone calls to all hospitals, physicians, and public health clinics on Tahiti and Moorea requesting the number of cases of dengue and influenza seen.

Reported cases peaked first on the western coast of Tahiti, south of Papeete, and then spread eastward along the northern coast. There were 6,778 reported cases of dengue on Tahiti (population, 97,100) and at least 471 cases on Moorea (population, 6,600) from January 1 through March 31, 1979. Although the overall incidence in this 3-month period was 6.98 per 100 persons on Tahiti, 2 areas had unusually high rates: Paea and Papara on the west coast (average cumulative incidence, 14.40 per 100) and Tiarei on the northeast coast, (12.81 per 100) (Figure 1). On Moorea the reported incidence was slightly over 7%. On Bora Bora the rate was 9.68 per 100 from mid-February through April 5.

There were less reported cases of influenza than of dengue. With the exception of a few reporting units (communes), the dates of onset and peaks in incidence for the 2 diseases were different. In another small group of communes, the incidence of 1 disease dropped as the other peaked, suggesting that the presence of 1 virus may have delayed the appearance of the other.

In this outbreak clinical dengue was characterized by fever, severe headache, retroorbital pain, myalgia, polyarthralgia, rash, and altered taste sensation. In addition, many

FIGURE 1. Reported incidence* of dengue per 100 inhabitants, by commune, Tahiti,
January 1-March 31, 1979

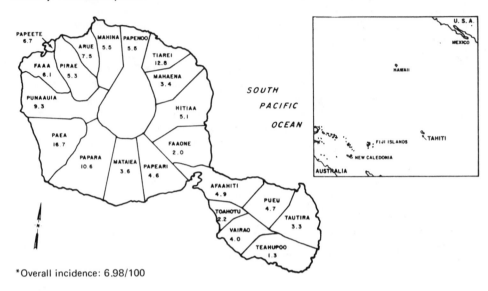

*Overall incidence: 6.98/100

patients reported nausea or cough. The illness was generally mild, and 77% of those questioned reported that the acute illness lasted 7 days or less. Approximately 35 persons were hospitalized in Papeete with suspected dengue. The majority of these were children, admitted because of fever, dehydration, or hemorrhage. One 3-year-old female, who had a single dengue titer of 1:640, died of a shock syndrome (without hemorrhage). Her illness was complicated by the possibility that she may have been treated before hospitalization with toxic local herbs; thus, the actual cause of death is not known.

Results of hemagglutination-inhibition tests in Papeete of 504 paired serum samples from patients suspected by their physicians to have dengue revealed 311 (62%) with confirmed dengue; 148 (29%) with probable dengue; 38 (8%) with confirmed influenza A; 2 (0.4%) with confirmed influenza B; and 5 (1%) with adenovirus infection.

As of May 2, the peak of the dengue epidemic has passed in Tahiti and Moorea; outbreaks continue to be reported in neighboring French Polynesian islands.

Reported by J Laigret, MD, F Parc, MD, Institut de Recherches Medicales, Louis Malarde, Papeete, Tahiti, French Polynesia; L Rosen, MD, DrPH, Pacific Research Unit, Research Corporation of University of Hawaii, Honolulu; Viral Diseases Div, Bur of Epidemiology, CDC.

Editorial Note: Dengue has caused sizeable outbreaks in the Western Hemisphere in recent years. On Tahiti, outbreaks were recorded in 1852, 1870, 1902, 1944 (type 1), 1964-1965 (type 3), 1969 (type 3), 1971 (type 2), and 1975 (type 1). The great majority of the island population probably has had at least 1 dengue infection before dengue 4 appeared this year, and dengue 1 is still endemic in the area. (There has been 1 confirmed isolate of dengue type 1 on Tahiti in 1979).

On Tahiti there are 2 species of Aedes of the subgenus Stegomyia; both (A. aegypti and A. polynesiensis) are known to transmit at least some types of dengue virus. Although the former is the most common vector worldwide, on Tahiti both species are considered capable of transmitting dengue virus to humans. A. aegypti breeds most commonly in artificial water containers, such as flower vases, old tires, and empty cans. This species was found only in the city of Papeete until recent years, but it has spread throughout Tahiti as the island population has expanded. *A. polynesiensis* breeds primarily in natural water reservoirs such as crabholes and tree trunks. It is found primarily in more rural areas, and until recently was, with few exceptions, the only 1 of the 2 species on Tahiti found outside Papeete.

The illness caused by the dengue 4 virus appears to be relatively mild. Perhaps the dengue 4 virus in Polynesia is inherently less virulent, or perhaps the population is partially protected against more severe disease because the 3 other dengue types have circulated there in the recent past.

It is not yet known which of the 2 *Aedes* species is the primary vector for dengue on Tahiti. Studies are underway to answer this question.

Travelers to Tahiti or other areas of French Polynesia are at increased risk of acquiring dengue both during and after an island outbreak (when the virus is almost certainly still circulating). The risk should be no higher than last year, however, when dengue 1 was circulating at low levels. All travelers to French Polynesia are advised to use commercially available mosquito repellant, whenever possible, and to report to their physicians any illness with fever and headache beginning within 2 weeks of leaving Polynesia.

MMWR 28:402 (8/31/79)

Dengue — Mexico

On August 2, 1979, the Mexican government notified the Pan American Health Organization that cases of dengue had been confirmed in persons in the states of Quintano Roo, Chiapas, and Oaxaca in southern Mexico. In the period January-June 1979, 524 cases of clinical dengue were reported; the majority of the tested cases were confirmed serologically in Mexico as dengue type 1. There have been no deaths reported.

Aedes aegypti, the mosquito vector for dengue, is found in these 3 states, as well as in Veracruz, Tabasco, and Campeche; in northeastern areas of Mexico; and along the Gulf Coast. *A. aegypti* are reportedly not found along Mexico's Pacific Coast.

Reported by Director General de Epidemiologia, Secretaria de Salubridad y Asistencia and Direccion General de Asuntos Internacionales, Mexico; Pan American Health Organization; Viral Diseases Div, Bur of Epidemiology, CDC.

Editorial Note: Dengue type 1 outbreaks occurred in 1978 throughout the Caribbean and in Central America. Although there has been no reported outbreak of dengue in the continental United States since 1934, the virus has spread northward during the past year and could possibly enter the United States at the southern border, where several of the Gulf states are known to have *A. aegypti*. These states have been notified of the recent confirmation of cases in Mexico.

Travelers to the small area in southern Mexico where dengue is occurring are advised to take precautions against mosquito bites, including using commercially-available mosquito repellant and wearing protective clothing, whenever possible.

CHAPTER 28

Hemorrhagic Fevers: Lassa, Ebola, and Rift Valley

MMWR 27:182 (5/26/78)

Suspected Lassa Fever — Washington, D.C.

Recently a suspected case of Lassa fever was reported from Washington, D.C. Laboratory studies subsequently failed to confirm this diagnosis.

The patient, a 42-year-old man who had lived for the past 7 years in Kenema, Sierra Leone, was hospitalized on May 16, 1978, at a hospital in Washington, D.C., with suspected Lassa fever. His wife had survived confirmed Lassa fever approximately 1 year ago, and his driver in Sierra Leone died of Lassa fever in March, 1978. The patient left Kenema on April 26, traveled to Freetown, Sierra Leone, and then flew to Paris, France; Zurich, Switzerland; and Colombo, Sri Lanka. He spent May 1-5 in Sri Lanka and, on May 4, developed cough, pharyngitis, and rhinitis, but no apparent fever. The patient's clinical illness did not change over the ensuing week. He departed from Colombo on the morning of May 6 and traveled to London where he stayed at his home 4 days. He left London for Washington, D.C., arriving on May 10. On May 15, he had a shaking chill, his sore throat worsened, and he felt febrile. On May 16, he was seen by a physician in Washington, D.C., who documented a temperature of 39 C (102 F) and a severe pharyngitis with plague-like lesions on the gums, tonsils, and posterior pharynx.

The same day the patient was placed in strict isolation in a hospital in Washington, D.C. The next day he developed headache and epigastric upset while being treated with Erythromycin* and chloroquine. Over the following 2 days, his condition improved; his oral lesions ulcerated and began to fade. Serum specimens collected on May 17, 18, 19, and 22 were negative for Lassa antibody by the indirect immunofluorescent antibody (IFA) test. The first 3 serum specimens were also tested for the presence of Lassa virus and were negative. No Lassa virus was found by immunofluorescence in conjuctival cells obtained on May 18. Thick and thin smears for malaria parasites were also negative.

Pending the results of these laboratory tests, the family members with whom the patient had been staying in Bethesda, Maryland, had been placed under daily surveillance with the assistance of the Montgomery County Health Department. Names of other contacts who were felt to be at high risk were also compiled. Following receipt of negative laboratory results, the patient was discharged from the hospital, and surveillance efforts were terminated. *Reported by MS Wolfe, MD; KH Acree, MD, State Epidemiologist, Maryland State Department of Health & Mental Hygiene; ME Levy, MD, District of Columbia Community Health & Hospital Administration; Special Pathogens Br, Virology Div, Bur of Laboratories, Field Services Div, and Viral Diseases Div, Bur of Epidemiology, CDC.*

Editorial Note: This case exemplifies the difficulty in making an early diagnosis of Lassa fever. The patient, who presented with a fever and sore throat and who has lived in an area highly endemic for the disease, would have to be considered suspect for Lassa fever on both clinical and epidemiologic grounds. The patient's mild clinical course is not inconsistent with what is now known about Lassa fever. The difficulty in precisely establishing the exact date of onset of illness for this patient made interpretation of serologic results difficult. Fluorescent antibody (FA) would be expected to be present 2 weeks into illness. If the patient's onset were May 4, serum collected on May 17-19 should have been FA-positive. On the other hand, if the onset had been May 15, then FA would probably not yet be detectable. Ruling out the diagnosis demanded both careful clinical follow-up of the patient as well as negative virologic studies, which required 3-5 days to complete.

Lassa fever does not now appear to be a highly communicable disease. Since the disease was first recognized in 1969, at least 5 patients with confirmed Lassa fever have traveled aboard commercial airliners, but no secondary cases among airline passengers have been detected. Nevertheless, until more is learned about the transmission of this disease, CDC recommends that confirmed or suspected Lassa fever patients not travel by commercial airliner.

Persons who have recently arrived from parts of the world known to be endemic for Lassa fever and who present with pharyngitis and fever should be considered suspected cases. Fever remains the most important clinical hallmark of the disease, and pharyngitis has been found in the majority of hospitalized patients. Such patients should be immediately hospitalized in strict isolation and the state

---

*Use of trade names is for identification only and does not constitute endorsement by the PHS, U.S. Dept. HEW.

health department and CDC alerted.   Specimens, includirg throat swab, clotted blood, and urine, should be collected by a physician wearing a mask and protective clothing. High-risk contacts (those known to have face-to-face, conversational, or other intimate exposure to the patient or exposure to his or her blood or other bodily secretions) should be identified. A decision to place such persons under surveillance needs to be made on an individual case basis. In most situations, active surveillance can await laboratory confirmation of the diagnosis.

Reference
1. Zweighaft RM, Fraser DW, Hattwick MAW, Winkler WG, Jordan WC, Alter M, Wolfe M, Wulff H, Johnson KM: Lassa fever: Response to an imported case. New Engl J Med 297:803-807, 1977

MMWR 28:557 (11/30/79)

Ebola Hemorrhagic Fever — Southern Sudan

An outbreak of Ebola hemorrhagic fever was recently reported in Southern Sudan (1). Surveillance measures rapidly instituted by the Sudanese Ministry of Health, with later cooperation from consultants from the World Health Organization, uncovered 69 suspected cases, including 27 deaths. All but 1 of these cases was investigated. Based on clinical, serologic, and epidemiologic data, the actual number of cases was determined to be 33; 22 were fatal. The outbreak was limited to the Yambio-Nzara District, the site where the first cases of this disease were identified in 1976 (Figure 1).

The present epidemic began in late July, when a 45-year-old man, who lived and worked in the Nzara area, had onset of fever, headache, sore throat, myalgia, vomiting, chest pain, and diarrhea. On August 2, he was admitted to the Nzara hospital, where he died in shock 3 days later after extensive gastrointestinal hemorrhage. A patient in the next bed, convalescing from an unrelated illness, and a visitor to another patient on that ward each developed a similar disease, 5 and 14 days, respectively, after the index patient died; these 2 patients also died. Two more cases occurred in hospital staff: a nurse and another hospital employee became ill after they came in contact with the index patient and other subsequently hospitalized patients. The last known case had onset on October 6.

Indirect fluorescent antibody tests on serum taken from suspected cases, performed in Sudan at the laboratory at Li-Rangu Sleeping Sickness Hospital, demonstrated the presence of Ebola virus antibody in the surviving patients and in some of those who eventually died. These results have been confirmed by CDC. Ebola virus has also been isolated from the blood of at least 1 of several patients from whom specimens were taken during the acute phase of the illness.

Preliminary evaluation of the epidemiologic and serologic data collected from this outbreak suggests that close physical contact in caring for patients or preparing bodies for burial resulted in a high risk of illness. Casual contact with patients did not appear to result in infection.

The source of infection for the index patient has not been determined. Ebola virus antibody was found in 3 of 51(6%) of asymptomatic contacts of hospitalized controls and in 11 of 152(7%) of asymptomatic workers in a large industrial and agricultural complex in Nzara. Both of these survey groups denied contact with cases during this epidemic, suggesting that the virus is endemic in the region.

FIGURE 1. Foci of outbreaks of Ebola hemorrhagic fever, Sudan and Zaire, 1976 and 1979

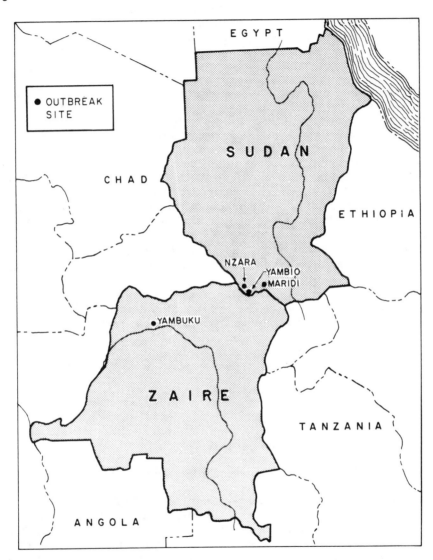

The following measures were recommended to control the present epidemic and to reduce the potential for future epidemics:

1. Because nosocomial transmission plays an important part in the amplification of the disease, rigid practice and supervision of isolation and barrier nursing techniques with suspected cases is essential. Hospital staff should be trained in decontamination techniques and in specific techniques for the use of simple isolation equipment, including gloves, gowns, caps, and masks.

2. A basic surveillance system to detect and report suspected cases of hemorrhagic fever should be implemented. The hospital and dispensary-based physicians and primary health workers should be asked to report any suspected cases of hemorrhagic fever to the surveillance team. In addition 2 or 3 public health officers should be assigned to regular bicycle routes to question families and local chiefs about persons who may be known to have fever and hemorrhagic symptoms.

Reported by the Regional Ministry of Health and Social Welfare, Juba, Sudan; the Sudanese Ministry of Health, Khartoum, Sudan; WHO Regional Office for the Eastern Mediterranean Region, Alexandria, Egypt; WHO Headquarters, Geneva, Switzerland; Virology Div, Bur of Laboratories, and Viral Diseases Div, Bur of Epidmiology, CDC.

Editorial Note: Two essential findings of this investigation need to be emphasized. First, the presence of Ebola antibody in persons unassociated with the current epidemic indicates that the disease is endemic and suggests that transmission occurs sporadically and possibly continuously from some natural source. Second, this outbreak, as with those that were well documented in 1976 in Maridi, Sudan, and in Yambuku, Zaire (2) (Figure 1), began with hospital spread which effectively amplified the transmission into the community. Because of cultural and social preferences, severely ill persons are rarely hospitalized. Thus, with infrequent, sporadic cases of hemorrhagic fever, transmission may be limited to a few family members living in compounds that are spread far apart in rural areas. Yet, it is the occasionally hospitalized, severely ill patient with hemorrhagic fever who may initiate transmission in the hospital; subsequently, the disease spreads throughout the community.

Continuous surveillance is essential in order to determine the frequency, location, and seasonal occurrence of sporadic cases, to recognize the potential threat of epidemic amplification of the virus, and to institute promptly hospital and community measures that will interrupt the chain of transmission.

References
1. World Health Organization: Viral haemorrhagic fever surveillance. Weekly Epidemiological Record 54:319, 1979
2. World Health Organization: Viral haemorrhagic fever — Zaire. Weekly Epidemiological Record 51:383, 1976

MMWR 28:607 (1/4/80)

Rift Valley Fever with Retinopathy — Canada

On January 29, 1979, a 41-year-old woman on safari in Mombasa, Kenya, became ill with fever, myalgia, dizziness, fatigue, and severe headache and neck regidity which lasted 2-3 days. The woman, a Canadian working in Jeddah, Saudi Arabia, had traveled from Jeddah with her son and husband on January 25 to Nairobi, Kenya, where they set out on safari to Mombasa. The family returned to Jeddah at the beginning of February, but the woman did not feel well and began to note a blurring and impairment of her vision early in February. Because her vision did not improve she was referred to an ophthalmologist in Jeddah on March 4; he diagnosed her illness as Rift Valley Fever (RVF).

The patient returned to Canada and was examined by an ophthalmologist and at the Tropical Disease Unit of Toronto General Hospital. Ophthalmologic examination on March 8 revealed normal external findings, motility, refraction, and intraocular pressures bilaterally. The right-eye vision was 20/20 and the media was clear; there was an opaque white exudative lesion 10° temporal to the fovea, 1.67mm in diameter. Angiography showed fluorescein leakage at the site of the lesion and retinal hemorrhage inferior to it. Adjacent vessels were normal, and there was no cellular reaction in the overlying vitreous. The left-eye vision was 20/600, and there was minimal aqueous flare, no cells, and clear vitreous. A white exudative lesion involved the left fovea and extended nasally. Fluorescein angiography revealed multiple foci of leakage within the lesion and retinal hemorrhage inferiorly. Adjacent vessels were patent.

Examination of serum specimens collected on March 8, March 18, and June 29 showed antibody titers of 1:320 by the hemagglutination inhibition test to RVF antigen. Plaque reduction neutralization tests done by the U.S. Army Medical Research Institute of Infectious Diseases showed neutralizing antibody titers of 1:5,120 and 1:10,240 (in the sera collected March 8 and 18), respectively. The patient had no detectable antibodies to many of the other arboviral antigens when tested by the hemagglutination inhibition and complement fixation tests; no antibodies were detected to cytomegalovirus and toxoplasmosis by complement fixation and immunofluorescence testing.

Reported by Canada Diseases Weekly Report, Vol. 5-42, October 20, 1979

Editorial Note: The serologic results, the clinical diagnosis based on ophthalmologic examination, and the history of travel and disease are all consistent with a diagnosis of RVF.

The recent epidemics in Egypt may serve as the foci from which RVF could spread to other areas. The extensive travel between this part of the world and North America emphasizes the possibility of importation of this disease. Because of the high concentration of virus in the blood during the viremia, humans can become a vehicle for spreading this virus into new geographic areas. The potential for spread is increased because of the large number of mosquito species reported as possible vectors of RVF virus.

MMWR 28:617 (1/4/80)

Rift Valley Fever Studies — Egypt

Rift Valley Fever (RVF) was first reported in Egypt in 1977. This outbreak which occurred primarily in the Sharqiya Governorate north of Cairo, continued from October to December of 1977 and included at least 317 human cases. Livestock were found to be infected, primarily sheep. A second outbreak was reported in Egypt, first in Sharqiya in March 1978 and later in other areas of the north and south in the Nile River Valley. A clinical history from over 200 of the cases revealed that most cases were characterized by hemorrhagic manifestations, including subcutaneous hemorrhage, epistaxis, hemoptysis, melena, and hematuria. A small percentage of cases showed ocular manifestations, primarily retinal degeneration, and a small percentage showed encephalitic disease.

Laboratory confirmation by virus isolation was obtained for 64 of the human cases. Serologic investigations revealed a seropositivity rate of 26% in areas where the disease was recognized and 9% in areas where no human cases were reported. The serologic surveys suggest the outbreak may have been far more extensive than indicated by the number of recognized cases. RVF virus was also isolated from several mosquito pools.

Reported by the World Health Organization in the Weekly Epidemiological Record, Vol. 54, No. 38, September 21, 1979.

CHAPTER 29

Yellow Fever

MMWR 27:520 (12/22/78)

Yellow Fever — The Gambia

An outbreak of yellow fever is in progress in the interior of The Gambia (Figure 1). Clinical cases have been observed since mid-November, and 78 deaths have been reported by the government of The Gambia (GOTG) through December 12. All cases have occurred in areas of the Gambia River basin upriver from the capital city, Banjul. The diagnosis of yellow fever is based on increased hemagglutination inhibition and neutralization antibody titers in convalescent serum specimens from survivors and on histologic morphology of liver specimens from fatal cases. Results of virus isolation studies from specimens are pending.

On December 12 the GOTG Ministry of Health requested emergency assistance from the U.S. Government, and the next day the U.S. Ambassador in Banjul issued a disaster declaration, paving the way for U.S. assistance in supplying vaccine, equipment, and technical aid to support the GOTG in mounting an extensive vaccination campaign. The World Health Organization and the U.S. Agency for International Development are assisting the GOTG in obtaining 500,000 doses of yellow fever vaccine, and CDC has provided equipment and technical assistance for vaccine administration.

FIGURE 1. The Gambia, West Africa

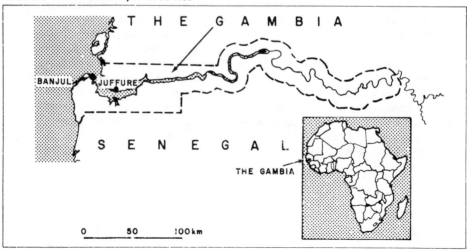

Reported by Office of Foreign Disaster Assistance, Agency for International Development; Bur of Smallpox Eradication, Viral Diseases Div, Bur of Epidemiology, CDC.
Editorial Note: Although small, The Gambia has become a major destination for U.S. travelers as the town of Juffure was the home of Kunta Kinte, protagonist of the novel "Roots." Yellow fever is endemic in West Africa, and although human cases are reported only infrequently, persons who plan to travel extensively in these countries should receive yellow fever vaccination. Senegal currently requires that all travelers over the age of 12 months entering the country possess a valid yellow fever vaccination certificate except those who arrive from a non-infected area and stay less than 2 weeks. In view of the present outbreak, CDC recommends that all travelers to The Gambia and to adjacent areas of Senegal be vaccinated.

MMWR 28:279 (6/22/79)

Yellow Fever — Trinidad

According to the Ministry of Health, Trinidad and Tobago, as of June 5, 1979, the island of Trinidad was no longer officially classified as infected with yellow fever. The date of onset of the last case on Trinidad was March 6, 1979.

The Ministry of Health has maintained an intensive surveillance program of yellow fever in humans and monkeys since November 1978, when a yellow fever outbreak was detected in forest monkeys. Eight persons with febrile illness were found to have had yellow fever infections; the infections were confirmed by isolation of yellow fever virus in 7 cases and by characteristic histopathologic changes in autopsy specimens in the remaining case. Six of the 8 persons with confirmed yellow fever recovered. None of the 8 patients had been immunized before onset of illness.

A mass immunization program has been conducted throughout the entire country. As of April 20, a total of 832,000 persons were immunized—75% of the entire population. Additionally, 200,000 persons in high-risk groups had already been immunized from 1972 to November 1978, when the mass immunization program began.

Surveillance of Trinidad's monkey population has shown no evidence of spread of the epizootic beyond the original focus of activity in forested areas of southern Trinidad. Measures to control *Aedes aegypti* and surveillance for suspected human yellow fever cases are continuing in all populated areas.

Reported by the Caribbean Epidemiology Centre in the CAREC Surveillance Report 5(4), April 1979; the Pan American Health Organization; Quarantine Div, and the Enteric and Neurotropic Viral Diseases Br, Viral Diseases Div, Bur of Epidemiology, CDC.
Editorial Note: Because of the apparent cessation of yellow fever activity in humans and monkeys, the high level of yellow fever immunization in the population, and the official removal of "yellow fever infected" status, the Public Health Service no longer recommends yellow fever vaccination for all U.S. travelers to Trinidad. Such vaccination continues to be recommended, however, for U.S. travelers who will visit the forested areas of Trinidad, where jungle yellow fever may remain endemic.

MMWR 28:439 (9/21/79)

Yellow Fever — Trinidad, Colombia

Trinidad: On September 11, the Ministry of Health, Trinidad and Tobago, officially notified the Pan American Health Organization and the World Health Organization (WHO) that an outbreak of jungle yellow fever had been confirmed in howler monkeys from the Mamural Forest of central Trinidad. In addition, 7 suspected human cases—all sylvatic—were under investigation.

A similar outbreak of jungle yellow fever in the Guayaguayare Forest of southeast Trinidad occurred in the fall of 1978 and spring of this year (*1-3*). As a result of that outbreak, more than 75% of the population of Trinidad was immunized in a mass immunization program in the spring of 1979.

Control measures for *Aedes aegypti* and surveillance for suspected human cases are continuing throughout the island.

The island of Tobago remains free of yellow fever infection.

Colombia: A recently reported outbreak of yellow fever (*4*) appears to be spreading north from Valledupar toward the more populated coastal areas. Several cases have been reported in Fundación and Ciénaga, about 40 miles east of Barranquilla on the coast. Health officials are vaccinating persons in the Fundación area and other coastal areas to the west. Although it has not been determined that the *A. aegypti* vector is involved in the outbreak, this species is known to be prevalent throughout the affected area.

Currently, the following areas of Colombia are officially included in those listed by WHO as being infected with jungle yellow fever: Caquetá Intendencia, Cesar Department, Magdalena Department, Meta Intendencia, Norte de Santander Department, Santander Department, and Vaupés Comisaria.

Reported by the Pan American Health Organization; Office of Foreign Disaster Assistance, U.S. Department of State; Quarantine Div, Viral Diseases Div, Bur of Epidemiology, CDC.

Editorial Note: Because of the official declaration that the island of Trinidad is infected with yellow fever, CDC now recommends yellow fever vaccination for all travelers to the island of Trinidad. There is no evidence of risk for visitors who limit their activities to urban areas, such as cruise ship passengers visiting Port of Spain. Nevertheless, even visitors with such limited travel in Trinidad may be subject to quarantine restrictions in other Caribbean and Central American ports of entry in view of Trinidad's "yellow fever infected" status.

In view of the current yellow fever activity in Colombia, all travelers to the northern coast of that country should be vaccinated against yellow fever. Travelers to other areas of Colombia listed as infected with yellow fever should be vaccinated, unless their activities are limited to urban areas.

References
1. MMWR 27:509, 1978
2. MMWR 28:72, 1979
3. MMWR 28:279, 1979
4. MMWR 28:371, 1979

CHAPTER 30

Hepatitis

MMWR 28:157 (4/13/79)

Non-A, Non-B Hepatitis Infection
Transmitted via a Needle — Washington

On November 27, 1978, the Epidemiology Section of the Washington Department of Social and Health Services was notified of a case of hepatitis in a nurse, possibly acquired by accidental inoculation of the virus by a needle. Laboratory studies on the nurse were consistent with non-A, non-B (NANB) hepatitis.

The patient whom the nurse was attending at the time of the accident was a 57-year-old woman, who was hospitalized because of terminal pancreatic carcinoma with biliary obstruction. During a surgical procedure on October 26, she received 5 units of whole blood obtained from 5 volunteers. She was markedly jaundiced throughout her hospitalization and had had liver enzyme elevations consistent with obstructive jaundice. Tests for the hepatitis B surface antigen (HBsAg) were negative.

On October 31, 5 days after the patient received her transfusions, the nurse attending her pushed the needle of an albumin infusion setup through the soft rubber infusion site on the intravenous (IV) bottle and into the palm of her hand, causing bleeding from the puncture site. In retrospect, the nurse noted that blood would frequently back up into the IV tubing when the patient moved. This had happened earlier during the shift when the patient was being transferred from a bed to a chair. The nurse did not report the accidental prick from the needle to her supervisor, nor did she receive immune globulin.

In mid-November the nurse, who was 41 years old, had onset of an influenza-like illness with fatigue, nausea, vomiting, and malaise. On November 18, her urine was noted to be turning darker, and on November 20 her sclerae were yellow. She was seen in a local emergency room and admitted to the hospital. Admission laboratory studies revealed an SGOT of 130 IU/L, alkaline phosphatase of 310 IU/L, and total bilirubin of 2.6 mg/dl. A test for hepatitis B surface antigen was negative. By December 7, her enzymes and bilirubin had returned to normal. She returned to work on December 8. There were no secondary cases in the hospital or in the nurse's family.

The nurse had no known history of hepatitis and was not taking any known hepatotoxic drugs. In the preceding 6 months she had not cared for any other jaundiced patients, nor had she been exposed to anyone subsequently diagnosed as having hepatitis. Follow-up tests on the nurse continue.

Serum from the nurse was sent to the Hepatitis Laboratories Division in Phoenix for antibody testing. The serum was negative for HBsAg and for antibody to HBsAg. The test for antibody to hepatitis A virus (anti-HAV) was positive, but the differential test for immunoglobulin class showed the anti-HAV activity to be IgG-mediated, which is consistent with a previous, but not current, HAV infection (1-3). NANB hepatitis, a diagnosis of exclusion, was thus made. The most probable source of the nurse's infection was the inadvertent, percutaneous inoculation of the patient's blood.

The donors of the suspect blood were contacted through the local blood bank. None had had clinical hepatitis, or had donated blood to other persons.

Reported by W Herron, MD, MPH, E Peterson, RN, Tacoma-Pierce County Health Dept; JW Taylor, MD, MPH, State Epidemiologist, Washington Dept of Social and Health Services; Hepatitis Laboratories Div, Field Services Div, Bur of Epidemiology, CDC.

Editorial Note: Based on these data, it appears that the nurse's infection was NANB hepatitis with an incubation period of 2 weeks. A similar case has been reported with onset 6 weeks after accidental, percutaneous exposure (4). NANB hepatitis, the major cause of post-transfusion hepatitis in the United States (5), resembles hepatitis B epidemiologically. As with hepatitis B, the agent (or agents) apparently causes a chronic viremia (1,2,5) from which virus can be transmitted to susceptible individuals through transfusion or other percutaneous routes.

References

1. Alter HJ, Holland PV: Transmissible agent in non-A, non-B hepatitis. Lancet 1:457-465, 1978
2. Bradley DW, Cook EH, Maynard JE, et al: Experimental infection of chimpanzees with antihemophilic (factor 8) materials: Recovery of virus-like particles associated with non-A, non-B hepatitis. J Med Virol 3:4 (in press), 1979
3. Bradley DW, Fields HA, McCaustland KA: Serodiagnosis of viral hepatitis A by a modified competitive binding radioimmunoassay for immunoglobulin M anti-hepatitis A virus. J Clin Microbiol 9:120-127, 1979
4. Tabor E, Gerety RJ, Drucker JA, et al: Transmission of non-A, non-B hepatitis from man to chimpanzee. Lancet 1:465-466, 1978
5. Seeff LB, Zimmerman JH, Wright EC, et al: A randomized, double blind controlled trial of the efficacy of immune serum globulin for the prevention of post-transfusion hepatitis. Gastroenterol 72:111-121, 1977

MMWR 28:373 (8/17/79)

Hepatitis B — New Bern, North Carolina

Since July 12, 9 persons with hepatitis B have been hospitalized in New Bern, North Carolina, a town of 18,000 people in eastern North Carolina. Six of the patients have died.

All but 1 of the patients were male; they ranged in age from 18 to 26 years. All were hepatitis B surface antigen (HBsAg) positive. Four were subtypable; all 4 were subtype ayw.

Five of the 6 deaths occurred during the first week of hospitalization as a result of fulminant hepatitis. The sixth death occurred after 25 days of hospitalization, during which the patient manifested hepatic coma requiring intensive supportive care, including assisted ventilation. Autopsies performed on fatal cases revealed complete hepatic necrosis with little or no normal hepatic tissue visable on histologic sections. Significant abnormal pathologic findings were limited to the liver.

All 9 patients admitted to using or were reported to use illicit drugs intravenously. The drug use among patients varied from occasional to regular. None of the patients was an addict, and none used known hepatotoxic drugs. The intravenous drugs most commonly used were MDA (3, 4 methylene dioxyamphetamine) and cocaine.

The outbreak occurred among 2 groups of friends who socially gathered at separate locations in New Bern. There were rare social interactions between the 2 groups.

To define the extent of hepatitis in the communities of social and household contacts of the cases, over 300 individuals have been tested for liver enzyme (alanine aminotransferase [ALT]) elevations and serologic evidence of infection with hepatitis B virus, namely, HBsAg, antibody to the hepatitis B surface antigen (anti-HBs), and antibody to the hepatitis B core antigen (anti-HBc). Seven individuals were identified with ALT values 2 times the upper limit of normal. One of these was HBsAg positive, and 2 others were anti-HBc positive. Fifteen additional people with normal ALT values had serologic evidence of infection with hepatitis B surface antigen: 9 had anti-HBs, 3 had anti-HBc, and 3 had both anti-HBs and anti-HBc.

Reported by V Barefoot, MD, B Golec, RN, Craven County Health Dept, New Bern; J Overby, MD, JP Mahaney, MD, J Burnett, MD, Craven County Hospital, New Bern; JN MacCormack, MD, MP Hines, DVM, State Epidemiologist, P Hudson, MD, H Tilson, MD, PhD, North Carolina Division of Health Services; H Fales, MD, National Heart and Lung Institute, Bethesda, Maryland; Field Services Div, Chronic Diseases Div, and Hepatitis Laboratories Div, Bur of Epidemiology, Clinical Chemistry Div, Bur of Laboratories, CDC.

Editorial Note: Hepatitis B is usually a relatively mild disease. Most patients are not hospitalized; of those that are, the mortality rate is generally 1%. The usual cause of death is fulminant hepatitis. It is not yet clear why there was such a high mortality associated with this outbreak. It may have been caused by a particularly virulent strain of the virus, although this seems unlikely since the mortality from hepatitis B has been quite constant worldwide. Another possibility is that there was some potentiating factor. There has been 1 previous report of a hepatitis B outbreak with a high mortality rate (37%); it occurred among psychiatric patients who were taking multiple drugs (1). Intensive epidemiologic and laboratory investigations are continuing.

Reference
1. Dougherty WJ, Altman R: Viral hepatitis in New Jersey, 1960-1961. Am J Med 32:704-716, 1962

MMWR 28:581 (12/14/79)

Viral Hepatitis Outbreaks — Georgia, Alabama

Ten recent cases of probable hepatitis A associated with consumption of raw oysters from Florida have been identified in Albany, Georgia, and Mobile, Alabama.

An investigation of 3 Albany residents in whom hepatitis was diagnosed during the week of October 28 disclosed that 2 had eaten raw oysters on October 13, and the other had eaten raw oysters on October 15. The oysters had all come from a single sack purchased in Florida.

An investigation of 5 Mobile residents with onset of hepatitis from November 5-7 found that their only common exposure was having eaten raw oysters at a club dinner on October 11. Two other Mobile hepatitis patients who had eaten raw oysters purchased from the same store at the same time as the oysters purchased to serve at the club dinner, were also identified.

The Food and Drug Administration, CDC, and state and local health authorities are trying to trace the source of the oysters for both outbreaks. Preliminary results suggest that the oysters came from a single area in Florida. The investigation is continuing.

Reported by D Smith, Georgia Dept of Human Resources; J Cutts, DVM, Mobile County Health Dept; T Chester, MD, State Epidemiologist, Alabama Dept of Public Health; R Gunn, MD, State Epidemiologist, Florida Dept of Health and Rehabilitative Services; U.S. Food and Drug Administration; Enteric Diseases Br, Bacterial Diseases Div, and Epidemiology Section, Hepatitis Laboratories Div, Bur of Epidemiology, CDC.

Editorial Note: Raw oysters have been implicated as the vehicle for transmission of hepatitis in several outbreaks in the United States, most recently in 1973, when 285 people became ill after eating raw oysters harvested in Louisiana (1). The number of cases involved in the 2 outbreaks reported here is small compared with such previous outbreaks, although there may be cases which have not yet been identified. Physicians are urged to report all cases of hepatitis to the appropriate public health authorities and to be particularly alert to possible oyster-associated cases.

Reference
1. Portnoy BL, Mackowiak PA, Caraway CT, Walker JA, McKinley TW, Klein CA: Oyster-associated hepatitis. Failure of shellfish certification programs to prevent outbreaks. JAMA 233:1065-1068, 1975

MMWR 28:594 (12/21/79)

Follow-up on Viral Hepatitis Outbreaks — Alabama, Georgia

The origin of oysters associated with 7 cases of hepatitis in Mobile, Alabama, and 3 cases of hepatitis in Albany, Georgia (1), has been traced to Apalachicola Bay, Florida.

By obtaining descriptions of oyster packaging and studying invoices of oyster dealers, the investigators traced shucked oysters consumed in the Mobile hepatitis outbreak to dealers that handled oysters harvested exclusively from Apalachicola Bay. Oysters associated with the Georgia outbreak had been purchased as shell stock from a different dealer, who also used Apalachicola Bay oysters exclusively. In neither investigation were any persons who were involved in the harvesting or handling of the oysters before their consumption identified as having hepatitis. The exact growing area of the incriminated oysters in Apalachicola Bay cannot be identified. The most probable dates of harvesting of the incriminated oysters were September 25-26 for the Georgia cases and October 6-8 for the Alabama outbreak. No cases of hepatitis related to the consumption of raw oysters from Apalachicola Bay have been identified with dates of onset after November 8.

During the last week of September and first week of October, fecal coliform counts transiently exceeded the recommended standard of 14 coliforms* per 100 ml of water (2) at several stations of the bay that were open for oyster harvesting. These counts ranged from 23 to 240 coliforms MPN* with a median of 49. One area of the bay was subsequently closed to oyster harvesting on October 4 by the Florida Department of Natural Resources because of these high coliform counts.

Reported by PC White, MD, District 8, D Smith, JS Terry, MD, Acting State Epidemiologist, Georgia Dept of Human Resources; J Cutts, DVM, Mobile County Health Dept; T Chester, MD, State Epidemiologist, Alabama Dept of Public Health; R Gunn, MD, State Epidemiologist, Florida Dept of Health and Rehabilitative Services; U.S. Food and Drug Administration; Enteric Diseases Br, Bacterial Diseases Div, and Epidemiology Section, Hepatitis Laboratories Div, Bur of Epidemiology, CDC.

Editorial Note: This investigation illustrates the problems of identifying the precise cause of contamination of shellfish so that preventive measures can be taken. It was difficult to trace the oysters to Apalachicola Bay and impossible to locate the exact growing area in the bay since Florida does not require labeling of oysters to indicate their place of harvesting.

Several hypotheses can be advanced to explain transient contamination of oyster beds in the bay: increased run-off associated with heavy rains caused by hurricane Frederic during mid-September, illegal dumping of sewage from passing boats, and illegal disposal of waste from land sources. Since large numbers of oysters are harvested from the bay, and only a few cases of oyster-associated hepatitis have been recognized, it seems likely that only a small proportion of oysters from the bay harbored hepatitis virus. The apparent lack of new cases suggests that the problem may have abated.

---

*Most probable number (MPN) index.

Fecally contaminated shellfish have been associated with outbreaks of typhoid fever, cholera, and viral (Norwalk agent) gastroenteritis *(3-5)* in addition to hepatitis; in all these outbreaks the shellfish were eaten raw or undercooked. Well-cooked shellfish do not appear to be associated with a risk of acquiring hepatitis. Strict enforcement and scrupulous compliance with all shellfish sanitation regulations should minimize the risk of disease caused by fecally contaminated shellfish.

References

1. MMWR 28:581, 1979
2. Food and Drug Administration: National Shellfish Safety Program: Proposed rulemaking. Federal Register 40:25930, 1975
3. Lumsden LL, Hasseltine HE, Leake JP, et al: A typhoid-fever epidemic caused by oyster-borne infection (1924-1925). Public Health Rep 50(suppl):1-102, 1975
4. Blake PA, Rosenberg ML, Bandeira Costa J, et al: Cholera in Portugal, 1974. 1. Modes of transmission. Am J Epidemiol 105:337-343, 1977
5. Murphy AM, Grohmann GS, Christopher PJ, et al: An Australia-wide outbreak of gastroenteritis from oysters caused by Norwalk virus. Med J Aust 2:329-333, 1979

MMWR 28:106 (3/9/79)

Morbidity Trends for Viral Hepatitis — United States, 1977

The downward trend in hepatitis A cases, which has been observed since 1971 in the United States, continued in 1977. The case rate for 1977 (14.40 cases/100,000) was one-half that observed 6 years earlier (28.90 cases/100,000). The actual decrease is even larger, however, because the earlier figure for hepatitis A included unspecified cases, which account for approximately 3.44-3.99 cases/100,000 per year. By contrast, the long-term trend for heightened hepatitis B morbidity continued, reaching its highest case rate (7.78 cases/100,000) since 1966, when hepatitis B was first reported separately.

The total number of cases of viral hepatitis reported to the MMWR for 1977 was 56,623—slightly more than the annual total reported for 1976 and 1975 (Table 2). The increase of 874 cases over the 1976 total can be attributed to the additional 1,858 hepatitis B and 1,151 unspecified cases, which exceeded the decrease of 2,135 reported hepatitis A cases.

TABLE 2. Reported cases of viral hepatitis, by type and year, United States, 1966-1977*

Year	Hepatitis A		Hepatitis B		Unspecified		Total	
	No.	Rate §	No.	Rate	No.	Rate	No.	Rate
1966	32,859	16.77	1,497	1.79	†	†	34,356	18.56
1967	38,909	19.67	2,458	1.28	†	†	41,367	20.95
1968	45,893	22.96	4,829	2.49	†	†	50,722	25.45
1969	48,416	23.98	5,909	3.02	†	†	54,325	27.00
1970	56,797	27.87	8,310	4.08	†	†	65,107	31.95
1971	59,606	28.90	9,556	4.74	†	†	69,162	33.64
1972	54,074	25.97	9,402	4.52	†	†	63,476	30.49
1973	50,749	24.18	8,451	4.03	†	†	59,200	28.21
1974	40,358	19.54	10,631	5.15	8,351	3.95	59,340	28.07
1975	35,855	16.82	13,121	6.30	7,158	3.44	56,134	26.34
1976	33,288	15.51	14,973	7.14	7,488	3.57	55,749	25.97
1977	31,153	14.40	16,831	7.78	8,639	3.99	56,623	26.17

*Source: CDC: Reported Morbidity and Mortality in the United States, 1977. MMWR (53 Annual Suppl):2, 1978

§ Cases per 100,000 population

†Not reported nationally until 1974

TABLE 3. Average incidence of hepatitis A and B, by U.S. Census Division, May 1976 through May 1978

| Division | Hepatitis A | | Hepatitis B | |
	Average incidence†	Trend	Average incidence	Trend
New England	0.49	Down	0.29	Up
Middle Atlantic	0.73	Down	0.60	Down
East North Central	0.84	No change	0.43	No change
West North Central	0.80	No change	0.37	No change
South Atlantic	0.98	Down	0.55	Up
East South Central	1.17	Down	0.52	No change
West South Central	1.15	Up	0.37	Up
Mountain	2.02	Up	0.57	No change
Pacific	2.07	Down	1.08	No change
United States	1.09	Down	0.56	No change

†4-week incidence/100,000 population is based on 4-week totals of cases reported to MMWR in 1976-1978.

For the 2-year period from May 1976 to May 1978, reported hepatitis A morbidity trends within the 9 U.S. Census Divisions varied considerably. For the entire United States the incidence of such cases for the 27, 4-week report periods has decreased. In the New England, Middle Atlantic, and both North Central Divisions the average incidence was significantly lower than that for the nation as a whole. On the other hand, the Mountain and Pacific states reported significantly higher than average incidence (Table 3). Areas with case rates below the U.S. average formed a contiguous region, as did the areas with above average and average rates. In terms of trends over the 2-year period, the North Central areas showed little change, and the West South Central and Mountain areas increased sharply, contrary to the morbidity in the more populous parts of the nation.

For the same 2-year period, hepatitis B incidence has shown little monthly change, although the annual rate for 1977 is the highest recorded to date. As with type A hepatitis, there were substantial geographic differences in morbidity (Table 3). New England, while exhibiting the lowest average 4-week incidence, had a notable increase in cases. Another area with an upward trend, the West South Central Division, also exhibited a relatively low average incidence. The South Atlantic Division also showed an increase, although not as steep a one as in the 2 previously mentioned areas. The Middle Atlantic Division was the only area with a downward trend in reported hepatitis B incidence. The Pacific Division continued to demonstrate the highest average 4-week incidence, 1.08/100,000 cases—a figure that is nearly twice the national average. The average incidence for the New England, East North Central, West North Central, and West South Central Divisions was significantly lower than the U.S. average.

Reported by the Viral Hepatitis Surveillance Activity, Hepatitis Laboratories Div, Bur of Epidemiology, CDC.

MMWR 27 (A.S., 1978): 29

HEPATITIS — Reported Case Rates by Year, United States, 1952—1978

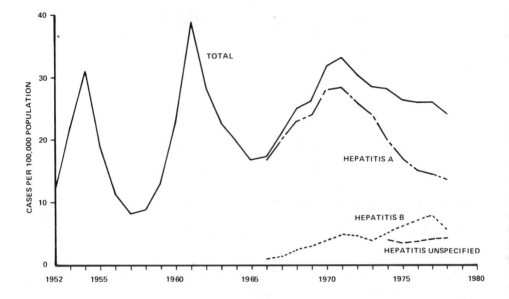

Viral hepatitis continues to be one of the 5 most frequently reported infectious diseases in the United States. The total number of viral hepatitis cases reported for 1978, however, was the lowest since 1968; the case rate, the lowest reported since 1967. Decreases were found in 1978 in the case rates and in the number of cases of both hepatitis A and hepatitis B. Persons from 15 through 29 years of age continue to be the group most affected by hepatitis.

CHAPTER 31

Smallpox and Monkeypox

MMWR 27:319 (9/1/78)

Laboratory-Associated Smallpox — England

England has reported a case of laboratory-associated smallpox. This is the first small-pox case reported in the world since October 26, 1977, when a case occurred in Somalia.

The patient is a 40-year-old female medical photographer employed at Birmingham Medical School; her office is located on the floor above the Department of Virology, where work on variola viruses is done. She developed fever on August 11 and rash 2 days later. She was hospitalized on August 24; the same day she was transferred to a small-pox infectious disease hospital.

Electron microscopy (EM) was positive for pox virus on August 25; on August 27, variola major virus was isolated.

Thirty-nine close and 196 casual contacts of the patient have been identified. Three contacts who have become ill have been admitted to isolation as a precautionary measure. EM results on one such contact, who had rash and fever, showed *Herpes* virus. As of August 30, all other contacts are well.

One contact, a 20-year-old British woman, traveled to North Dakota on August 18. When it was learned that her co-worker had smallpox, state and local health officials were notified, and CDC dispatched a medical epidemiologist to the farm where she is staying. She is afebrile and has no symptoms. She had been vaccinated 5 years ago. Daily surveillance is being maintained by local health authorities.

As of August 30, the patient is still hospitalized but improving. She has a confluent rash on her face and discrete lesions on her extremeties. The medical school labora-tory has been closed.

Reported by PA Hyzler, MD, National Health Div, Dept of Health and Social Security, London; K Mosser, State Epidemiologist, North Dakota State Dept of Health; Bur of Smallpox Eradication, CDC.

Editorial Note: This patient was presumably infected by airborne transmission of vari-ola virus from the smallpox laboratory on the ground floor to the patient's normal work area on the first floor. The ability of variola virus to transmit from 1 floor to another via external air currents has been previously documented in a hospital out-break of smallpox in Meschede, Germany (1). Investigation will be required to iden-tify the specific safety breakdown in the Birmingham laboratory.

As smallpox laboratories hold the only known reservoir of smallpox virus, the World Health Organization (WHO) has urged that storage of the reference virus strains be restricted to the 5 WHO Pox Virus Reference Centers (2). Since 1975, 62 of 76 labora-tories with known variola virus have destroyed or transferred their virus stocks. The

Birmingham incident emphasizes the continuing risk of laboratory-acquired infection and the need to ensure maximum security at every facility holding the virus.

The British contact now in the United States is not believed to be at risk of developing smallpox because her exposure to the case occurred 2-3 days before the patient had become infectious and 21 days have elapsed since exposure—more than the maximum expected incubation period. U.S. and British vaccination requirements for international travelers remain unchanged (3). However, Malta and Jamaica are now requiring valid vaccination certificates for anyone who has been in Birmingham in the previous 14 days.

References
1. Wehrle PF, Posch J, Richter KH, Henderson DA: An airborne outbreak of smallpox in a German hospital and its significance with respect to other recent outbreaks in Europe. Bull WHO 43:669-679, 1970
2. WHO: Laboratories retaining variola virus. Weekly Epidemiological Record 53:221-222, 1978
3. MMWR 27:295, 1978

MMWR 27:346 (9/15/78)
Follow-up on Smallpox — England

The English medical photographer who contracted smallpox in August (1) died on September 11 of renal failure and bacteremia. One close contact, the mother of the deceased patient, has had a pox virus visualized on electron microscopy. She was vaccinated on August 14; culture results to differentiate between variola and vaccinia viruses are pending. Over 250 persons are still under surveillance.

Reported by International Health Div, Dept of Health and Social Services, London; Bur of Smallpox, CDC.
Reference
1. MMWR 27:319, 1978

MMWR 27:364 (9/22/78)
Follow-up on Smallpox — England

The mother of the English smallpox patient (1) has been confirmed by culture as having smallpox. She is in quarantine in a smallpox hospital with mild "modified" type disease. She was vaccinated on August 25, not August 14, as previously reported (1), and was prophylactically treated with vaccinia immune globulin and methisazone. Her 1 contact, an ambulance driver, is under surveillance.

Reported by International Health Div, Dept of Health and Social Services, London; Bur of Smallpox Eradication, CDC.
Reference
1. MMWR 27:346, 1978

MMWR 27:415 (10/27/78)
Smallpox Surveillance — Worldwide

October 26, 1978, marks the first anniversary of the last case of endemic smallpox. The last known case occurred in Merka, Somalia. The recent laboratory-associated outbreak in Birmingham, United Kingdom, has not altered plans of the World Health Organization (WHO) for final certification of global eradication. Intensive surveillance continues in Somalia, Ethiopia, Kenya, Djibouti, and the Yemen Arab Republic with plans for Certification Commissions in the fall of 1979.

A reward of $1,000 has been established by the Director-General of WHO for the first person who reports an active case of smallpox resulting from person-to-person transmission and confirmed by laboratory tests (1).

Reference
1. Resolution WHA 31.54, World Health Assembly, 1978

MMWR 28:265 (6/15/79)

Adverse Reactions to Smallpox Vaccination — 1978

Adverse reactions to smallpox vaccination continued to be noted by CDC during 1978.

Case 1, California: On August 15, 1978, a 53-year-old man with chronic lymphocytic leukemia was vaccinated with vaccinia virus as proposed therapy for a presumed herpes simplex infection. Over the next week, increasing inflammation and eventually necrosis were noted at the vaccination site. Peripheral vaccinial lesions appeared; vaccinia virus was identified from several lesions by fluorescent antibody (FA) testing. The patient recovered after 3 courses of vaccinia immune globulin (VIG) and 1 course of methisazone.

Case 2, California: On the advice of airline personnel and a military recruiting officer, a 29-year-old woman received a smallpox vaccination in June 1978 for travel to Germany. Nine days later, she was hospitalized with fever and a necrotic ulcer at the vaccination site. FA staining of scrapings from a chin pustule was positive for vaccinia. She recovered without use of VIG.

Case 3, New Jersey: A 56-year-old U.S. Army reservist, who was taking cyclophosphamide for chronic lymphocytic leukemia, received a smallpox vaccination on May 7, 1978, at a military vaccination clinic. Within 2 weeks, a painful ulcer was noted at the vaccination site. Because of the appearance of an increasing number of peripheral lesions (from 1 of which vaccinia virus was eventually isolated), and because of continued enlargement of the initial ulcer, he was treated with VIG, methisazone, adenine arabinoside, transfer factor, and vaccinia hyperimmune plasma. Eventual recovery was complicated by *Pseudomonas* sepsis and the need for a skin graft at the vaccination site.

Case 4, Australia: A woman, 8 weeks pregnant, received a smallpox vaccination. A 500-gm infant, born at 24 weeks gestation, survived for 1 hour. Vaccinia virus was isolated from 1 of multiple skin lesions and from a lesion found in the lung at the postmortem examination.

Reported by JH David, MD, Mountain View, California, C Brass, MD, Stanford University Medical Center, R Roberto, MD, LG Dales, MD, and J Chin, MD, State Epidemiologist, California Dept of Health, in California Morbidity, No. 33, August 25, 1978, and No. 37, September 23, 1978; FJ Brescia, MD, Millburn, New Jersey; R Altman, MD, State Epidemiologist, New Jersey State Dept of Health; Australia Communicable Disease Intelligence Bulletin, April 6-19, 1978; Immunization Div, Bur of State Services, Bur of Smallpox Eradication, and Field Services Div, Bur of Epidemiology, CDC.

Editorial Note: The hospitalization charges for cases 1 and 3 totaled $22,010.

These cases illustrate several important points:

1. Smallpox vaccine, a live virus vaccine, is contraindicated in persons with hematologic or other malignancies, in persons on immunosuppressive therapy, and in pregnant women (1).

2. Smallpox vaccine apparently continues to be used by physicians for treatment of herpetic infections despite the failure to demonstrate efficacy (*1,2*) and the proven danger of this therapy (*2,3*).

3. Airlines, travel agents, health facilities, and others who provide advice to travelers should be certain that their information regarding need for smallpox vaccination conforms to the latest international travel regulations.

4. Health-care providers should be aware that smallpox vaccination of active duty and active reserve U.S. military personnel is continuing. In addition, the military is not yet actively discouraging smallpox vaccination of dependents (*4*).

5. Fetal vaccinia, although very rare, can occur in offspring of vaccinees.

These cases and most of the others reported to CDC were avoidable. The United States no longer requires smallpox vaccination of any travelers (*5*). There are no current medical or epidemiologic reasons for countries to require smallpox vaccine for anyone except the few laboratory workers likely to have contact with the variola virus (*6*). The number of countries which still, for administrative reasons, require vaccination as a condition of entry is steadily decreasing.*

Routine smallpox vaccination of U.S. children was discontinued in 1971. Routine smallpox vaccination of U.S. hospital employees was discontinued in 1976. Despite this, more than 4.4 million doses of smallpox vaccine were distributed in the United States during 1978 (*7*).

Public health officials should ensure that smallpox vaccine providers in their areas are aware of the most current recommendations for its use. Use of vaccinia virus should be limited to persons with valid indications. The vast majority of U.S. travelers go to Mexico, Canada, Europe, Japan, the Caribbean Islands, and Israel. None of these areas require smallpox vaccination for entry. When counseling persons traveling to a country still requiring smallpox vaccination for administrative reasons, health-care providers should be aware that the World Health Organization's International Health Regulations provide for smallpox vaccination waiver letters to be issued to travelers for whom vaccination is contraindicated for health reasons. In view of the apparent success of the smallpox eradication effort, some authorities have advocated giving such letters, signed by a physician and validated by a health agency, to all travelers. The only country that had been refusing to accept such letters (*8*)—except for rare individual actions by an immigration officer acting contrary to national policy—recently stopped requiring certificates for travelers from the United States. As with other vaccinations, complications of smallpox vaccination should continue to be reported to local and state health departments and to CDC.

References

1. Advisory Committee on Immunization Practices: Smallpox vaccine. MMWR 27:156, 1978
2. Kern AB, Schiff BL: Smallpox vaccinations in the management of recurrent herpes simplex: A controlled evaluation. J Invest Dermatol 33:99-102, 1959
3. Lane JM, Ruben FL, Abrutyn E, Millar JD: Deaths attributable to smallpox vaccination, 1959 to 1966 and 1968. JAMA 212:441-444, 1970
4. Departments of the Army, the Navy, the Air Force, and Transportation: Medical Services Immunization Requirements and Procedures. Washington, D.C., 7 Jun 1977, p 6
5. MMWR 27:295, 1978

---

*As of June 7, 1979, the following countries require smallpox vaccination for direct travel from the United States: **Africa:** Angola, Benin (for stay >2 weeks), Botswana, Cameroon, Central African Republic, Chad, Comoros, Congo, Djibouti, Egypt, Equatorial Guinea, Ethiopia, Guinea, Ivory Coast, Lesotho, Libyan Arab Jamahariya, Madagascar, Mali, Mozambique, Namibia, Rhodesia, Sao Tome and Principe, Seychelles, Sierra Leone, South Africa, Sudan Uganda, Upper Volta, Zaire. **Asia:** Brunei, Democratic Kampuchea, East Timor, Iran, Lao People's Democratic Republic, Mongolia, Nepal, Philippines, Ryukyu Islands (unofficial), Saudi Arabia (during pilgrimage), Viet Nam. **Americas:** Belize, Bolivia.

6. World Health Organization: Functioning of the International Health Regulations (1969) for the period 1 January to 31 December 1977. Weekly Epidemiological Record 53:354-355, 1978
7. CDC: Biologics Surveillance Report No. 76. Annual Summary 1978. Mar 1979
8. California Department of Health: Smallpox vaccination requirements for international travel. California Morbidity (11), 23 Mar 1979

MMWR 28:497 (10/26/79)

Smallpox Certification — East Africa

Two years ago today the world's last known patient with endemic smallpox had onset of rash (Figure 1). Ali Maow Maalin, a cook at the district hospital in Merka, Somalia, developed smallpox on October 26, 1977. Since then, intensive surveillance has failed to identify any additional cases of naturally transmitted smallpox.*

Separate International Commissions have been assessing campaigns in the last 4 countries requiring certification of eradication: Somalia, Kenya, Ethiopia, and Djibouti. Today in Nairobi, the chairpersons of these commissions will make their reports to the Director-General of the World Health Organization. It is anticipated that the Horn of Africa will be certified to be smallpox free.

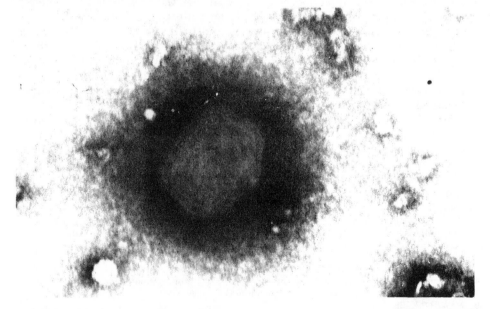

FIGURE 1. Variola minor virus isolate from world's last endemic case, Merka, Somalia, 1977. Magnification, 115,000 X.

*Two cases of laboratory-acquired smallpox occurred in Birmingham, United Kingdom, on August 13 and September 8, 1978, but the World Health Organization's Global Commission for Smallpox Eradication has determined that these cases should not alter the plans for certification of naturally transmitted smallpox.

MMWR 28:135 (3/30/79)

Monkeypox in Humans — West Africa

A 35-year-old man from Omifounfoun Village in Oyo State, Nigeria, developed a rash on November 24, 1978. On December 5 he went to the hospital in Parakou town, Borgou Province, Benin, where medical authorities suspected smallpox or monkeypox. They immediately placed the patient in isolation and took specimens for laboratory analysis. Typical poxvirus particles were seen on electron microscopic examination by the World Health Organization (WHO) Collaborating Center at CDC on December 24, and monkeypox virus was isolated on December 27.

Although the patient's residence is in the Republic of Benin, he reportedly had been visiting in Nigeria for 2 months before the onset of rash. He had no smallpox vaccination scar. There have been no secondary cases reported in Benin. Joint Benin/WHO and Nigeria/WHO investigations are in progress.

Editorial Note: Besides this case, 35 cases of monkeypox in humans have been reported from West and Central Africa since 1970; 27 have occurred in Zaire, 4 in Liberia, 2 in Nigeria, and 1 each in the Ivory Coast and Sierra Leone. Twenty-eight cases have been in children 9 years of age or younger. Six patients have died.

The disease is clinically indistinguishable from smallpox. The most important epidemiologic difference between the 2 is that monkeypox transmits poorly between humans; in only 2 instances has possible secondary transmission occurred in the same family. Among susceptible family members, the monkeypox secondary attack rate is less than 4%, in comparison to 30%-45% for smallpox.

Thirty-two of the 36 people with monkeypox had never been vaccinated. (Smallpox vaccination protects against monkeypox.) However, since over 50% of children in the areas reporting monkeypox are susceptible to smallpox, the absence of more monkeypox cases is yet another indication that the disease is rare and not very contagious.

Monkeypox virus is an orthopoxvirus that differs from variola virus in several biological characteristics. The source of human monkeypox is unknown, but it is thought to be a zoonosis. The virus was associated with 10 outbreaks in nonhuman primates among captive monkey colonies in European and North American laboratories between 1958 and 1968. Special study groups convened by WHO in 1973, 1976, and 1978 have concluded that monkeypox is not a public health problem. They have recommended that the epidemiology and ecology of this disease be further defined.

Reported by the WHO in the Weekly Epidemiological Record 54:12-13, 1979

CHAPTER 32

Rubella

MMWR 27:451 (11/17/78)

Rubella Vaccine

Changes in the ACIP recommendation for the use of rubella vaccine focus on more effective delivery of the vaccine to older individuals and, in particular, to females in the childbearing age group. All comments related to the vaccine and its use pertain both to the HPV-77 DE5 (Meruvax) and to the RA 27/3 (Meruvax II) strains of vaccine virus. The RA 27/3 vaccine—like the HPV-77 DE5 vaccine—is licensed for subcutaneous administration only and is expected to be available in January 1979.

INTRODUCTION

Rubella is a common childhood rash disease that is often overlooked or misdiagnosed. Signs and symptoms vary. The most common features—postauricular and suboccipital lymphadenopathy, arthralgia, and transient erythematous rash with low fever—may not be recognized as rubella. Moreover, subclinical infection occurs frequently. Transient polyarthralgia and polyarthritis sometimes accompany or follow rubella illness. This occurs in women in particular, but it is also seen in men and in children. Central nervous system disorders and thrombocytopenia have been reported, but they are rare.

By far the most important consequences of rubella are the fetal anomalies that frequently result from rubella infection in early pregnancy, especially in the first trimester. Preventing infection of the fetus and consequent congenital rubella syndrome is a major objective of rubella immunization programs.

Postinfection immunity appears to be long-lasting. However, as with other viral diseases, re-exposure to natural rubella occasionally results in reinfection without clinical illness. The only reliable evidence of rubella immunity is specific antibody, best determined by hemagglutination-inhibition (HI) antibody technique. Laboratories that regularly perform this test are generally the most reliable because of better standardization of reagents and procedures.

Before rubella vaccine was available, most cases of rubella occurred in school-age children. Now, most cases are in adolescents and young adults. In 1977, 70% of cases occurred in those 15 years of age and older. Of persons in these age groups, 10%-20% are susceptible. Since licensure of rubella vaccine in 1969, the incidence of reported rubella in adolescents and young adults has not decreased appreciably because vaccine was primarily used for preschoolers and elementary school children. Through 1977, more than 80 million doses of live attenuated rubella virus vaccine were distributed in the United States. Despite the considerable vaccination effort in young children, outbreaks of rubella continue to be reported in junior and senior high schools, colleges, the military, and places of employment—most notably hospitals.

LIVE RUBELLA VIRUS VACCINE

Live rubella virus vaccine* available in the United States is prepared either in duck embryo cell culture or human diploid cell culture. It is produced in monovalent (rubella only) form and in combinations: measles-rubella (MR) and measles-mumps-rubella (MMR) vaccines. MMR is encouraged for use in routine infant-vaccination programs. In all situations in which rubella vaccine is to be used, consideration should be given to using a combination vaccine if recipients are likely to be susceptible to measles and/or mumps as well as to rubella.

A single dose of rubella vaccine at 12 months of age or older induces antibodies in approximately 95% of susceptible persons. Although antibody titers are generally lower than those following rubella infection, vaccine-induced immunity protects against clinical illness from natural exposure. Antibody levels have declined little during the more than 9 years of follow-up of children who were among the first to receive the vaccine. Long-term, even life-long, protection against both clinical rubella and subclinical viremia is expected.

Rubella reinfection without illness can occur in persons with low levels of antibody whether the antibodies resulted from vaccination or from natural rubella. Reinfection, however, does not cause detectable viremia or significant pharyngeal excretion of virus and thus poses no recognized risk to susceptible contacts. Further study is needed to evaluate the clinical and epidemiologic significance of reinfection, but the apparent absence of viremia suggests that immune females reinfected during pregnancy would be unlikely to infect their fetuses.

VACCINE USAGE

General Recommendations

Rubella vaccine is recommended for all children, many adolescents, and some adults, particularly females, unless it is otherwise contraindicated. Vaccinating children protects them against rubella and prevents their subsequently spreading it. Vaccinating susceptible postpubertal females confers individual protection against rubella-induced fetal injury. Vaccinating adolescent or adult males and females in population groups such as those in colleges, places of employment, or military bases, protects them against rubella and reduces the chance of epidemics in partially immune groups.

Dosage: A single dose of vaccine in the volume specified by the manufacturer should be administered subcutaneously.

Individuals at Risk

Live rubella virus vaccine is recommended for all children when 12 months of age or older. It should not be administered to younger infants because persisting maternal antibodies may interfere with seroconversion. When the rubella vaccine is part of a combination vaccine that includes the measles antigen, it should be administered to children about 15 months of age or older to achieve the maximum rate of measles seroconversion. Children who have not received rubella vaccine at the optimum age should be vaccinated promptly. Because a history of rubella is not a reliable indicator of immunity, all children for whom vaccine is not contraindicated should be vaccinated.

Increased emphasis should be placed on vaccinating unimmunized prepubertal girls and susceptible adolescent and adult females in the childbearing age group. Because of the

---

*Official name: Rubella Virus Vaccine, Live

theoretical risk to the fetus, females of childbearing age should receive vaccine only if they are not pregnant and understand that they should not become pregnant for 3 months after vaccination. In view of the importance of protecting this age group against rubella, asking females if they are pregnant, excluding those who are, and explaining the theoretical risks to the others are reasonable precautions in a rubella immunization program. When practical, serologic testing of potential vaccinees in the childbearing age group may be undertaken to show susceptibility to rubella.

Educational and training institutions such as colleges, universities, and military bases should seek proof of rubella immunity (a positive serologic test or documentation of previous rubella vaccination) from all female students and employees in the childbearing age. Non-pregnant females who lack proof of immunity should be vaccinated unless contraindications exist.

When reliable laboratory services are available, routine premarital serology for rubella immunity would enhance efforts to identify susceptible females before pregnancy. Prenatal or ante partum screening for rubella susceptibility should be undertaken and vaccine administered in the immediate postpartum period—*prior* to discharge. Previous administration of anti-Rho (D) immune globulin (human) or blood products is not a contraindication to vaccination; however, 6- to 8-week postvaccination serologic testing should be done on those who have received the globulin or blood products to ascertain that seroconversion has occurred. Obtaining laboratory evidence of seroconversion in other vaccinees is not necessary.

In order to protect susceptible female patients and female employees, persons working in hospitals and clinics who might contract rubella from infected patients or who, if infected, might transmit rubella to pregnant patients should be immune to rubella.

Individuals Exposed to Disease

Use of vaccine following exposure: There is no evidence that live rubella virus vaccine given after exposure will prevent illness or that vaccinating an individual incubating rubella is harmful. Since a single exposure may not result in infection and postexposure vaccination would protect an individual in the event of future exposure, vaccination is recommended unless otherwise contraindicated.

Use of immune serum globulin following exposure: Immune serum globulin (ISG) given after exposure to rubella will not prevent infection or viremia, but it may modify or suppress symptoms. The routine use of ISG for postexposure prophylaxis of rubella in early pregnancy is not recommended. (Infants with congenital rubella have been born to women who were given ISG shortly after exposure.) The only time when ISG might be used is when rubella occurs in a pregnant woman who would not consider termination of pregnancy under any circumstances. Serologic testing for rubella immunity is useful if an exposure in early pregnancy is suspected.

SIDE EFFECTS AND ADVERSE REACTIONS

Vaccine side effects such as rash and lymphadenopathy occasionally occur in children. Joint pain, usually of the small peripheral joints, has been noted in up to 40% of vaccinees in large-scale field trials, although frank arthritis is reported in fewer than 1%. Arthralgia and transient arthritis occur more frequently and tend to be more severe in susceptible women than in children. When joint symptoms or non-joint-associated pain and paresthesia do occur, they generally begin 2-10 weeks after immunization, persist for 1-3 days, and rarely recur. The persistent arthritic symptoms that have occasionally been described probably represent coincidental disease rather than a vaccine complication. Transient peripheral neuritic complaints such as paresthesia and pain in the hands and feet have also occurred but are very uncommon.

Some vaccinees intermittently shed small amounts of virus from the pharynx 7-28 days after vaccination. However, studies of more than 1,200 susceptible household contacts have yielded no evidence that vaccine virus has been transmitted. These data strongly suggest that vaccinating susceptible children whose mothers or other household contacts are pregnant does not present a risk.

Although vaccine is safe and effective for all ages over 12 months, its safety for the developing fetus is not fully known. Thus, rubella vaccine is **NOT** suitable for pregnant women because of the theoretical risk of fetal abnormality caused by the vaccine virus, which does cross the placenta. Although no recognizable malformations attributable to rubella have been seen in infants born to more than 60 susceptible women who inadvertently received rubella vaccine during early pregnancy and continued their pregnancies to term, the theoretical risk remains.

PRECAUTIONS AND CONTRAINDICATIONS
Pregnancy

Pregnant women should not be given rubella vaccine. If a pregnant woman is inadvertently vaccinated or if she becomes pregnant within 3 months of vaccination, she should be counseled on the theoretical risks to the fetus.

Persons with febrile illness should not be vaccinated until they have recovered. Minor illnesses such as upper respiratory infections, however, do not preclude vaccination.

Allergies

Live rubella virus vaccine is produced in duck embryo cell culture or in human diploid cell culture. It has not been reported to be associated with allergic reactions and can be given to all who need it, including persons with allergies to eggs, ducks, and feathers. Live rubella virus vaccine does not contain penicillin. Some vaccines do contain trace amounts of other antibiotics, however, to which patients may be allergic. Those administering vaccines should review the label information carefully before deciding whether patients with known allergies to such antibiotics can be vaccinated safely.

Altered Immunity

Replication of the rubella vaccine virus may be potentiated in patients with immune deficiency diseases and by the suppressed immune responses that occur with leukemia, lymphoma, or generalized malignancy or with therapy with corticosteroids, alkylating drugs, antimetabolites, or radiation. Patients with such conditions should not be given live rubella virus vaccine.

Simultaneous Administration of Certain Live Virus Vaccines

See "General Recommendations on Immunization," MMWR 25:349-350, 355, 1976.

OUTBREAK MANAGEMENT

To prevent the spread of rubella in outbreaks, susceptibles at risk should be vaccinated promptly. Women at risk of exposure who are not aware of being pregnant and agree to prevent conception for 3 months should be vaccinated. Although prevaccination serologic testing is not necessary, it may be useful to collect a blood specimen at the time of vaccination. Later, it can be tested if the woman had been pregnant at the time of vaccination or should become pregnant in the next 3 months.

SURVEILLANCE

Accurate diagnosis and reporting of rubella, congenital rubella syndrome, and vaccine complications are of great importance in assessing the progress in rubella control. Furthermore, all cases of birth defects suspected of being related to rubella should be thoroughly investigated and reported to state health departments.

SELECTED BIBLIOGRAPHY

Cooper LZ, Krugman S: The rubella problem. DM, Feb 1969, pp 3-38

Farquhar JD: Follow-up on rubella vaccinations and experience with subclinical reinfection. J Pediatr 81:460, 1972

Hayden GF, Modlin JF, Witte JJ: Current status of rubella in the United States, 1969-1975. J Infect Dis 135:337, 1977

Herrmann KL, Halstead SB, Brandling-Bennett AD, et al: Rubella immunization. Persistence of antibody 4 years after a large-scale field trial. JAMA 235:2201, 1976

Horstmann D: Controlling rubella: Problems and perspective. Ann Intern Med 83:412, 1975

Kamin PB, Fein BT, Britton HA: Use of live, attenuated measles virus vaccine in children allergic to egg protein. JAMA 193:1125, 1965

Krugman S: Present status of measles and rubella immunization in the United States: A medical progress report. J Pediatr 90:1, 1977

Marymont JH, Herrmann KL: Rubella in pregnancy: Review of current problems. Postgrad Med 56:167, 1974

Modlin JF, Brandling-Bennett AD, Witte JJ, et al: A review of 5 years' experience with rubella vaccine in the United States. Pediatrics 55:20, 1975

Modlin JF, Herrmann KL, Brandling-Bennett AD, et al: Risk of congenital abnormality after inadvertent rubella vaccination of pregnant women. N Engl J Med 294:972, 1976

MMWR 28:325 (7/20/79)

Rubella in Hospital Personnel and Patients — Colorado

In the period January 27-February 26, 1979, 9 clinical cases of rubella were reported in employees and patients of a hospital and adjacent rehabilitation center in the Denver area (Figure 1) (1). The first 7 cases were in female employees, who ranged in age from 26 to 52 years and worked in various areas of the hospital. There was no known rubella activity in the community. Six of the 7 employees were confirmed as having rubella infection either by a ≥4-fold rise in rubella hemagglutination-inhibition (HI) titers or by the presence of rubella-specific IgM antibodies at a titer of ≥1:4. Two of these 6 individuals had previously been serologically tested for rubella immunity and found to be susceptible, but they had not been vaccinated. The last 2 reported cases, neither of which was serologically confirmed, were in male patients (aged 22 and 26 years) in the rehabilitation center.

On February 6, the Colorado State Department of Health and the hospital administration began a week-long rubella immunization program for all employees of both institutions (1,350 in the 318-bed hospital and 450 in the 80-bed rehabilitation center). Patients were not included, but their physicians were notified that an outbreak of rubella was occurring.

Rubella vaccine (HPV-77:DE-5) was administered to all employees except those with previous rubella serologic immunity, those with documentation of previous rubella vaccination, or those who were known to be pregnant. Rubella HI tests were run at the state health department laboratory, when requested by employees. Each female employee of childbearing age was asked if she was pregnant or contemplating pregnancy in the next 3 months. Those with affirmative responses were not vaccinated but did have a blood specimen drawn, held, and, if requested, processed. All other females of childbearing age were vaccinated immediately after a blood specimen was obtained; all remaining females and all males were simply vaccinated. A total of 1,211 vaccinations were given.

FIGURE 1. Rubella in a Denver-area hospital, by date of onset of rash, January 27-February 26, 1979

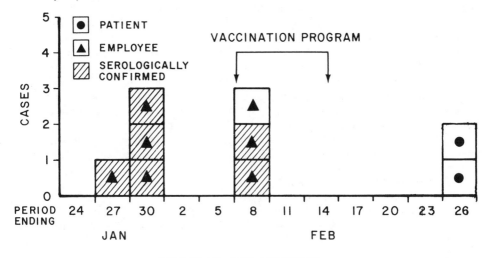

ONSET (3-DAY PERIODS)

All vaccinees were asked about adverse reactions in the 3 weeks after vaccination. The 37 (3.1%) employees who reported reactions had mild symptoms of short duration. Twenty-seven reported that they had experienced joint involvement (17 with arthralgia, 10 with arthritis), 11 had noted rash, and 9 had had low-grade fever.

Prevaccination serum from 10 of the 37 persons who had reported reactions was available for serologic testing; 6 of these persons had been susceptible to rubella and 4, immune. Based on these numbers, an estimated 22 of the 37 persons who had reactions were susceptible, and 15 were immune. In an attempt to stratify reaction rates by prevaccination immunity status, 114 blood specimens were randomly selected from those obtained just before vaccination. Since 13 (11.4%) of these were found to lack HI rubella antibodies, 138 of the 1,211 vaccinees are estimated to have been susceptible. The estimated reaction rate for susceptibles (22/138=15.9%) was significantly higher than that for immune individuals (15/1,073-1.4%) (relative risk=11.4, 95% confidence interval, 6.8-19.0).

A total of 41 workdays, over a 4-week period, were missed by 21 of the 37 employees who reported a vaccine-associated reaction. (Breakdown of the data by immunity status is unavailable.) Assuming a 5-day workweek for the 1,211 vaccinees (24,220 person-days for 4 weeks), the absenteeism rate was less than 0.2% (41/24,220). The background absenteeism rates per 4-week period for the hospital were 4% and 5% for the 3-month period from February through April in 1978 and 1979, respectively. Thus, the absenteeism rate was not noticeably affected by the vaccination program.

Reported by TA Edell, MD, C Howard, RN, Denver; SW Ferguson, PhD, Acting State Epidemiologist, B Harrel, J Connor, Colorado State Dept of Health; Immunization Div, Bur of State Services, CDC.

Editorial Note: Outbreaks of rubella in hospital employees have been receiving increased attention (2-4). The only effective way to minimize the possibility of employees introducing and spreading rubella is to have a highly immune employee population (5). This protects both the female employees and the patients. Employee-to-patient spread apparently did occur in this outbreak (Figure 1).

Concern has been raised that vaccination of large numbers of hospital employees might be associated with many vaccine-associated complications and increased absenteeism. The results of this vaccination program for hospital employees indicate that these problems are minimal. The overall reaction rate, which probably includes some non-vaccine-associated complaints, was low. The estimated reaction rate for susceptible vaccinees (15.9%) is within the reported range (6). Even if all 37 persons who reported reactions had been susceptible, the calculated rate would be only 26.8% (37/138). In large-scale field trials of rubella vaccine, up to 40% of adult vaccinees reported arthralgia alone (7). The estimated rate of joint complaints, rash, or fever for immune persons (1.4%) would be expected to be small and no greater than that among non-vaccinees (8-10). The unchanged absenteeism rate is further evidence that such vaccination programs do not interfere appreciably with work. In contrast, all employees with diagnosed rubella must be kept out of work for the duration of their contagious period (until the fifth or sixth day after onset of rash (11), and, if ill, some may be expected to be bed-ridden for 3-5 days or even hospitalized (12,13).

References

1. Colorado State Dept of Health: Hospital rubella outbreak. Colorado Disease Bulletin 7(10), March 10, 1979
2. MMWR 27:123, 1978
3. Rubella testing and immunization of health personnel. California Morbidity, No. 37 (Suppl): 1-4, September 22, 1978
4. McLaughlin MD, Gold LH: The New York rubella incident: A case for changing hospital policy regarding rubella testing and immunization. Am J Public Health 69:287-289, 1979
5. Public Health Service Advisory Committee on Immunization Practices: Rubella vaccine. MMWR 27:451-454, 459, 1978
6. CDC: Rubella Surveillance Report. July 1973 - December 1975. Issued August 1976
7. Spruance SL, Smith CB: Joint complications associated with derivatives of HPV-77 rubella virus vaccine. Am J Dis Child 122:105-111, 1971
8. Lerman SJ, Nankervis GA, Heggie AD, Gold E: Immunologic response, virus excretion, and joint reactions with rubella vaccine. A study of adolescent girls and young women given live attenuated virus vaccine (HPV-77:DE-5). Ann Intern Med 74:67-73, 1971
9. Landrigan PJ, Stoffels MA, Anderson E, Witte JJ: Epidemic rubella in adolescent boys. Clinical features and results of vaccination. JAMA 227:1283-1287, 1974
10. Reidenberg MM, Lowenthen DT: Adverse non-drug reactions. N Engl J Med 279:678-679, 1968
11. American Academy of Pediatrics: Report of the Committee on Infectious Diseases. 18th ed., Evanston, Illinois, AAP, 1977, p 243
12. Peczenik A, Gauld JR: Rubella at a military installation. Arch Environ Health 6:657, 663, 1963
13. Tarasov VI: Some complications of rubella in adults. Sov Med 12:82-85, 1978

MMWR 28:374 (8/17/79)

Rubella — United States, 1977-1979

As of August 4, 1979, 10,342 cases of rubella were reported to CDC compared to 16,021 cases reported in the same 31-week period in 1978. This 36.1% decrease in rubella activity represents a continuation of the decline noted in 1978 (Figure 1).

The provisional 1978 total of 18,243 cases was 10.6% less than the 1977 total of 20,395 (Table 1). Age data were available for 10,277 (56.3%) of the reported 1978 cases. That year, the proportion of cases and the risk of disease declined in those less than 20 years of age, when compared to 1977. Fifteen- to nineteen-year-olds continued to

FIGURE 1. Reported rubella, by year, United States, 1966-1979*

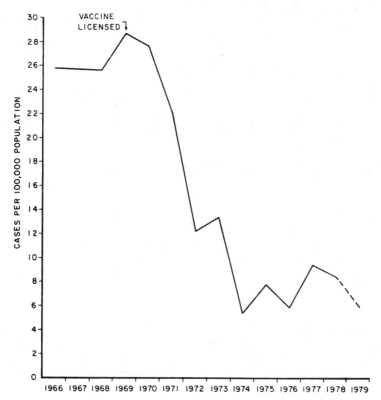

*1979 annual incicence rate for rubella was extrapolated from the number of cases for the first 31 weeks of 1979. The 1978 figure is provisional.

account for the greatest percentage of reported cases and had the highest incidence rate (1). However, the rate in this age group did decrease by 18.7% from 1977 to 1978 and was only 3.8% greater than the rate for 1975 (36.8 per 100,000), the first year in which reporting by age became available from a large number of states. The 1978 rates in those less than 5, 5-9, and 10-14 years old were less than those for 1975 by 28.9%, 41.3%, and 18.5%, respectively.

Individuals 20 years of age and older made up a greater proportion of reported cases of known age in 1978 (32.0%) as compared to both 1977 (21.9%) and 1975 (15.7%). Only the 20- to 24-year age group, which alone accounted for 24.7% of such cases, experienced an increased risk (36.7%) of acquiring rubella between 1977 and 1978. However, the risk of rubella for those 20 years and older is still greater than that in 1975: almost 2.5 times as great for those 20-24 years old, and approximately 1.5 times as great for those 25 years of age and older.

Reported by Surveillance and Assessment Br, Immunization Div, Bur of State Services, CDC.

Editorial Note: Reported rubella activity fluctuates, but at a level approximately 70% less than that reported in prevaccine years (1). If the currently observed reduction in reported rubella cases continues throughout 1979, not only will the number of rubella cases have declined for 2 consecutive years, but also the total will approach the lowest number of

TABLE 1. Percent distribution of reported rubella cases and incidence rate,* by age group, United States, 1977-1978

Age (years)	1977			1978†			Percent change 1977-1978	
	Number	Percent	Rate	Number	Percent	Rate	Percent	Rate
<1-4	941	7.8	10.4	781	7.6	9.1	−2.6	−12.5
5-9	1,012	8.4	10.0	616	6.0	6.4	−28.6	−36.0
10-14	1,610	13.3	14.2	1,047	10.2	9.7	−23.6	−31.7
15-19	5,867	48.6	47.0	4,542	44.2	38.2	−9.1	−18.7
20-24	1,950	16.1	16.6	2,538	24.7	22.7	+53.4	+36.7
25-29	346	2.9	4.0	362	3.5	3.6	+20.7	−10.0
30+	352	2.9	0.6	391	3.8	0.6	+31.0	0.0
Total with known age	12,078	59.2	−	10,277	56.3	−	−	−
Unknown age	8,317	40.8	−	7,966	43.7	−	−	−
TOTAL	20,395	100.0	9.4	18,243	100.0	8.4	−	−10.6

*Incidence rate = cases per 100,000 population (1977 U.S. census) extrapolated from the age distribution of cases from 40 reporting areas.
†Provisional total.

cases ever recorded—11,917, in 1974.

A continuous reduction in rubella from 1975 to 1978 occurred only in those less than 15 years of age. It is clear that there must be more effective vaccination of older individuals, especially childbearing-aged females, to decrease further their risk of rubella infection (1,2).

References
1. MMWR 27:495-497, 1978
2. Advisory Committee on Immunization Practices: Rubella vaccine. MMWR 27:451-454, 1978

MMWR 27 (A.S., 1978): 54

RUBELLA (German Measles) — Reported Case Rates by Month, United States, 1976—1978

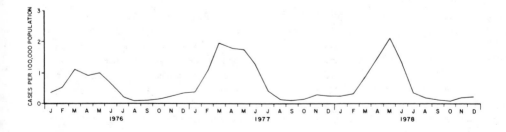

CHAPTER 33

Measles

MMWR 27:427 (11/3/78)

Measles Prevention

These revised ACIP Measles Prevention recommendations represent an effort to address more directly some of the key issues in measles prevention and control.

The issues discussed in previous statements on Measles Vaccine (MMWR 25:359-360, 365, 376, 1976) and Measles Outbreak Control (MMWR 26:294, 299, 1977) have been combined in this statement. The relative increase in reported measles cases in adolescents prompted an extension and clarification of recommendations for immunization of adolescents, both males and females. The usefulness of school immunization requirements has been emphasized. The definition of measles susceptibles and revaccination recommendations for them have been more clearly established.

INTRODUCTION

Measles (rubeola) is often a severe disease, frequently complicated by middle ear infection or bronchopneumonia. Encephalitis occurs in approximately 1 of every 1,000 cases; survivors often have permanent brain damage and mental retardation. Death, predominantly from respiratory and neurologic causes, occurs in 1 of every 1,000 reported measles cases. The risks of encephalitis and death are known to be greater in infants, and suspected to be greater in adults, than in children and adolescents.

Measles illness during pregnancy increases fetal risk. Most commonly, this involves premature labor and moderately increased rates of spontaneous abortion and of low birth weight (1). One retrospective study in an isolated population suggests that measles infection in the first trimester of pregnancy was associated with an increased rate of congenital malformations (2).

Before measles vaccine was available, more than 400,000 measles cases were reported annually in the United States. Since the introduction of vaccine in 1963, the collaborative efforts of professional and voluntary medical and public health organizations in vaccination programs have resulted in a 90% reduction in the reported incidence of measles. In 1977, 57,345 cases were reported. In the pre-vaccine era, the majority of measles cases occurred in preschool and young, school-age children. In 1977, more than 60% of cases in which the age was known occurred in persons 10 or more years old. More than 20% were reported in the 15- to 19-year-old age group.

With the highly effective, safe measles vaccines now available, the degree of measles control in the United States depends largely on the effectiveness of the continuing effort to vaccinate all susceptible persons who can safely be vaccinated.

MEASLES VIRUS VACCINE

Live measles virus vaccine* available in the United States is prepared in chick embryo cell culture. The vaccine virus strain primarily used at present has been attenuated beyond the level of the original Edmonston B strain and is therefore known as a further attenuated strain. Vaccine prepared with the further attenuated measles virus is generally preferred, in part because it causes fewer reactions than its predecessor. It is available in monovalent (measles only) form and in combinations: measles-rubella (MR) and measles-mumps-rubella (MMR) vaccines. All vaccines containing measles antigen are recommended for use at about 15 months of age. MMR is encouraged for use in routine infant vaccination programs. In all situations where measles vaccine is to be used, consideration should be given to using a combination vaccine when recipients are likely to be susceptible to rubella and/or mumps as well as to measles. Edmonston B measles vaccine is not available in combined form and is now rarely used.

Measles vaccine produces a mild or inapparent, non-communicable infection. Measles antibodies develop in at least 95% of susceptible children vaccinated at about 15 months of age or older with the current further attenuated vaccine. Evidence now extending to 15-year follow-up indicates that, although titers of vaccine-induced antibodies are lower than those following natural disease, the protection conferred appears to be durable.

Vaccine Shipment and Storage

Failure of protection against measles may result from the administration of improperly stored vaccine. During shipment and storage prior to reconstitution, measles vaccine must be kept at a temperature between 2-8 C (35.6-46.4 F). It must also be protected from light, which may inactivate the virus.

VACCINE USAGE

General Recommendations

Persons can be considered immune to measles only if they have documentation of:

(1) Physician-diagnosed measles or laboratory evidence of measles immunity, or

(2) Adequate immunization with live measles vaccine when 12 or more months of age.

Most persons born before 1957 are likely to have been infected naturally and generally need not be considered susceptible. All other children, adolescents, and adults are considered susceptible and should be vaccinated, if not otherwise contraindicated.

Dosage

A single dose of live measles vaccine (as a monovalent or combination product) should be given subcutaneously in the volume specified by the manufacturer. Immune serum globulin (ISG) should **NOT** be given with further attenuated measles virus vaccine. It is indicated only if Edmonston B vaccine is used.

Age at Vaccination

Measles vaccine is indicated for persons susceptible to measles, regardless of age, unless otherwise contraindicated. Current evidence indicates that for a maximum rate of seroconversion, measles vaccine should preferably be given when children are about 15 months of age. Whenever there is likely exposure to natural measles, infants as young as 6 months should be vaccinated. However, to ensure protection of infants vaccinated before 12 months of age, they should be revaccinated when they are about 15 months old. It is particularly important to vaccinate infants before they might encounter measles in day-care centers or other such environments.

Because of the *upward* shift in age distribution of reported cases, the immune status of all adolescents should be evaluated. Complete measles control will require protection

*Official name: Measles Virus Vaccine, Live, Attenuated

of all susceptibles; therefore, increased emphasis must be placed on vaccinating susceptible adolescents and young adults. Susceptible persons include those who received inactivated vaccine or who were given live measles virus vaccine before they were 12 months of age, as well as those who were never vaccinated or never had measles.

Revaccination of Persons Vaccinated According to Earlier Recommendations

Persons vaccinated with live measles vaccine before 12 months of age and those vaccinated at any age with inactivated vaccine (available from 1963 to 1967) should be identified and revaccinated. Persons who are unaware of their age at vaccination or who were vaccinated prior to 1968 with a vaccine of unknown type should also be revaccinated. In addition, persons who received live measles vaccine in a series within 3 months of inactivated measles vaccine should be revaccinated.

There has been some confusion concerning the immunity of children vaccinated against measles at 12 months of age. This is because some recent data have indicated a slightly lower rate of seroconversion among children vaccinated at 12 months of age than among those vaccinated at 13 months or later. This difference is not sufficient to warrant routinely revaccinating persons in the former group; the vast majority are fully protected. If, however, the parents of a child vaccinated when 12 to 15 months old request revaccination for the child, there is no immunologic or safety reason to deny the request.

Individuals Exposed to Disease

Use of vaccine: Exposure to measles is not a contraindication to vaccination. Available data suggest that live measles vaccine, if given within 72 hours of measles exposure, may provide protection. If the exposure does not result in infection, the vaccine should induce protection against subsequent measles infection.

Use of ISG: To prevent or modify measles in a susceptible person exposed less than 6 days before, ISG, 0.25 ml/kg (0.11 ml/lb) of body weight, should be given (maximum dose—15 ml). ISG may be especially indicated for susceptible household contacts of measles patients, particularly contacts under 1 year of age, for whom the risk of complications is highest. Live measles vaccine should be given about 3 months later, when the passive measles antibodies should have disappeared, if the child is then at least 15 months old. *ISG should not be used in an attempt to control measles outbreaks.*

SIDE EFFECTS AND ADVERSE REACTIONS

Experience with more than 100 million doses of measles vaccine distributed in the United States through early 1978 indicates an excellent record of safety. About 5%-15% of vaccinees may develop fever $\geqslant$103 F ($\geqslant$39.4 C) beginning about the sixth day after vaccination and lasting up to 5 days. Most reports indicate that persons with fever are asymptomatic. Transient rashes have been reported rarely. Central nervous system conditions including encephalitis and encephalopathy have been reported approximately once for every million doses administered. Limited data indicate that reactions to vaccine are not age-related.

Subacute sclerosing panencephalitis (SSPE) is a "slow virus" infection of the central nervous system associated with a measles-like virus. Results from a recent study indicate that measles vaccine, by protecting against measles, significantly reduces the chance of developing SSPE (3,4). However, there have been reports of SSPE in children who did not have a history of natural measles but did receive measles vaccine. Some of these cases may have resulted from unrecognized measles illness in the first year of life or possibly from the measles vaccine. The recent decline in numbers of SSPE cases in the presence of careful surveillance is additional strong presumptive evidence of a protective effect of measles vaccination.

Revaccination Risks

There is no evidence of enhanced risk from receiving live measles vaccine for one who has previously received live measles vaccine or had measles. Specifically, there does not appear to be any enhanced risk of SSPE. The previously cited study showed no association between SSPE and either receiving live measles vaccine more than once or receiving it after having had measles.

On exposure to natural measles, some children previously inoculated with inactivated measles virus vaccine have developed atypical measles, sometimes with severe symptoms. Reactions, such as local edema and induration, lympadenopathy, and fever, have at times been observed when live measles virus vaccine was administered to recipients of inactivated vaccine. However, despite the risk of local reaction, children who have previously been given inactivated vaccine (whether administered alone or followed by a dose of live vaccine within 3 months) should be revaccinated with live vaccine to avoid the severe atypical form of natural measles and to provide full and lasting protection.

PRECAUTIONS AND CONTRAINDICATIONS

Pregnancy: Live measles vaccine should not be given to females known to be pregnant. This precaution is based on the theoretical risk of fetal infection, which applies to administration of any live virus vaccine to females who might be pregnant or who might become pregnant shortly after vaccination. Although no evidence exists to substantiate this theoretical risk from measles vaccine, concern about it has constrained measles vaccination programs for adolescent girls. Considering the importance of protecting adolescents and young adults against measles with its known serious risks, asking females if they are pregnant, excluding those who are, and explaining the theoretical risks to the others are reasonable precautions in a measles immunization program.

Febrile illness: Vaccination of persons with febrile illness should be postponed until recovery. Minor illnesses such as upper respiratory infections, however, do not preclude vaccination.

Allergies: Live measles vaccine is produced in chick embryo cell culture. It has not been reported to be associated with allergic reactions and can be given to all who need it, including persons with allergies to eggs, chickens, and feathers. Some vaccines contain trace amounts of antibiotics to which patients may be allergic. Those administering vaccines should review the label information carefully before deciding whether patients with known allergies to such antibiotics can be vaccinated safely. Live measles virus vaccine does not contain penicillin.

Recent Administration of ISG: Vaccination should be deferred for about 3 months after a person has received ISG because passively-acquired antibodies might interfere with the response to the vaccine.

Tuberculosis: Tuberculosis may be exacerbated by natural measles infection. There is no evidence, however, that the live measles virus vaccine has such an effect. Therefore, tuberculin skin testing need not be a prerequisite for measles vaccination. The value of protection against natural measles far outweighs the theoretical hazard of possibly exacerbating unsuspected tuberculosis. If there is a need for tuberculin skin testing, it can be done on the day of vaccination and read 48 to 72 hours later. If a recent vaccinee proves to have a positive skin test, appropriate investigations and, if indicated, tuberculosis therapy should be initiated.

Altered immunity: Replication of the measles vaccine virus may be potentiated in patients with immune deficiency diseases and by the suppressed immune responses that occur with leukemia, lymphoma, or generalized malignancy or with therapy with corticosteroids, alkylating drugs, antimetabolites, or radiation. Patients with such conditions should not be given live measles virus vaccine. Their risks of being exposed to measles may be reduced by vaccinating their close susceptible contacts. Management of such persons, should they be exposed to measles, can be facilitated by prior knowledge of their immune status.

Management of Patients with Contraindications to Measles Vaccine

If immediate protection against measles is required for persons for whom live measles virus vaccine is contraindicated, passive immunization with ISG, 0.25 ml/kg (0.11 ml/lb) of body weight, should be given as soon as possible after known exposure (maximum dose—15 ml). It is important to note, however, that ISG, which will usually prevent measles in normal children, may not be effective in children with acute leukemia or other conditions associated with altered immunity.

Simultaneous Administration of Certain Live Virus Vaccines

See "General Recommendations on Immunization," MMWR 25:349-350, 355. 1976.

MEASLES CONTROL

Ongoing Programs

The best means of reducing the incidence of measles is by having an immune population. Universal immunization as part of good health care should be accomplished through routine and intensive programs carried out in physicians' offices and public health clinics. Programs aimed at vaccinating children against measles at about 15 months of age should be established by all communities. In addition, all other persons, regardless of age, thought to be susceptible should be vaccinated when they are identified, unless vaccine is otherwise contraindicated.

Official health agencies should take whatever steps are necessary, including development and enforcement of school immunization requirements, to assure that all persons in schools and day-care settings are protected against measles. Enforcement of such requirements has been correlated with reduced measles incidence.

Measles outbreaks have been and continue to be reported from places where young adults are concentrated, such as colleges and military bases. Measles control in these places may require careful evaluation of susceptibility and vaccination of those who are susceptible.

Concern is often expressed because of observations during outbreaks that cases occur in persons with a history of proper vaccination. Even under optimal conditions of storage and use, measles vaccine may have a 5% failure rate. A 90% or greater reduction in attack rates has been demonstrated consistently in appropriately vaccinated persons when compared to others. As greater numbers of susceptibles become vaccinated and as measles incidence is further reduced, there will be a relative increase in the proportion of cases seen among appropriately vaccinated persons.

Outbreak Control

The danger of a measles outbreak exists whenever a measles case is reported in a community. Once an outbreak occurs, preventing dissemination of measles depends on promptly vaccinating susceptible persons. Ideally, they will have been identified before the outbreak (by school record reviews, for example); if not, they must be quickly identified.

Speed in implementing control programs is essential in preventing the spread of measles. All persons who cannot readily provide a *documented* history of measles or of vaccination with live measles virus vaccine when more than 12 months of age should be vaccinated or excluded from school. If a person's measles immunity is in doubt, he/she should be vaccinated.

An effective means of terminating outbreaks and increasing rates of immunization quickly is to exclude from school all children or adolescents who cannot present valid evidence of immunity through vaccination or prior disease. Exclusion should include pupils who have been exempted from measles vaccination because of medical, religious, or other reasons. Exclusion should continue until at least 2 weeks after the onset of the last case of measles in the community. Less rigorous approaches such as voluntary appeals for vaccination have not been effective in terminating outbreaks.

ISG should not be used in an attempt to control measles outbreaks.

SURVEILLANCE

Known or suspected measles cases should be reported immediately to local health departments. Effective surveillance of measles and its complications can delineate inadequate levels of protection, further define groups needing special attention, and assess the effectiveness of control activities. Continuous and careful review of adverse reactions is also important. All serious reactions in vaccinated children should be evaluated and reported in detail to local and state health officials as well as to the manufacturer.

References
1. Siegel M, Fuerst HT: Low birth weight and maternal virus diseases: A prospective study of rubella, measles, mumps, chicken-pox, and hepatitis. JAMA 197:680-684, 1966
2. Jesperson CS, Lettauer J, Sagild U: Measles as a cause of fetal defects. Acta Paediatr Scand 66:367-372, 1977
3. Modlin JF, Jabbour JT, Witte JJ, et al: Epidemiologic studies of measles, measles vaccine, and subacute sclerosing panencephalitis. Pediatrics 59:505-512, 1977
4. Center for Disease Control: Subacute sclerosing panencephalitis and measles. MMWR 26:309, 1977

SELECTED BIBLIOGRAPHY

Albrecht P, Ennis FA, Saltzman EJ, et al: Persistence of maternal antibody in infants beyond 12 months: Mechanism of measles vaccine failure. J Pediatr 91:715-718, 1977

Barkin RM: Measles mortality. Analysis of the primary causes of death. Am J Dis Child 229:307-309, 1975

Berkovich S, Starr S: Use of live-measles-virus vaccine to abort an expected outbreak of measles within a closed population. N Engl J Med 269:75-77, 1963

Center for Disease.Control: Atypical measles—California. MMWR 25:245-246, 1976

Horowitz O, Grunfeld K, Lysgaard-Hansen B, et al: The epidemiology and natural history of measles in Denmark. Am J Epidemiol 100:136-149, 1974

Kamin PB, Fein BT, Britton HA: Use of live, attenuated measles virus vaccine in children allergic to egg protein. JAMA 193:1125, 1965

Krugman RD, Rosenberg R, McIntosh K, et al: Further attenuated measles vaccines: The need for revised recommendations. J Pediatr 91:766-767, 1977

Landrigan PJ, Witte JJ: Neurologic disorders following live measles vaccination. JAMA 223:1459-1462, 1973

Langmuir AD: Medical importance of measles. Am J Dis Child 103:34-56, 1962

Linnemann CC: Measles vaccine. Immunity reinfection and revaccination. Am J Epidemiol 97:365-371, 1973

Marks JS, Halprin TJ, Orenstein WA: Measles vaccine efficacy in children previously vaccinated at 12 months of age. Pediatrics (in press)

Orenstein WA, Halsey NA, Hayden GF, et al: Current status of measles in the United States 1973-1977. J Infect Dis 137:847-853, 1978

Shasby DM, Shope TC, Downs H, et al: Epidemic measles in a highly vaccinated population. N Engl J Med 296:585-589, 1977

Shelton JD, Jacobson JE, Orenstein WA, et al: Measles vaccine efficacy: The influence of age at vaccination versus duration of time since vaccination. Pediatrics (in press)

Wilkins J, Wehrle PF: Evidence for reinstatement of infants 12 to 14 months of age into routine measles immunization programs. Am J Dis Child 132:164-166, 1978

Yeager AS, Davis JH, Ross LA, et al: Measles immunization successes and failures. JAMA 273:347-351, 1977

MMWR 28:298 (6/29/79)

Death from Measles, Possibly Atypical — Michigan

A 13-year-old girl died on February 18, 1978, after being hospitalized at University Hospital, Ann Arbor, Michigan, with a diagnosis of measles encephalitis and pneumonia. The patient had been vaccinated in 1966 or 1967 with 3 injections of killed measles vaccine.

One week before admission, and 10 days after a known measles exposure, she developed fever, headache, chills, cough, rhinorrhea, and severe vomiting. A fine rash appeared on her arms and spread to her trunk and face. She was seen by her physician, who diagnosed atypical measles. A week later, on January 23, her fever increased, and she had her first seizure. She was seen in the emergency room of a community hospital and treated with intravenous diazepam, but seizures persisted, and she required intubation. Because of the character of the rash, a diagnosis of meningococcal meningitis was considered, and the patient was transferred to University Hospital in Ann Arbor.

Upon arrival, she was treated with intravenous penicillin and hydrocortisone. Despite anticonvulsant therapy, she continued to have focal and then generalized seizures. Examination was remarkable for rales throughout both lung fields, a petechial rash over the face, and a fine, blanching, maculopapular rash over the entire body. A pustular component was also noted. Admission laboratory findings included a white blood cell count (WBC) of 14,500/mm^3 and a normal platelet count. Lumbar puncture (LP) revealed 2 red and 9 white blood cells/mm^3. The total protein level was 104 mg/dl, and the glucose level was 50 mg/dl. Chest X ray showed left lower lobe and perihilar infiltrates. Repeat LP 1 day after admission was essentially unchanged. A final LP on the 14th hospital day showed normal chemistries and cellular elements.

On January 23 and again on February 9, 1978, measles antibody titer in the patient's serum, determined by immunofluorescent antibody testing (IFA), was 1:4,096. Measles antibody titer from her cerebral spinal fluid, also determined by IFA, was 1:32 on January 23 and February 4. Attempts to isolate virus from throat washings, urine, and from unstimulated lymphocytes were unsuccessful. Over the next several days, the rash began to fade, but the patient remained comatose. She died on the 21st hospital day.

Reported by JV Baublis, MD, PhD, Dept of Pediatrics, University of Michigan Hospital, Ann Arbor; VJ Turkish, DO, Ypsilanti; N Hayner, MD, State Epidemiologist, Michigan State Dept of Public Health; Immunization Div, Bur of State Services, CDC.

Editorial Note: A large number of cases of what has come to be called atypical measles have been reported since its first description in 1965 (*1*). Most cases have occurred in persons who had previously received inactivated (killed) measles vaccine, 1.8 million doses of which were distributed in 1963-1967 (*2*). Killed vaccine was usually given in a series of 2 to 4 doses at monthly intervals; the final dose was often live (Edmonston B) measles vaccine (for example, killed-killed-live sequence).

Atypical measles characteristically consists of a prodrome of high fever, usually without cough or coryza, followed by development of a polymorphic rash, which begins on the distal extremities and spreads centrally (*1,3*). Pneumonia is common, as is abdominal pain (*1,3*). Although these patients have appeared ill, association with encephalitis or with fatal outcome has not previously been reported.

Inactivated (killed) measles vaccine was withdrawn from use in part because of reports of atypical measles but also because immunity after this vaccine series was found to wane rapidly (*4*). Waning immunity has not been noted in persons who received only the live Edmonston B measles vaccine (with or without simultaneous immune serum globulin), which also became available in 1963, or in those persons who have received the more recent, further attenuated virus vaccines. These persons do not need reimmunization provided they were immunized at or after 12 months of age (5,6). Persons who received only the killed vaccine series should be reimmunized unless they have already received a dose of live measles vaccine *at least 3 months after their last dose of killed vaccine* (5,6). This recommendation is made, despite the occasional occurrence of marked local reactions in revaccinees, because of the potential severity of atypical measles (7). This teenager had not been reimmunized.

Physicians and clinics should continue efforts to ensure that their pediatric and adult patients have proof of adequate immunization against measles. None of 6 children previously reported to have fatal measles in 1978 (8) had been immunized according to current recommendations.

References
1. Rauh LW, Schmidt R: Measles immunization with killed virus vaccine. Am J Dis Child 109:232-237, 1965
2. CDC: Measles Surveillance Report No. 10, 1973-1976. Issued July 1977
3. Nichols EM: Atypical measles syndrome: A continuing problem. Am J Public Health 69:160-162, 1979
4. Fulginiti VA, Arthur JH: Altered reactivity to measles virus. J Pediatr 75:609-616, 1969
5. Advisory Committee on Immunization Practices: Measles prevention. MMWR 27:427-430, 435-437, 1978
6. American Academy of Pediatrics: Report of the Committee on Infectious Diseases, 8th ed. Evanston, Illinois, AAP, 1977
7. Krause PJ, Cherry JD, Naiditch MJ, Deseda-Tous J, Walbergh EJ: Revaccination of previous recipients of killed measles vaccine: Clinical and immunologic studies. J Pediatr 93:565-571, 1978
8. MMWR 27:424-425, 1978

MMWR 28:553 (11/23/79)

Measles in Air Force Recruits — Texas

During the 5-year period ending October 1979, 3,323 cases of measles were seen in recruits at Lackland Air Force Base, Texas. This contrasts sharply with the preceding 5-year period, when 70 cases occurred. The years of highest activity were 1977 (1,356 cases) and 1978 (992 cases). Although cases occurred throughout the year, seasonal peaks occurred in March and April. Complications were frequent and included pneumonia (4.3%), otitis media (4.3%), sinusitis (2.2%), and encephalitis (2 cases).

Since March 1979, all susceptible recruits (that is, those with hemagglutination inhibition tests ≤1:10) have been immunized with live, further attenuated vaccine on their eighth day of training, and there has been a subsequent sharp decline in measles cases.

Because of concern about potential reactions to the vaccine in young adults, 220 aircraft personnel who were immunized against measles and 435 who were not but were vaccinated against other diseases, were surveyed by questionnaire 4 weeks after immunization for local and systemic reactions. These aircraft personnel, who were all from the same training group, complained of less pain and local swelling at the measles vaccination site than at the tetanus-diphtheria, influenza, and meningococcal polysaccharide vaccination sites. There was no significant difference in the incidence of dispensary visits, hospitalizations, eye pain, pharyngitis, coryza, cough, myalgias, joint pain, diarrhea, or headache in those who received measles vaccine compared with those who did not; there was a small increase in reports of fever.

Reported by V Martinez, MD, G Crawford, MD, D Gremillion, MD, Wilford Hall Medical Center, Lackland Air Force Base, Texas; Immunization Div, Bur of State Services CDC.

FIGURE 1. Cases of measles in U.S. Air Force recruits, by quarter, January 1975-September, 1979

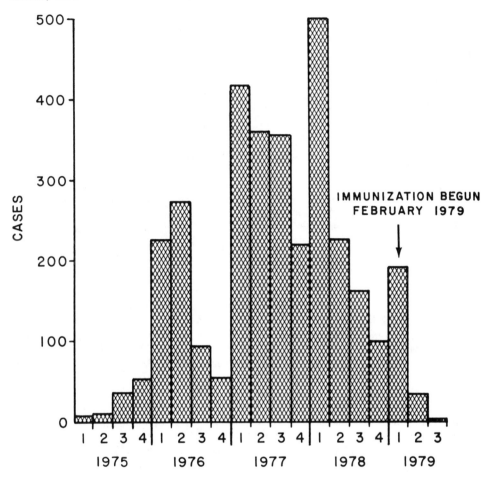

Editorial Note: In this population of young military recruits, selective immunization of susceptibles is proving to be an effective method of measles control that is not associated with serious reactions.

MMWR 28:410 (8/31/79)

Measles — United States, 1977-1979

As of August 25 (the thirty-fourth week of 1979), 12,000 cases of measles were reported in the United States. This is a 48.8% decrease from the number of cases reported for the comparable time period in 1978 and a 40.3% decrease from the total cases reported in the first 34 weeks of 1974, the year with the lowest total number of recorded cases (22,094).

FIGURE 3. Reported measles cases, United States, 1970-1979*

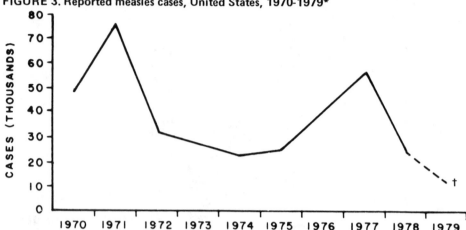

*Provisional data have been used for 1978.
†1979 annual total was extrapolated from the number of cases reported for the first 34 weeks of 1979.

The provisional 1978 number of reported measles cases (25,859) was a 54.9% decline from the final 1977 total (57,345) (Figure 3). Ages were available for 14,779 cases (57.2%) from 47 reporting areas (Table 2). A large proportion of cases of known age continued to occur in older children (1). In 1978, as in 1977, approximately 60% of reported cases occurred in children 10 years of age and older. Before 1976, less than 50% of cases occurred in this age group (2). Those under 5 and more than 20 years old made up a greater proportion of cases in 1978 than in 1977. Significant decreases in incidence rates were noted for all age groups; however, the 10- to 14-year age group remained at highest risk for measles infection (42.8 cases per 100,000 population) followed by those 5-9 years of age (36.1 per 100,000).

Reported by Surveillance and Assessment Br, Immunization Div, Bur of State Services, CDC.

Editorial Note: If reported measles activity continues to decline at the current rate, the projected 1979 total will be between 13,000 and 14,000 reported cases, an all-time low for the United States (Figure 3).

Several factors contributed to the sharp decline noted in 1978 and mid-1979, including intensive measles vaccination programs and increased measles activity during 1977, both of which diminished the number of susceptibles. In 1977, public programs administered 55% more measles vaccine than was used during the comparable period in 1976. The amount of measles vaccine currently being administered approximates the 1977 level. Several states have enforced school immunization laws and have excluded from school those children who did not have an adequate documentation of measles vaccination. Rigorous review of school records and vaccination of those without previous immunization have led to a marked decrease in the number of children at risk (3,4).

While the age-specific data illustrate the continued need to vaccinate susceptible elementary, junior, and senior high school students, they also point out the significant proportion of cases contributed by those less than 5 years old. There obviously is a need to increase measles prevention activities in nursery and day-care settings.

TABLE 2. Percent distribution of reported measles cases and incidence,* by age group, United States, 1977-1978

Age (years)	1977			1978†			Percent changes for 1977 to 1978	
	Total cases	Percent distribution	Cases per 100,000	Total cases	Percent distribution	Cases per 100,000	Percent	Cases per 100,000
<5	5,843	14.1	52.7	2,619	17.7	30.0	+25.5	−43.1
5-9	10,498	25.2	83.3	3,552	24.0	36.1	−4.8	−56.7
10-14	14,231	34.2	99.8	4,703	31.8	42.8	−7.0	−57.1
15-19	9,447	22.7	61.6	3,263	22.1	27.1	−2.6	−56.0
20+	1,582	3.8	1.3	642	4.3	0.8	+13.2	−38.5
Total with known age	41,601	72.5	−	14,779	57.2	−	−	−
Unknown age	15,744	27.5	−	11,080	42.8	−	−	−
TOTAL	57,345	100.0	26.5	25,859	100.0	11.9	−	−55.1

*Incidence = cases per 100,000 population extrapolated from the age distribution of known cases from 49 reporting areas in 1977 and 47 in 1978.
†Provisional total.

References
1. MMWR 27:235-237, 1978
2. Orenstein WA, Halsey NA, Hayden GF, et al: Current status of measles in the United States, 1973-1977. J Infect Dis 137:847-853, 1978
3. MMWR 27:303-304, 1978
4. Preblud SR, Brandling-Bennett AD, Hinman AR: An update of measles, mumps, and rubella. Presented at the Fourteenth Immunization Conference, St. Louis, Missouri, March 1979

MMWR 27 (A.S., 1978): 38

MEASLES (Rubeola) – Reported Case Rates by Year, United States, 1950–1978

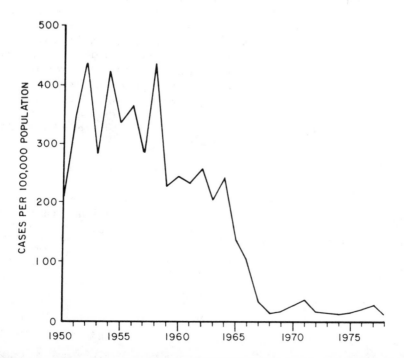

CHAPTER 34

Various Viral Diseases

MMWR 27:507 (12/15/78)

Aseptic Meningitis — Maryland

An outbreak of aseptic meningitis occurred in a tri-county area of eastern Maryland between July 16 and August 20, 1978. The outbreak peaked during the week of August 7-13. Through active case finding, 55 patients with aseptic meningitis were identified: 25 were considered to be definitive cases, 26 presumptive, and 4 suspected.* Twenty-three of the cases were located in a predominantly non-white area of County A; 8, including adults and children, could be linked epidemiologically to a local day-care center; and 15 were clustered in a group of homes adjacent to a migrant labor camp, which had no contact with the day-care center. Of the 55 patients, 36 (65.5%) were between the ages of 5 and 19 years. The attack rate for meningitis among white patients was 58/100,000 population; that for non-whites was 251/100,000. The overall attack rate was 107/100,000.

From January 1-October 13, 1978, Maryland reported 233 patients with aseptic meningitis, including the 55 from the tri-county area who were identified through active case finding. During the summer outbreak period, the state laboratory reported that 69 of 77 non-polio enteroviral isolates were echovirus 9.

This year's report records the largest number of aseptic meningitis cases associated with a single enteroviral agent since aseptic meningitis became reportable in the state in 1963. During the past 10 years, the average reported number of patients with aseptic meningitis has been 86 per year. The number of echovirus 9 isolations this year is nearly triple the number from 1971, the most recent year with major echovirus 9 activity in Maryland.

Reported by DL Sorley, MD, MPH, State Epidemiologist, Maryland State Dept of Health and Mental Hygiene; Field Services Div, Viral Diseases Div, Bur of Epidemiology, CDC.

---

*A definitive case of aseptic meningitis was defined as fever, headache and/or stiff neck, cerebrospinal fluid pleocytosis with negative bacterial cultures, and recovery without antibiotics. A presumptive case was one with fever, headache and/or stiff neck, recovery without antibiotics, known contact of a patient with definitive meningitis, and no lumbar puncture performed. A suspected case was one with fever, headache and/or stiff neck, plus 2 of the following: sore throat, abdominal cramping, and rash; no known contact with meningitis patients; and no lumbar puncture.

MMWR 27 (A.S., 1978): 19

ASEPTIC MENINGITIS — Reported Cases per 100,000 Population by State, United States, 1978

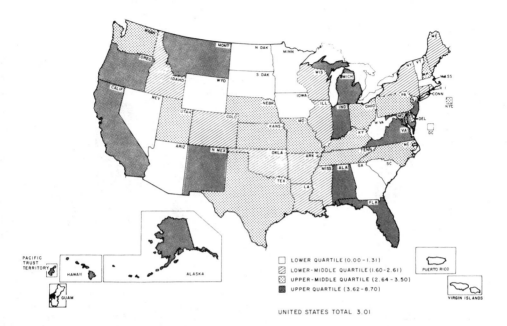

LOWER QUARTILE (0.00 - 1.31)
LOWER-MIDDLE QUARTILE (1.60 - 2.61)
UPPER-MIDDLE QUARTILE (2.64 - 3.50)
UPPER QUARTILE (3.62 - 8.70)

UNITED STATES TOTAL 3.01

MMWR 28:530 (11/9/79)

Adenovirus Type 16 — Long Island, New York

From January 16 to March 12, 1979, adenovirus type 16 (AV-16) was isolated from 12 Long Island, New York, patients by the Nassau County Medical Center (NCMC). In the previous 10 years, AV-16 had been isolated from only 3 patients at NCMC; all 3 isolations were in 1977.

The first patient this year had onset of symptoms on January 12. Most of the subsequent cases occurred in the fourth through eighth week of 1979 (Figure 1). Eighty-three percent (10/12) were children <6 years of age (mean age, 5.5 years; age range, 1-18 years). Seven patients were boys, and 5 were girls. A review of medical records for the 12 patients showed that the most common findings were a history of fever (100%), injected pharynx (92%), nausea and/or vomiting (67%), lymphadenopathy (58%), and nasal congestion (58%). Conjunctivitis was present in 6 cases. Cough, myalgia, abdominal pain, headache, diarrhea, rash, hypertrophied tonsils, injected tympanic membranes, and rhonchi were noted, but less frequently. The average recorded temperature was 38.6 C (range 36.6-40.6 C), and the white blood cell count was mildly elevated in 3 of 5 patients tested. Three persons required hospitalization. AV-16 was recovered from the pharynx of 11 patients and from the rectum of 2 of 3 persons cultured. Nine persons resided in southern Nassau County and 3 in nearby Suffolk County. Telephone interviews in September with 8 of the 12 patients' mothers failed to identify any common exposure.

The secondary attack rate among household contacts was 28% (7 of 25 persons at risk). Three of the 7 were parents of the cases, and 4 were siblings. The incubation period for the secondary cases was 1 to 6 days (mean, 2.5 days).

FIGURE 1. Persons culture positive for adenovirus type 16, by week of onset of illness, Long Island, New York, January 1-March 24, 1979

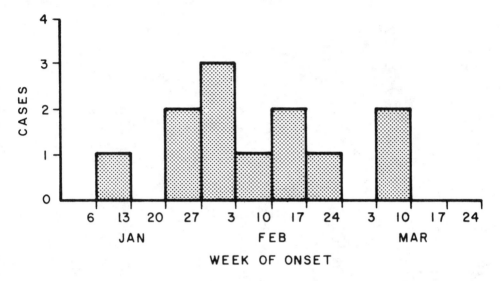

Reported by SW Klein, MD, J McPhee, Virology Laboratory, NCMC: TC Abruzzot, MD, MPH, Nassau County Health Dept; Bureau of Disease Control, New York State Dept of Health; Viral Diseases Div, Bur of Epidemiology, CDC.

Editorial Note: AV-16 was first isolated in Saudi Arabia in persons with conjunctivitis (*1*). Although little information is available regarding the occurrence of this virus, it appears to be uncommon. It only rarely causes conjunctivitis (*2-4*), and it was cultured from only 6 of 7,509 patients with pharyngitis over a 4-year period (*5*). The 3 AV-16 isolates at NCMC in 1977 occurred in persons who had conjunctivitis (in 2 persons) and pharyngitis (in 1). Since the cases detailed here, NCMC has isolated AV-16 from 4 other persons with conjunctivitis or fever. There have been no other reported isolates of AV-16 in New York this year.

References
1. Murray ES, Chang RS, Bell SD, et al: Agents recovered from acute conjunctivitis case in Saudi Arabia. Am J Ophthalmol 43:32-35, 1957
2. Bell SD, McComb DE, Murray ES, et al: Adenoviruses from Saudi Arabia (Part I). Am J Trop Med Hyg 9:492-500, 1959
3. Feng M, Chang RS, Smith TR, Snyder JC: Adenoviruses from Saudi Aradia (Part II). Am J Trop Med Hyg 9:500-506, 1959
4. Jackson GG, Muldoon RL: Viruses causing common respiratory infection in man. IV. Reoviruses and adenoviruses. J Infect Dis 128:811-866, 1973
5. Vargosko AJ, Kim HW, Parrott RH, et al: Recovery and identification of adenovirus in infections of infants and children. Bacteriol Rev 29:487-495, 1965

MMWR 27 (A.S., 1978): 22

CHICKENPOX — Reported Case Rates by Month, United States, 1974—1978

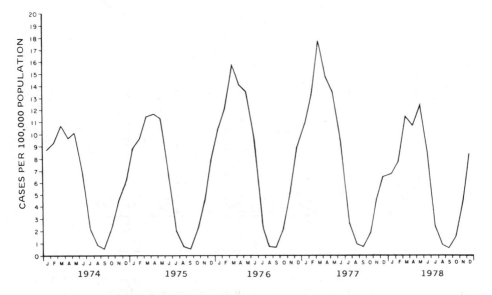

MMWR 27:392 (10/13/78)

Echovirus Type 9 Outbreak — New York

An outbreak of echovirus type 9 infection is occurring on Long Island, New York. Between April 20 and September 23, 1978, 158 viral isolates have been obtained from 106 persons ages 1 day to 30 years (Figures 1 and 2). The outbreak peaked during the summer months and currently appears to be declining.

Several patients presented with aseptic meningitis, but the vast majority have had upper respiratory tract involvement, primarily pharyngitis (Table 1). Twenty-eight of the 106 persons were hospitalized. Seventeen patients (16%) presented with meningitis. Of the 89 patients who did not have meningitis, 68 (76%) had clinical pharyngitis. The 21 (24%) without meningitis or apparent pharyngitis had fever or sepsis (8), rash (4),diar-rhea (4), or other respiratory findings (5). Nearly half of these (10/21) were younger than 1 year.

Of the 17 patients with aseptic meningitis, 88% were age 9 or older. Significantly more males (15/17) than females had aseptic meningitis ($p < 0.05$). The clinical presentation was typical of that generally seen with meningitis; rash and/or pharyngitis were also found in several patients. Echovirus type 9 was isolated from all 17 aseptic meningitis cases, 60% from throat swabs, 60% from cerebrospinal fluids. Virus was isolated from both sources in only 2 patients.

Ninety-two percent of the patients this year were children under 15 years of age. A comparison of the age distributions of ECHO 9 cases from this outbreak with cases from 1970-1977 on Long Island and with cases from 1967-1970 among 20 nations (1) reveals that patients were generally older in previous outbreaks.

Reported by SW Klein, MD, J McPhee, MS, Nassau County Medical Center, New York; DO Lyman, MD, State Epidemiologist, New York Dept of Health; Viral Diseases Div, Bur of Epidemiology, CDC.

FIGURE 1. Onset of illness, by week, in ECHO 9 cases,* Long Island, New York, 1978

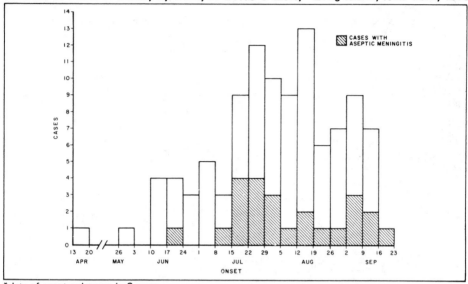

*date of onset unknown in 2 cases

FIGURE 2. Clinical presentation of ECHO 9 cases with either pharyngitis or aseptic meningitis, by age, Long Island, New York, April 20-September 23, 1978

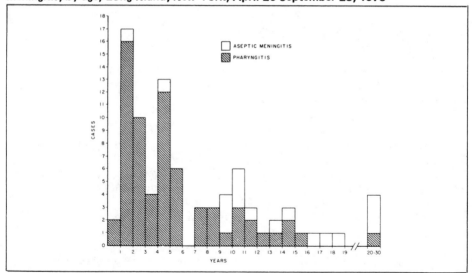

Editorial Note: ECHO 9 is classically associated with infection of the central nervous system (CNS) (2,3); it is primarily seen in older children and adolescents. In this outbreak only 16% of patients had CNS infection, in comparison with 79% of patients in the 20-nation study by the World Health Organization (1).

The Nassau County Medical Center actively encouraged specimen collection for pur-

TABLE 1. Clinical findings among ECHO 9 patients, Nassau County, 1978 and 1970-1977

Clinical finding	Percent with finding	
	1978 (n=106)	1970-1977 (n=86)
Fever	83	77
Pharyngitis (total)	67	33
Pharyngitis with exudate	20	0
Nausea/vomiting	39	26
Headache	34	32
Rash	24	25
Nasal congestion	22	22
Diarrhea	16	3
Otitis media	16	4
Cough	13	15
Nuchal rigidity	6	22
Photophobia	6	4

poses of virus isolation of all febrile pediatric patients and all patients suspected of having an illness of viral etiology. Because of this, several cases of pharyngitis or upper respiratory tract infection were identified as probably due to ECHO 9.

Whereas pharyngitis without evidence of Group A β-hemolytic *Streptococcus* is often presumed to be "viral"—without further definition—active surveillance and laboratory evaluation, in this instance, identified ECHO 9 as one such viral agent that can cause pharyngitis in children.

References
1. Assaad F, Cockburn WC: Four-year study of WHO virus reports on enteroviruses other than poliovirus. Bull WHO 46:329-336, 1972

MMWR 28:422 (9/7/79)

Mumps — United States, 1978-1979

As of August 25 (the 34th week of 1979), 11,015 cases of mumps were reported to CDC. This represents a 16.6% decrease in mumps activity compared to the same time period in 1978.

The 1978 total of mumps cases (16,817) was 21.5% less than the 1977 total (21,436) (Figure 3). Thirty-three reporting areas provided age data on 6,173 (36.7%) of the cases. Between 1977 and 1978, there were declines in reports of mumps for all age groups except for the ≥20-year group, which experienced no change. Mumps continues to be a disease primarily of elementary school children (Table 2). Children 5-9 years of age accounted for 50% of the cases and had the highest incidence rate (49.1 cases per 100,000 population). Approximately one-fourth of the cases occurred in the 10- to 14-year age group, which had the next highest incidence rate (21.8 cases per 100,000 population).

Children less than 5 years old made up only approximately 10% of the cases and had an incidence rate of 13.8 cases per 100,000 population, which was below that of the 10- to 14-year-olds. In prevaccine and early postvaccine years, the less than 5-year-olds made up a greater proportion of the cases and had a greater risk of acquiring mumps than the 10- to 14-year-olds (1).

FIGURE 3. Reported cases of mumps, United States, 1922-1978

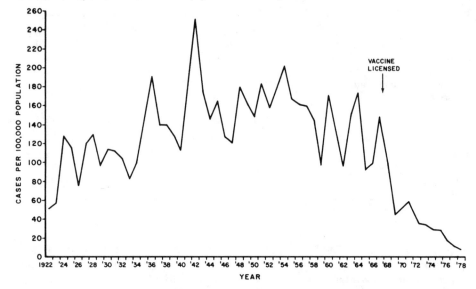

TABLE 2. Percent distribution of reported mumps cases and incidence rate,* by age group, United States, 1978†

Age group (yrs)	Number of cases	Percent distribution	Incidence rate
<5	774	12.5	13.8
5-9	3,092	50.1	49.1
10-14	1,526	24.7	21.8
15-19	400	6.5	5.2
20+	381	6.2	0.7
Total with age known	6,173	36.7	—
Total with age unknown	10,644	63.3	—
TOTAL	16,817	100.00	7.8

*Incidence rate = cases per 100,000 population extrapolated from the age distribution of known cases from 33 reporting areas.
†Provisional total.

Reported by Immunization Div, Bur of State Services, CDC.

Editorial Note: Reported mumps activity has declined fairly steadily since 1971, 4 years after licensure of mumps vaccine (Figure 3). This has been accompanied by decreases in the reported mumps-associated complications (aseptic meningitis, encephalitis, and death) (1).

The changes in age-specific epidemiology are undoubtedly secondary to current practices of vaccine distribution. These changes have also been observed with measles and rubella (2,3).

References
1. CDC: Mumps Surveillance Report, July 1974 - December 1976. Issued 1978
2. MMWR 28:410-411, 1979
3. MMWR 28:374-375, 1979

MMWR 28:589 (12/14/79)

Varicella-Zoster Immune Globulin

Varicella-Zoster Immune Globulin (VZIG) continues to be available for immunodeficient children exposed to chickenpox. It is being released at no cost through the Division of Clinical Microbiology, Sidney Farber Cancer Institute (SFCI), 44 Binney Street, Boston, Massachusetts (617-732-3121). The Immunization Division, CDC (404-329-3747), the SFCI, and former VZIG consultants are available for consultation regarding alternative modes of therapy.

Since VZIG is still an investigational drug and its supply is limited, several criteria for release apply. These 5 criteria have been previously published in the MMWR in tabular form (1), but this year several clarifications are needed.

First, the term "newborn contact" (See Table 2, II-D) was previously described as a "newborn whose mother contracted varicella *within 4 days* before delivery or within 48 hours after delivery." In the revised table, the italicized term has been changed to "less than 5 days" because an appropriate newborn contact includes infants whose mothers develop the varicella rash up to but not including the fifth day before delivery. (Such infants have a 30% mortality rate [2,3].) No mortality has been associated with infants whose mothers contract varicella 5 or more days before delivery.

Second, the criterion concerning the age of patients, as listed on the table (item IV), is for patients less than 15 years old. However, on an *individual* basis, VZIG will be made available for certain patients between 15 and 21 years old.

Finally, the fifth criterion indicates that the request for treatment must be initiated within 72 hours of exposure. While any request for treatment must be initiated within this time period, treatment may be expected to modify or even prevent disease if started within 96 hours of exposure.

Reported by the Sidney Farber Cancer Institute, Boston, Massachusetts; and the Immunization Div, Bur of State Services, CDC.

References
1. MMWR 27:508, 1978
2. Meyers JD: Congenital varicella in term infants: Risk reconsidered. J Infect Dis 129:215-217, 1974
3. Gershon AA: Varicella in mother and infant: Problems old and new, in Drugman S, Gershon AA (eds): Symposium on Infections of the Fetus and the Newborn Infant. New York, Alan R. Liss, Inc., 1975, pp 88-89

TABLE 2. Five criteria for release of Varicella-Zoster Immune Globulin (VZIG) for the prophylaxis of varicella

I. One of the following underlying illnesses or conditions
    A. Leukemia or lymphoma
    B. Congenital or acquired immunodeficiency
    C. Under immunosuppressive medication
    D. Newly born of mother with varicella
II. One of the following types of exposure to varicella or zoster patient
    A. Household contact
    B. Playmate contact (>1 hour play indoors)
    C. Hospital contact (in same 2- to 4-room bedroom or adjacent beds in a large ward)
    D. Newborn contact (newborn whose mother contracted varicella less than 5 days before delivery or within 48 hours after delivery)
III. Negative or unknown prior disease history
IV. Age of less than 15 years
V. The request for treatment must be initiated within 72 hours of exposure.

MMWR 27:403 (10/20/78)

Viral Gastroenteritis — Pennsylvania

Two recent waterborne outbreaks of gastroenteritis totaling at least 423 cases have occurred in Pennsylvania summer camps. Serologic evidence from 6 patients has implicated parvovirus-like agents as the cause.

Outbreak 1: In June 1978, CDC was notified of a gastrointestinal illness occurring in visitors at a camp in northeastern Pennsylvania. Fifty-seven of the 74 groups visiting this camp between May 1 and June 16 were questioned, and 13 reported illness in over 15% of their members. A total of 350 persons were reported to have been ill. All but 1 of the 13 groups with illness stayed at the camp between either May 12 and May 21 or June 5 and June 14. The attack rate among the 8 groups that had illness and also completed questionnaires ranged from 17%-73%.

Serum and stool specimens were collected from the members of the last group that visited the camp and reported illness. Studies for bacterial pathogens were negative, but 3 of 5 ill persons had a 4-fold titer rise in antibody to a Norwalk-like agent; 2 controls were negative. The illness in this group was characterized by vomiting (81%), abdominal pain (74%), nausea (67%), and diarrhea (56%). A questionnaire administered to this group showed no association between illness and performing activities, eating food, occupying a particular cabin, or drinking water from a stream that flows through the camp. However, a significant association was found between quantity of camp water consumed and illness. A similar questionnaire, administered to 2 other ill groups, showed no association between illness and activities performed, food eaten, cabin occupied, or exposure to stream water. In 1 of the 2 groups, however, a significant association between quantity of camp water consumed and illness was shown.

The initial study of the water system demonstrated the presence of coliforms (38/dl), inadequate chlorination (0 ppm), and several sites of possible contamination. These problems were corrected, and no further illness has been reported from the camp.

Outbreak 2: On July 27, 1978, an outbreak of gastroenteritis was reported from another summer camp in northeastern Pennsylvania. The cases were characterized by abdominal pain (80%), nausea (73%), and vomiting (53%). Headache (47%), diarrhea (38%), and chills (38%) were also prominent findings. The median duration of illness was 2 days.

Review of the infirmary records revealed 73 cases of gastroenteritis during the first session of the summer camp, which lasted from June 6-July 23. This is approximately 10 times the rate reported from last year. A sharp increase in cases began 48 hours after the arrival of the second-session campers. As determined from questionnaire data, the attack rate in the second session was 61.5% (120/195). Food was not incriminated. However, consumption of 5 or more glasses a day of water or water-containing beverages was significantly associated with illness (p<.05). Bacterial samples from the camp water supply revealed fecal coliforms from well water. Although the camp water supply was chlorinated, tests for residual chlorine level revealed 0 ppm until July 28, when an adequate chlorination level was achieved. No new cases have been reported since July 29.

Laboratory studies of stools from 10 patients and 10 controls revealed no bacterial pathogens. Three of 3 paired serum specimens, however, showed 4-fold or greater rises to Norwalk agent by radioimmunoassay. Electron microscopy of stools is pending.

Reported by M van Ouiverkerk, South Brunswick Township, New Jersey; R Altman, MD, State Epidemiologist, H Ragazzoni, DVM, W Weisgarber, New Jersey Dept of Health; J LaCoe, Pennsylvania Dept of Environmental Resources; D Arbott, RN, M Castello, RN, M Grumbine, RN, WE Parkin,

DVM, DrPH, State Epidemiologist, I Ratliff, RN, Pennsylvania Dept of Health; Enteric Virology Br, Virology Div, Bur of Laboratories, Environmental Health Services Div, Bur of State Services, Enteric Diseases Br, Bacterial Diseases Div, Enteric and Neurotropic Viral Diseases Br, Viral Diseases Div, Bur of Epidemiology, CDC.

Editorial Note: Parvovirus-like agents (for example, Norwalk, Montgomery County, Hawaii) have been suspected of causing waterborne outbreaks of gastroenteritis (*1*). The agents responsible for 2 outbreaks previously reported have been confirmed as Norwalk-like viruses (*2,3*). These 2 Pennsylvania outbreaks further illustrate that parvovirus-like agents may contribute to gastrointestinal disease. Newer techniques, such as radioimmunoassay, have made diagnosis of outbreaks easier as long as proper specimens have been collected.

These 2 outbreaks also substantiate previous reports that a high attack rate, predominance of upper gastrointestinal symptoms, and a relatively short duration of illness are compatible with viral gastroenteritis (*2,4*).

References
1. Zweighaft RM, Morens DM, Bryan JA: Viral gastroenteritis, in Practice of Medicine, Vol. IV. New York, Harper and Row, 1978
2. MMWR 26:13-14, 1977
3. MMWR 26:176, 1977
4. Christopher PJ, Grohman GS, Millsom RH, Murphy AM: Paravovirus gastroenteritis—a new entity for Australia. Med J Aust 1:121-124, 1978

CHAPTER 35

Diseases of Uncertain Etiology

MMWR 28:217 (5/18/79)

Erythema Chronicum Migrans and Lyme Disease — Nine Probable Cases Diagnosed Outside the Northeastern United States

Erythema chronicum migrans (ECM) is an unusual, expanding annular rash known to physicians in Europe for many years (1). At least since 1976, a clustering of cases of ECM has occurred each summer in 3 contiguous towns adjacent to the lower Connecticut River (Lyme, Old Lyme, and East Haddam, Connecticut) in conjunction with the meningo-encephalitis and oligoarthritis of Lyme disease (2,3). Epidemiologic evidence for its transmission by ticks is convincing, even though no infectious agent has been isolated.

Presumptive cases of Lyme disease have also been noted in other areas in southern New England and near Long Island Sound (3,4). However, probable cases in persons residing in the United States but outside of the Northeast have only recently received attention. Below are details on 9 such cases occurring in the past decade. All 9 patients had recently traveled or spent leisure time in wooded areas, but only 3 in the places where ECM has been repeatedly observed.

Patient 1: In January 1969, a 57-year-old Wisconsin man complained of erythema on 1 side of his body, preceded by headache, malaise, and dull pain over 1 hip (5). An inflamed, punctate lesion was found above the iliac crest, an area in which he recalled having been bitten by a tick when he was hunting near Medford, in northwest Wisconsin, 3 months earlier. A welt, initially 2 cm in diameter, spread outward and cleared centrally; it then became an annular area of erythema, extending from the mid-chest to the mid-back and from the axilla to below the iliac crest. A biopsy was consistent with ECM. The patient became asymptomatic within 48 hours of receiving a single parenteral injection of penicillin; he had no sequelae in the succeeding year.

Patient 2: During the last 10 days of June 1974, a 46-year-old man traveled in rural northern Europe, hiking and picnicking (6). On July 1, he noted headache and pain over the upper spine. Two weeks later, after returning to California, he experienced right-sided tongue paresthesia and bilateral facial weakness over a 1-week period. During hospitalization an erythematous lesion, 22 cm in diameter, developed on his posterior chest wall. The typical manifestations of meningoencephalitis also appeared. Extensive microbiologic and serologic studies were unrevealing. The lesion soon expanded and cleared centrally. The patient was given oral penicillin therapy, and his symptoms subsided within a week. Recovery of neurologic function was more prolonged. There was a history of exposure to ticks but no bite.

Patient 3: A 32-year-old hiker was bitten on the thigh by a tick in Sonoma County,

California, in June 1975 (7). After 1 week, the man noted a pruritic, erythematous ring at the location of the bite. Four weeks after the bite, a physician found a large, erythematous, macular, non-scaling, centrifugally spreading ring; it had a trailing bluish cast. During the next month the ring expanded to 35 cm in diameter and faded. A tick, removed from the area of the bite hours after it was noted, was identified as *Ixodes*, most likely *I. pacificus*. In the next 2½ years the man experienced 2 brief episodes of stiffness in the hip related to walking; he had no other inflammatory symptoms.

Patient 4: A 13-year-old boy noted a red lesion on his thigh during the week before he returned home to Florida from Mystic, Connecticut, where he had spent the summer of 1975 (8). As the lesion grew and cleared centrally, several similar ones developed on 1 arm and both legs. Shortly after he arrived in Florida, he was treated with an antibiotic, and the lesions disappeared. One month later he developed a recurrent inflammatory joint condition. A knee effusion was aspirated and injected with a corticosteroid. A rheumatologist subsequently diagnosed the illness as juvenile rheumatoid arthritis and recommended salicylate therapy. Between May 1976 and the fall of 1977, the patient had 3 more attacks of arthritis.

Patients 5-7: A 30-year-old woman, a 23-year-old man, and the man's 2½-year-old niece were 3 of 11 persons camping in June 1977 near Sarona, in northwestern Wisconsin (9). All 3 removed ticks from the neck, back, or upper extremities and recalled being bitten. Soon afterward, each patient developed a combination of fever, headache, stiff neck, myalgia, anorexia, lethargy, somnolence, confusion, and periorbital edema. One of the patients had meningitis, and another had meningoencephalitis. Within 2 to 4 days, each patient had a single skin lesion, initially called cellulitis but subsequently recognized as ECM. Over the next 6 months each patient experienced pain and swelling of the shoulders, elbows, and knees on several occasions before becoming symptom free.

Patient 8: An 18-year-old Atlanta resident camped in the Lyme area for 3 days in late July 1977. On approximately August 10, he developed fever to 39.4 C, malaise, headache, neck pain, myalgia, and mild, watery diarrhea. He consulted a physician in Maine, who noted 3 to 4 erythematous, circular skin lesions on the back and arms. Blood and cerebrospinal fluid (CSF) studies and an EEG were not diagnostic. As the systemic symptoms subsided, the skin lesions grew larger and less distinct. When the patient returned to Atlanta at the end of August, a physician recognized the fading lesions as ECM. The man had only 1 other brief episode of headache, malaise, and myalgia about 10 days later. He remembered tick exposure but no bite during his travel.

Patient 9: A 26-year-old Florida woman traveled by air to and from Nantucket Island, Massachusetts, where she spent 2 weeks backpacking in November 1978. At 1 point she removed and discarded a tick attached to her upper left arm. For the next 3 weeks, after she had returned to Florida, she noted aching and 2 papules in the region of the tick bite. In a few days a round, reddish-purple, burning lesion, 9-10 cm in diameter, developed and expanded over her left shoulder and back. A dermatologist made no diagnosis but prescribed erythromycin and a topical steroid preparation. The lesion improved slightly but then evolved into concentric rings. Meanwhile, during the next 2 weeks, the patient experienced myalgia and fatigue. Physical examination, chest X ray, and routine laboratory tests were unremarkable. During the next several weeks she had 2 episodes of fever, headache, photophobia, stiff neck, and aching, culminating in hospitalization for meningoencephalitis with facial paralysis. She was treated with corticosteroids. Symptomatic improvement has been gradual. She has had arthralgia but no discrete joint pain or swelling.

Reported by CW Davidson, MD, Atlanta, Georgia; JN Lewis, MD, MPH, State Epidemiologist, Con-

necticut State Dept of Health; and the Arthritis and Immunologic Diseases Activity, Chronic Diseases Div, Bur of Epidemiology, CDC.

Editorial Note: The diagnosis of ECM can generally be made clinically, although there are helpful dermatopathologic changes (3). The rheumatic and neurologic illness that often follows ECM, known as Lyme arthritis or Lyme disease, cannot easily be distinguished from other similar inflammatory conditions in the absence of the skin lesion. Cryoglobulins are frequently present in the serum of patients who develop Lyme arthritis (3), but no laboratory test is diagnostic. The purported effectiveness of antimicrobial therapy has not been adequately evaluated.

The cases summarized here are typical of the disease as elucidated by the Yale investigators (2,3). Four of the cases emphasize the need for physicians remote from the endemic area to consider travel and recreational opportunities for exposure in their diagnostic approach.

Patient 9 is the first reported from Nantucket despite heavy infestation of that island with *I. dammini*, a newly proposed species heretofore not distinguished from *I. scapularis*. *I. dammini* is also the vector in human babesiosis on Nantucket. The case of patient 3 is the only known occurrence of ECM in California. Patients 5-7 from northwestern Wisconsin prominently displayed the major features of ECM and Lyme disease and are noteworthy for their clustering in an area where both ECM (Patient 1) and *I. dammini* (*10*) had apparently been observed in the past.

References

1. Goltz RW: The unusual figurate erythemas, in Fitzpatrick TB, Arndt KA, Clark WH Jr (eds): Dermatology in General Medicine. New York, McGraw-Hill, 1971, pp 709-711
2. Steere AC, Malawista SE, Snydman DR, et al: Lyme arthritis: An epidemic of oligoarticular arthritis in children and adults in three Connecticut communities. Arthritis Rheum 20:7-17, 1977
3. Steere AC, Malawista SE, Hardin JA, Ruddy S, Askenase PW, Andiman WA: Erythema chronicum migrans and Lyme arthritis: The enlarging clinical spectrum. Ann Intern Med 86:685-698, 1977
4. Calabro JJ, Dell'Italia LJ, Leers SA, Yunus M, Kilduff FJ, Hazard GW: Lyme arthritis. Arthritis Rheum 21:167, 1978
5. Scrimenti RJ: Erythema chronicum migrans. Arch Dermatol 102:104-105, 1970
6. Wagner L, Susens G, Heiss L, Ganz R, McGinley J: Erythema chronicum migrans: A possibly infectious disease imported from northern Europe. West J Med 124:503-505, 1976
7. Naversen DN, Gardner LW: Erythema chronicum migrans in America. Arch Dermatol 114:253-254, 1244, 1978
8. Zakem JM, Germain BF: Lyme arthritis in Florida. J Fla Med Assoc 66:281-283, 1979
9. Dryer RF, Goellner PG, Carney AS: Lyme arthritis in Wisconsin. JAMA 241:498-499, 1979
10. Spielman A, Clifford CM, Piesman J, Corwin MD: Human babesiosis on Nantucket Island, USA: Description of the vector, *Ixodes dammini*, n. sp. (Acarina: Ixodidae). J Med Entomol 15:218-234, 1979

MMWR 27:9 (1/13/78)

Kawasaki Disease — United States

Since 1975, 232 suspect cases of Kawasaki disease (formerly referred to as mucocutaneous lymph node syndrome, MCLS, MLNS, or MCLNS) have been reported to CDC. Kawasaki disease was documented* in 112 of 117 patients about whom information sufficient to confirm or rule out the diagnosis was provided.

---

*CDC diagnostic criteria and features of the illness are detailed elsewhere (*1*).

Cases have been reported from 31 states, Puerto Rico, and the District of Columbia — areas that together contain 80% of the total U.S. population. The male-to-female ratio was 1.5 to 1.0; 57% were white, 18% black, and 25% oriental or part oriental. The mean age was 3.8 years and the modal age 3 years, with an age range from 3 months to 13 years.

Reported by the Enteric and Neurotropic Viral Diseases Br, Viral Diseases Div, Bur of Epidemiology, CDC.

Editorial Note: Kawasaki disease is an acute febrile illness of prepubertal children associated with a characteristic picture of erythema of the conjunctivae and mucous membranes of the upper respiratory tract, erythema and indurative edema of the peripheral extremities, maculopapular rash, desquamation, and usually lymphadenopathy, often confined to the anterior cervical chain. Thrombocytosis (from 500,000 to 2,000,000/mm^3) and elevated white blood cell count and erythocyte sedimentation rates are usual. Meningitis, arthralgia, arthritis, proteinuria, sterile pyuria, diarrhea, and elevated liver enzymes are also seen. Throat culture, antistreptolysin-O titers, streptozyme test, and culture and serologic examination for rubeola, rubella, rickettsiae, and other infectious agents are negative. Deaths are almost always related to cardiac involvement, notably infarction secondary to diseased coronary arteries, or myocardial failure or arrhythmia due to myocarditis. It has recently been demonstrated that infantile periarteritis nodosa (IPN) is a severe and often fatal form of Kawasaki disease in the first few months of life (2). Cases of IPN have been described in the United States by pathologists for decades, suggesting that Kawasaki disease may have long existed but gone unrecognized. IPN was not seen in Japan prior to 1960, when Kawasaki disease cases were first noticed.

Since instituting disease surveillance in 1975, CDC has received a steadily increasing flow of reports of children with Kawasaki disease. As in Japan, where it is epidemic, disease in the United States does not appear to be limited by geographic, seasonal, socioeconomic, or environmental barriers. In addition to Japan and the United States, cases have also been diagnosed in Korea, Taiwan, the Philippines, Australia, Canada, Mexico, England, Scotland, Belgium, the Netherlands, Spain, Italy, Greece, West Germany, Sweden, and Turkey.

Because of well-organized biannual nationwide surveys, Japanese investigators have compiled detailed information on more than 10,000 cases. In Japan, the male-to-female ratio is 1.5 to 1.0, the median age 1 year, and the case-fatality ratio less than 2% (1). The Japanese have also observed small geographic clusters, recurrences, and second cases within families.

The etiology of Kawasaki disease has not been determined. Working independently, 3 laboratories have reported organisms (1 in spleen, 1 in buffy coat, and 1 in lymph nodes) morphologically similar to rickettsiae, but the evidence is inconclusive. Seroconversion to antigenic determinants of a number of infectious agents has been noted in cases initially suspected but deleted because the case definition specifies that other infectious diseases be ruled out. These agents include varicella-zoster virus, rubella, rubeola, para-influenza 2, and leptospira. Although HLA typing of patients and controls has been unrewarding (3), the disease has been reported with disproportionate frequency from Hawaii, where a majority of children are oriental or part oriental. Only 1 of 45 known cases from that state has been of purely Caucasian background. (Thirty-seven percent of the population of Hawaii is Caucasian.)

References
1. Morens DM, O'Brien RJ: Kawasaki disease in the United States. J Infect Dis 137:91-93, 1978
2. Landing BH, Larson EJ: Are infantile periarteritis nodosa with coronary artery involvement and fatal mucocutaneous lymph node syndrome the same? Comparison of 20 patients from North America with patients from Hawaii and Japan. Pediatrics 59:651-662, 1977
3. Matsuda I, Hattori S, Nagata N, Fruse A, Nambu H, Itakura K, Wakisaka A: HLA antigens in mucocutaneous lymph node syndrome. Am J Dis Child 131:1417-1418, 1977

MMWR 28:97 (3/9/79)

Reye Syndrome — United States

Since December 1978, 159 cases of Reye syndrome have been reported to CDC (*1-3*), including 6 clusters in areas with concurrent widespread influenza A activity. Eighteen deaths have been reported in 98 patients where the outcome is known.

Utah: Four children from the Salt Lake City area were hospitalized with Reye syndrome in a 2-week period in early December. One Reye syndrome patient had a 4-fold rise in hemagglutination inhibition (HI) antibody titer to influenza A (H1N1), and a second had a single convalescent titer of 1:64; serologic results are pending on 2 patients.

Arizona: Eight patients with Reye syndrome, 5 from the Phoenix area, were hospitalized in a 5-day period in mid-December. In 4 patients evidence of recent influenza A infection was demonstrated by a 4-fold rise in HI titers; in 2 patients single HI titers $\geq$128 were demonstrated. Two deaths occurred, both in 12-year-old females.

Colorado: Sixteen cases of Reye syndrome, including 3 deaths, have been confirmed. Fifteen of these cases occurred during the 6-week period from mid-December through January. Nine had a 4-fold rise in HI antibody titers to influenza A (H1N1). Laboratory results are pending on additional cases.

Michigan: Thirty-two cases have been confirmed since January 27. Most of these cases are from the southeastern section of the state, where influenza activity has been reported. Influenza A (H1N1) has been isolated from the nasopharyngeal swab of a 20-month-old boy with Reye syndrome. There have been 3 deaths.

Ohio: Since the beginning of December, 19 cases have been reported, 14 with onset in February. These 14 cases occurred in a 3-county area in northwestern Ohio that borders the area in Michigan where most of the cases of Reye syndrome have occurred.

Minnesota: Seven cases of Reye syndrome following respiratory prodromes and 1 following chicken pox were reported in a 10-day period in January; 6 were residents of the Twin Cities area, where increased influenza activity was concurrently reported. Two 10-year-old boys died.

Georgia: Since January 1, 14 cases of Reye syndrome have been reported, including a cluster of 6 cases from the northwestern portion of the state and 4 (1 following chicken pox) from 1 county in southern Georgia. Two patients had a 4-fold rise to influenza A (H1N1), and 1 patient had a single convalescent titer of 1:128. Four deaths were reported.

Oklahoma: Nine cases have been reported since mid-January, 6 following influenza-like prodromes and 3 following chicken pox. Seven are from the Tulsa area, where influenza activity was also reported. The ages of these patients ranged from 7 to 15 years; 1 death has been reported in a 12-year-old boy.

Investigations of these clusters are continuing.

Reported by T Fukushima, MD, State Epidemiologist, Utah State Dept of Social Services; A Kelter, MD, State Epidemiologist, W Stromberg, MA, Arizona State Dept of Health Services; T Edell, MD, Acting State Epidemiologist, N Halsey, MD, G Meiklejohn, MD, Colorado State Dept of Health; NS Hayner, MD, State Epidemiologist, Michigan State Dept of Public Health; TJ Halpin, MD, State Epidemiologist, F Holtzhauer, BS, Ohio State Dept of Health; A Dean, MD, State Epidemiologist, M Osterholm, MS, J Washburn, BA, Minnesota State Dept of Health; JE McCroan, PhD, State Epidemiologist, D Smith, Georgia Dept of Human Resources; S Fennell, MD, MA Roberts, MPH, Acting State Epidemiologist, Oklahoma State Dept of Health; Bur of State Services, Bur of Laboratories, Enteric and Neurotropic Viral Diseases Br, Viral Diseases Div, Bur of Epidemiology, CDC.

Editorial Note: The clusters which have been reported suggest a temporal and geographic association with influenza A (H1N1) activity. Laboratory data now available from patients in 4 clusters (Arizona, Utah, Colorado, and Georgia) demonstrate evidence of recent infection with influenza A. Continued surveillance and investigation of clusters during this period of influenza A activity are needed to determine the extent of this association.

References
1. MMWR 28:39, 1979
2. MMWR 28:64, 1979
3. MMWR 28:81, 1979

MMWR 27 (A.S., 1978): 92

In the 1977-78 period, the majority of cases of Reye syndrome occurred between December and March, when epidemic respiratory diseases are usually seen in children. Using data collected through 59 WHO collaborating laboratories as a measure of influenza activity, a temporal association is seen between the occurrence of Reye syndrome and the reporting of both the H3N2 and H1N1 influenza viruses. However, this association is not clear-cut; Reye syndrome cases dropped in frequency before a decrease in isolations of influenza A, and clusters of Reye syndrome cases were not reported in association with local outbreaks of influenza A. This is in contrast to the patterns in 1973-74 and 1976-77, when the epidemic curve for Reye syndrome cases more closely paralleled reported isolations of influenza B nationally, and outbreaks which were temporally and geographically associated with influenza B were reported in several states.

REYE SYNDROME — Reported Cases and Percentage of Influenza A Virus Isolates from Respiratory Specimens by Week of Isolation, United States, December 3, 1977—November 18, 1978

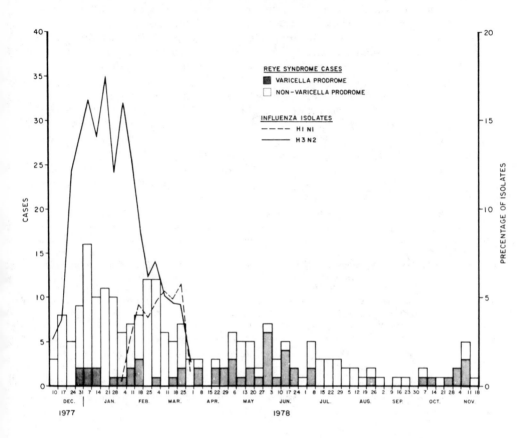

Part III

Diseases Caused by Fungi

CHAPTER 36

Mycoses

MMWR 26:375 (11/11/77)

Histoplasmosis — Northern Louisiana

An outbreak of acute pulmonary disease, presumptively identified as histoplasmosis, occurred in early September 1977 in northwest Louisiana. The outbreak involved all 6 men who cleared a field of bamboo cane on August 25 and 26. The field was known to be a blackbird roosting site and was located in an area considered to be heavily endemic for histoplasmosis (1).

Although no birds were present when the work was done, the grounds and a doghouse in the middle of the field were covered with several inches of bird droppings. One man, in addition to clearing the cane, cleaned off the roof of the doghouse while the others stood nearby. After the cane was bulldozed, it was burned and buried, and a fresh topping of soil was applied to the field.

The first person to become ill was the oldest participant, a 38-year-old man, whose illness began with low-grade fever and generalized aching 6 days after exposure. Over the next few days he had abdominal cramps and diarrhea followed by increasing fever, cough, chest pain, and dyspnea. His chest X ray showed widespread miliary infiltrates. The patient was hospitalized and improved over the next 2 weeks. The other 5 workers, all college students in their early 20s, developed acute illness with symptoms of fever, body aches, cough, and dyspnea 11-13 days after exposure. Chest X rays on all showed widespread miliary infiltrates. Bacterial and fungal cultures of sputum and blood were negative.

One patient developed respiratory failure, was treated with amphotericin B, and recovered. The others all recovered without specific anti-fungal therapy. Five had 4-fold or greater rises in titer to *Histoplasma capsulatum* yeast-phase complement fixation (CF) antigen, reaching a level of $\geq$ 1:64 in 4 patients and 1:32 in the fifth. The other man had a single titer of 1:16. Histoplasmin skin tests on 4 people, placed at the same time that the acute-phase serum specimens were drawn, were all negative. An aqueous suspension of the bird droppings from the doghouse showed structures identified as the tuberculate macroconidia of *H. capsulatum*. Cultures of the soil and the bird droppings from the doghouse roof are pending.

Reported by ES Butler, MD, Haynesville, Louisiana; RB George, MD, E Kotcher, ScD, AD Oberle, MS, LSU Medical School, Shreveport; CT Caraway, DVM, MPH, State Epidemiologist, Louisiana State Health and Human Resources Administration; Field Services Div, Special Pathogens Br, Bacterial Diseases Div, Bur of Epidemiology, CDC.

Editorial Note: As is often the case with this disease, the organism was not cultured from any of the patients in this outbreak. The diagnosis is supported, however, by the clinical illness, X rays, and serologic and epidemiologic findings. Numerous reports have indicated that a single histoplasmin skin test may stimulate humoral antibodies to *H. capsulatum* antigens in histoplasmin-hypersensitive individuals. In one study of 139 individuals who were skin-tested and later bled, none of the 25 who had negative skin tests had measurable antibodies, while 12 of the 114 who were skin-test positive had CF titers $\geq$ 1:8. Those 12 included 10 who responded to a level of $\geq$ 1:8 to the mycelial phase CF antigen and 2 who responded to a 1:8 level to the yeast-phase CF antigen. The highest titers observed were in 2 patients who had levels of 1:32 to the mycelial phase antigen (2).

In this outbreak the patients skin-tested were all skin-test negative and showed high titer serologic responses to the yeast-phase antigen. Thus, it is unlikely that the serologic responses are the result of skin-testing. As a general rule, however, skin-testing plays no role in the diagnosis of acute histoplasmosis since it usually does not provide helpful diagnostic information and potentially confuses the interpretation of serologic tests.

The danger of working with soil containing *H. capsulatum* organisms can be minimized if only workers with positive histoplasmin skin tests are involved and if the soil is decontaminated beforehand with 3% formalin.

References
1. Edwards LD, Acquaviva FA, Livesay VT: An atlas of sensitivity to tuberculin, PPD-B, and histoplasmin in the United States. Am Rev Respir Dis 99:1-132, 1969
2. Kaufman L, Terry RT, Schubert JH, and McLaughlin D: Effects of a single histoplasmin skin test on the serological diagnosis of histoplasmosis. J Bacteriol 94:798-803, 1967

MMWR 27:55 (2/17/78)

Coccidioidomycosis — California

A violent windstorm in the San Joaquin Valley on December 20 and 21, 1977, created extensive dust clouds which spread to many areas of California. State and local health officials became concerned that dust bearing the arthrocondia of *Coccidioides immitis* would expose people outside the regions endemic for coccidioidomycosis to the disease (*1*). During the first 24 days of January, 11% of 656 sera obtained from persons with suspected coccidioidomycosis and submitted to the Kern County (Calif) Health Department for tube precipitin tests were positive for *C. immitis;* by comparison, 2% of 300 sera submitted in January 1977, 9% of 400 sera submitted in January 1976, and 6% of 250 sera submitted in January 1975 were positive. During the same period, the University of California at Davis reported that 18% of 356 sera submitted were positive compared with 4% of 206 sera tested in January 1977. Several of these patients lived outside endemic regions of the state.

Reported by J Leonard, R Talbot, Kern County Health Dept Laboratory; Demosthenes Pappagianis, PhD, University of California, Davis; SB Werner, MD, California State Dept of Health; Bacterial Diseases Div, Bur of Epidemiology, CDC.

Editorial Note: Persons who traveled through the San Joaquin Valley during the storm and those who were subsequently exposed to dust clouds from the area may have been exposed to *C. immitis*. Because the incubation period is 1-3 weeks, physicians should suspect the diagnosis in exposed persons who developed flu-like symptoms in January. The diagnosis can be confirmed by the early appearance of *C immitis* precipitins or by the later appearance of antibodies detected by complement-fixation or immunodiffusion tests or skin-test conversion (*2*).

References
1. California State Dept of Health: The December 20-21, 1977, Central Valley dust storm and coccidioidomycosis. California Morbidity, supplement to No. 3, Jan 27, 1978
2. Smith CD, Saito MT, Simmons S: Pattern of 39,500 serologic tests in coccidioidomycosis. JAMA 160:546, 1956

MMWR 27:243 (7/14/78)

Follow-up on *Rhizopus* Infections Associated with Elastoplast* Bandages — United States

Since the February 1978 report on *Rhizopus* infections associated with Elastoplast bandages in Minnesota (*1,2*), 10 hospitals elsewhere in the United States have reported to CDC that 17 additional patients have had cutaneous infections caused by *Rhizopus* species. Several patients were identified by retrospective review; the earliest patient was seen in April 1977. Of the 17 patients, 14 had undergone surgical procedures and had had Elastoplast bandages placed over sterile gauze pads which covered the operative wound. The bandages and dressings remained in place for varying periods of time post-operatively, and lesions were usually present upon removal of the dressing. Lesions ranged from vesiculo-pustular eruptions to ulceration with eschar formation, and in some patients, skin necrosis was present and required debridement. Three other patients had similar cutaneous lesions after Elastoplast was applied over sterile gauze covering central venous line insertion sites (2 patients) and a bite wound (1 patient). One patient had diabetes mellitus, one had a malignancy, and one was on steroids for rheumatoid arthritis.

In 4 of the 10 hospitals, *Rhizopus* species have been isolated from either unused or partially used Elastoplast. Isolates from Elastoplast available from 3 of the 4 hospitals as well as isolates available from 8 of the 17 patients have been identified as *R. rhizopodiformis* by the Northern Regional Research Laboratory (NRRL), U. S. Department of Agriculture (USDA). The isolates originally reported (*1,2*) had been identified as *R. oryzae,* but these isolates are no longer available to confirm that identification.

Reported by Beiersdorf, Inc., South Norwalk, Connecticut; JJ Ellis, PhD, Agricultural Research Culture Collection, NRRL, USDA; Bur of Laboratories, Hepatitis Laboratories Div, Hospital Infections Laboratory Section, Epidemiologic Investigations Laboratory Br, Hospital Infections Br, Bacterial Diseases Div, Bur of Epidemiology, CDC.

Editorial Note: Infections with *Rhizopus* species are not routinely reported to CDC, and there is no information about patients with *Rhizopus* infections who have not been exposed to Elastoplast or who have been exposed to other wound-dressing materials. Approximately 1 million Elastoplast bandages per year are used in hospitals and, based upon the number of cases of *Rhizopus* infection reported to CDC, the risk of adverse reaction appears to be low. However, the characteristic clinical reactions reported (superficial cutaneous infection only at skin sites that had contact with the bandage) for the majority of patients and the recovery of *Rhizopus* species from the unused product suggest an association between use of the product and disease in patients.

The manufacturer does not guarantee a sterile product but does report that Elastoplast bandages are now being treated with cobalt irradiation before they are released to hospital suppliers. Preliminary studies conducted by CDC suggest that ethylene oxide sterilization of rolled bandages intrinsically or artificially contaminated with *Rhizopus,* vegetative bacteria, or bacterial spores is not effective. The manufacturer and CDC recommend that Elastoplast bandages should not be used over open wounds and should not come in contact with sterile fields if the maintenance of sterility is vital.

References
1. MMWR 27:33-34, 1978
2. MMWR 27:190, 1978

---

*Use of trade names is for identification only and does not constitute endorsement by the Public Health Service, U.S. Department of Health, Education, and Welfare.

MMWR 28:450 (9/28/79)

Blastomycosis in Canoeists — Wisconsin

In late July, 1979, 3 members of a southeastern Minnesota family developed fever, chills, night sweats, anorexia, weight loss of 6-14 lbs, headache, and pleuritic chest pain. Cough was present in only 1 individual. The diagnosis of pulmonary blastomycosis was made, based on pulmonary infiltrates and sputum cultures positive for *Blastomyces dermatitidis*. Subsequent epidemiologic investigation revealed that the 3 patients were part of a group of 8 who had taken a canoe trip on a northwestern Wisconsin river near Hayward on July 2. A common exposure may have occurred when the group stopped at a campsite along the river and gathered wood to build a fire and eat lunch.

Seven of the 8 group members had chest X-ray changes consistent with those seen in pulmonary blastomycosis; 4 were ill. Sputum from 3 of the symptomatic individuals and 2 of the cases with a positive X-ray grew *B. dermatitidis*. Serologic testing for blastomycosis, using complement-fixation and immunodiffusion methods, has been negative thus far in the 6 individuals tested. There has been no evidence of dissemination beyond the pulmonary tract in any of those infected, and the disease process is resolving without specific therapy. Environmental specimens obtained from the suspect campsite on August 28 are being cultured.

Reported by NS Brewer, MD, KH Rhodes, MD GD Roberts, PhD, JE Rosenblatt, MD, and RE Van Scoy, MD, The Mayo Clinic, Rochester, Minnesota; J Utz, MD, Georgetown University Medical School, Washington, D.C.; JP Davis, MD, State Epidemiologist, Wisconsin State Dept of Health and Social Services; Field Services Div, Special Pathogens Br, Bacterial Diseases Div, Bur of Epidemiology, CDC.

Editorial Note: North American blastomycosis is a granulomatous fungal infection that occurs sporadically in parts of the central and southeastern United States. The disease may be limited to respiratory symptoms, or it may be disseminated. Cases can be fatal if untreated, but the acute respiratory syndrome has been noted to resolve without specific therapy (*1*).

This unusual outbreak of blastomycosis was notable for the high attack rate, the non-specific nature of the symptoms, and the brevity of the apparent common exposure. A previous outbreak at Big Fork, Minnesota, in 1972 also demonstrated the first 2 features, but was associated with exposure to a site over the course of several months (*1*). The incubation period of approximately 30 days is consistent with that seen in a laboratory-acquired case (*2*). The low sensitivity of serologic testing has also been noted previously (*1*).

Further studies are in progress to investigate the possibility of other cases associated with the Wisconsin site, and to rule out other sites where exposure may have occurred. Suspected cases of blastomycosis in persons who reside in or have visited the area around Hayward should be reported to the Wisconsin State Department of Health and Social Services, to other appropriate health departments, or to CDC.

References
1. Tosh FE, Hammerman KJ, Weeks RJ, Sarosi GA: A common source epidemic of North American blastomycosis. Am Rev Respir Dis 109:525-529, 1974
2. Baum GL, Lerner PI: Primary pulmonary blastomycosis: A laboratory-acquired infection. Ann Intern Med 73:263, 1970

Part IV

Diseases Caused by
Protozoa and Helminths

CHAPTER 37

Malaria

MMWR 27:463 (11/24/78)

Chloroquine-Resistant Malaria Acquired in
Kenya and Tanzania — Denmark, Georgia, New York

Three cases of *Plasmodium falciparum* malaria in travelers to Kenya and Tanzania not cured by chloroquine have recently been reported. During late spring of 1978,1 patient, a 49-year-old man who worked in southeast Kenya, developed *P. falciparum* malaria after his return to New York. He was treated with chloroquine on 2 occasions, and each time his malaria recrudesced. He was finally treated successfully with a drug effective against chloroquine-resistant *P. falciparum* (1). The 2 other cases, which occurred in residents of Denmark and Georgia, are reported in detail below.

Copenhagen, Denmark: A 37-year-old man took a tour to Nairobi, Thika, Mombasa, and Amboseli and Tsavo National Parks from November 27 to December 9, 1977. He took the recommended chloroquine prophylaxis* while in Kenya and for 2 weeks after returning to Denmark. On December 28 he developed headache, fever up to 40 C (104 F), and chills. He was hospitalized on January 6 and found to have *P. falciparum* malaria. He received 2.5 gm of chloroquine phosphate over 3 days and was discharged after an uneventful recovery. He became febrile again on January 30, was again found to have *P. falciparum* parasitemia, and was treated with 3 gm chloroquine over 3 days. After treatment, no parasites could be found on a thick film. The third recrudesence occurred on April 2. *P. falciparum* was again seen. Over a 3-day period, 3125 mg of chloroquine was given. No parasites were found 2½ days later. Chloroquine absorption was documented by positive tests of urinary excretion. The fourth recrudescence occurred on May 2. He was treated with pyrimethamine and sulfadoxine, and no parasites were seen 4 days later. After 4 months no recrudescence has been detected, and the patient is presumed cured.

Atlanta, Georgia: A 50-year-old man took a hunting safari in southern Tanzania from August 15-September 3, 1978. He did not take malaria chemoprophylaxis. On September 9, he was admitted to an Atlanta hospital for shaking chills and intermittent fever (40.5 C [105 F]). *P. falciparum* parasites were identified on the thick and thin films. He received 2.5 gm of chloroquine over 3 days and was then discharged, despite mild "sweats" and headache, since no parasite could be seen on the smears. A blood smear performed on September 17 was negative, as was one done on October 10, although at that time the

---

*The current recommendation is chloroquine phosphate 500 mg (300 mg base) orally, once a week, beginning 1-2 weeks before arrival and continued for 6 weeks after departure. Primaquine use is discussed in the MMWR Malaria Supplement (3).

patient complained of low-grade fever and malaise. On October 12, a blood smear showed 5,000 parasites per mm^3, and the patient was then treated for 7 days with a twice-daily dosage of 160 mg of trimethoprim and 800 mg of sulfamethoxazole. By the second day of therapy, the smears became negative. The patient remains asymptomatic.

Reported by S Fogh, MD, S Jepsen, MD, P Eftersφe, Rigshospital and Statens Seruminstitut, Copenhagen, Denmark; BH Kean, MD, New York City; J Marr, MD, New York City Epidemiologist, Bur of Preventable Diseases; P Dubose, MD, Atlanta; J McCroan, PhD, State Epidemiologist, Georgia State Dept of Human Resources; Vector Biology and Control Div, Bur of Tropical Diseases, and Parasitic Diseases Div, Bur of Epidemiology, CDC.

Editorial Note: The World Health Organization recognizes 3 degrees of drug resistance— R1, R2, R3. The lowest degree of resistance, R1, is defined as the clearance of *asexual* malaria parasites (though not gametocytes) from the blood within 7 days of initiation of specific drug therapy (chloroquine in this case) followed by *recrudescence* of asexual parasitemia within 28 days after treatment. R2 resistance is the marked reduction, but not clearance, of asexual parasitemia. R3 resistance indicates no marked reduction in asexual parasitemia. The cases reported here appear to be R1 resistant. Generally acceptable criteria for documenting *P. falciparum* chloroquine resistance include: (1) No other *Plasmodium* species present; (2) Asexual *P. falciparum* parasitemia; (3) Adequately supervised chloroquine therapy with standard dosage—2.5 gm (1.5 gm base) over 3 days for adults; (4) Documentation of clearance of parasitemia followed by recrudescence (for R1 resistance), as determined by follow-up blood films up to 28 days after therapy; (5) Strict protection from reinfection for the 28-day period; and (6) *In vitro* documentation (optional) (2).

Chloroquine-resistant *P. falciparum* malaria has previously been reported from Asia, South America, Panama, and Oceania. In the last few years there has been an increasing number of reports of possible chloroquine-resistant malaria from Africa. The 3 cases reported here present the strongest evidence to date that chloroquine-resistant *P. falciparum* malaria has appeared in Africa.

It is premature to alter recommendations for chloroquine prophylaxis for travelers to Kenya and Tanzania, since the relative frequency of chloroquine-resistant strains there is unknown, and the degree of resistance appears low (R1). It is well known that clinical malaria may occur after appropriate chemoprophylaxis even with chloroquine-sensitive *Plasmodium*. In addition, one must now recognize that patients coming from Africa might have chloroquine-resistant *P. falciparum* malaria regardless of whether they took chloroquine prophylaxis. These individuals may, therefore, require treatment with regimens for chloroquine-resistant malaria. CDC can provide *in vitro* sensitivity testing and would like to receive reports through state health departments of suspected cases of chloroquine-resistant *P. falciparum* from Africa.

References
1. Kean BH: Chloroquine-resistant *falciparum* malaria from Africa. JAMA (in press)
2. Rieckmann KH: Determination of the drug sensitivity of *P. falciparum*. JAMA 217:573-578, 1971
3. MMWR 27(Suppl):81-90, 1978

MMWR 28:570 (12/7/79)

Malaria — United States, 1978

In 1978, malaria in civilians continued its upward trend. The number of infected civilians was *585*, a *24.5%* increase over 1977 and a 4-fold increase over 1970. This total reflects the worldwide resurgence of malaria, the increased travel to malarious areas, and the increasing number of immigrants from malarious areas, particularly from the Indian subcontinent.

Of last year's 616 malaria cases with onset in the United States and Puerto Rico, 95% occurred in U.S. and foreign civilians (Table 1). Most of the 270 cases among U.S. civilians occurred in tourists, students or teachers, business people, and missionaries. Thirty-one cases occurred among military personnel.

Of the countries where the 616 patients contracted malaria, Asia accounted for 52.1% of the cases (India, alone, for 39%), Africa for 28.9%, Central America and the Caribbean for 12.0%, South America for 2.2%, Oceania for 1.8%, and North America for 3.0%.

After India (where 241 cases were acquired), the largest number of imported cases were acquired in Nigeria (47), the Philippines (24), Kenya (17), and El Salvador (16).

TABLE 1. Malaria cases, by category, 1969-1978

Category	Year									
	1969	1970	1971	1972	1973	1974	1975	1976	1977	1978
Military	3,914	4,096	2,975	454	41	21	17	5	11	31
Civilian	139	134	148	160	181	302	431	405	470	585
U.S.	90	90	79	106	103	158	199	178	233	270
Foreign	49	44	69	54	78	144	232	227	237	315

Six deaths attributed to malaria were reported, compared with 3 in 1977. Four of the deaths occurred in civilians who had traveled to Africa, 1 in a seaman who was infected in Brazil, and 1 in a civilian who received a transfusion in Mexico. The latter case was caused by *Plasmodium malariae*, the rest, by *P. falciparum*. The *P. falciparum* malaria case-fatality ratio of 4% was higher than the ratio of 1.6% for the 10-year period 1966-1975.

The states with the largest number of imported malaria cases in 1978 were California (222), Virginia (37), Pennsylvania (28), and Texas (27).

In 1978, as in 1977, the seasonal distribution of malaria cases showed a distinct pattern: a definite peak in cases* was apparent in the late spring and in the summer months. For cases in which the exact date of arrival and date of onset were available, clinical malaria developed within 30 days after arrival into the United States in 79.5% of persons with *P. falciparum* infection and in 30.9% of those with *P. vivax* infection; these figures are consistent with those of previous years. Within 6 months after returning to this country, 96.2% of patients with *P. falciparum* malaria and 70.2% of those with *P. vivax* malaria developed clinical symptoms. Twenty-one patients (4.1%) became ill with malaria 12 months or longer after their last possible exposure to malaria abroad.

An increase in imported malaria cases is being reported in Western Europe as well as the United States (*1,2*).

Reported by the Parasitic Diseases Div, Bur of Epidemiology, CDC.

References
1. Hatz B, Stahel E, Weiss N, Begremont A: La malaria importée en Suisse de 1974-1976. Schweiz Med Wochenschr 108:1495-1499, 1978
2. World Health Organization: Malaria surveillance. Weekly Epidemiological Record 54:223-225, 1979

▲A copy of this report from which these data were derived will be available on request from CDC, Attn: Malaria Surveillance, Parasitic Diseases Div, Bur of Epidemiology, Atlanta, Ga. 30333.

---

*excluding cases with unknown date of onset.

MMWR 27 (A.S., 1978): 37

MALARIA — Reported Cases by Year, United States, 1933–1978

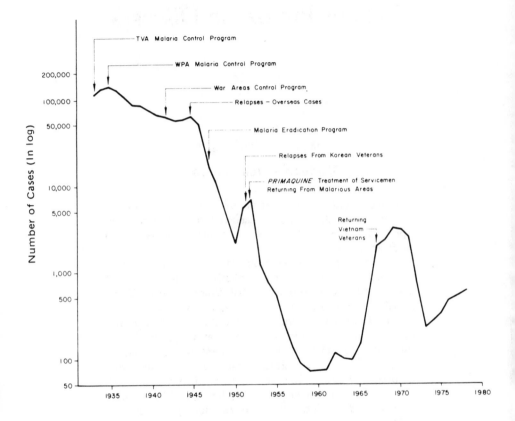

CHAPTER 38

Various Protozoan Diseases

MMWR 27:155 (5/12/78)

Giardiasis — Vail, Colorado

A multi-state outbreak of giardiasis in travelers to and residents of Vail, Colorado, occurred from March 14 to April 20, 1978. At least 38 confirmed cases have been reported, to date.

On April 13, a gastroenterologist in Petoskey, Michigan, reported the occurrence of giardiasis in 6 members of a family who had vacationed in Vail, Colorado, from March 23-25. All had epigastric pain, nausea, and weight loss. *Giardia lamblia* was confirmed in the stool specimen of 1 of the 6 patients. Additional information obtained from the Colorado State Health Department revealed that 13 cases of confirmed giardiasis had been reported from Colorado (7 from Colorado Springs, 6 from Denver), and 12 more confirmed cases from the state of New York— all in individuals who had visited Vail during the last week in March.

An epidemiologic investigation was begun by the Colorado Department of Health and CDC. Information was obtained on 777 long-term Vail residents by means of a questionnaire and stool survey. Of those surveyed, 465 (60%) gave a history of diarrheal illness within the past 3 months. A rise in the number of acute diarrheal illnesses began March 14-16 and reached a peak April 1-12 (Figure 1).

Preliminary analysis demonstrated no differences in attack rate by age or sex. Long-term ($\geqslant$7 days) and short-term ($<$7 days) diarrheal illness peaked at similar periods of time. The local hospital's routine examinations of stools for bacterial pathogens were negative. Stool and serum examinations by CDC for special bacterial and viral pathogens are pending.

Because contaminated water is a frequent cause of outbreaks of giardiasis, the Environmental Protection Agency

(EPA) and CDC reviewed the city's recent records of weekly sewage output. During the week of March 28-April 3, the number of gallons of sewage produced had dropped approximately 50%. This coincided with a sewer-line obstruction and leak into the creek supplying water to the city that had been previously discovered on March 31 and corrected.

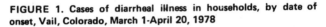

FIGURE 1. Cases of diarrheal illness in households, by date of onset, Vail, Colorado, March 1-April 20, 1978

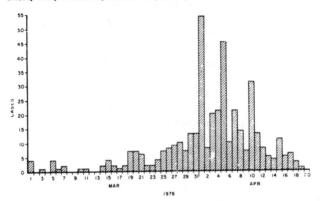

Meter readings of gallons of sewage had returned to normal by the next week. Cases continued to occur, however, up to the day of the survey, but at a much reduced level. Water from the creek and the storage tanks was filtered for *Giardia* cysts and viral pathogens by the EPA. The results are pending.

Reported by T Gietzan, MD, Petoskey, Mich; NS Hayner, MD, State Epidemiologist, Michigan State Dept of Public Health; P Landis, MD, St. Joseph's Hospital, Denver; Eagle County Health Dept, Vail; TM Vernon, MD, State Epidemiologist, Colorado State Dept of Health; DO Lyman, MD, State Epidemiologist, New York State Dept of Health; Environmental Protection Agency; Parasitic Diseases Div, Bur of Epidemiology, CDC.

Editorial Note: The fact that many cases occurred after discovery of the sewer-line obstruction is probably a reflection of the long incubation period of giardiasis (variable, but approximately 7 days) and the continued use of water from contaminated storage tanks. As dilution with fresh water occurred, illness disappeared.

Physicians examining patients who have recently traveled to Vail should be alert for symptoms compatible with giardiasis—diarrhea, abdominal cramps, gas, anorexia, and weight loss. Because the *Giardia* organism is intermittently excreted, 3 stool specimens obtained on different days may be needed to confirm the diagnosis.

MMWR 26:409 (12/16/77)

Toxoplasmosis — Georgia

One of the largest reported outbreaks of acute toxoplasmosis in the United States occurred among patrons of an
Atlanta, Georgia, riding stable in October.

The illness was characterized by fever, lymphadenopathy,
and headache. The initial diagnosis of toxoplasmosis was
made serologically on 2 of the patients and was confirmed
on follow-up of stable patrons. A total of 29 people were ill
with a constellation of symptoms consistent with toxoplasmosis; most cases occurred in mid-October (Figure 1).
Twenty-eight of the 29 had serologic evidence of acute
toxoplasmosis (All were >1:1024 by indirect fluorescent
antibody [IFA] for IgG and ≥1:256 by IFA for IgM.) Five
additional persons at the stable had serologic evidence of
acute toxoplasmosis but remained asymptomatic. Thirty
of the 34 persons identified were women. Twenty-four
were between 16 and 30 years old.

FIGURE 1. Toxoplasmosis cases, by week of onset, Georgia, 1977

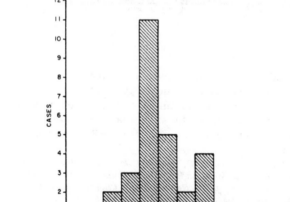

Another 48 patrons of the stable were interviewed and
were not ill. Twenty-nine serum specimens were obtained
from these 48 persons; 10 revealed evidence of previous
toxoplasmosis with low titers (<1:256), and 19 had no
serologic evidence of past or recent infection.

In a community immediately adjacent to the stable, 19
persons were interviewed and bled. Two gave histories of a
clinical disease compatible with toxoplasmosis; however,
their serum specimens, as well as those of the other 17 persons, were within the normal range for persons without
recent history of disease (<1:256).

Twenty people at another stable in the Atlanta area were interviewed and were tested for toxoplasmosis antibodies. None had evidence of clinical illness consistent with toxoplasmosis, and the serologic tests did not reveal titers diagnostic of acute infection.

Cats from the stable associated with the outbreak were bled. Serologic tests revealed that 2 of 3 cats had elevated toxoplasmosis titers (1:256, 1:1024). Rodents were obtained from both stables; histologic and parasitic results on them are pending. Soil samples from the stables have also been obtained to see if they contain oocysts, the cysts passed by cats which, after 3-4 days in the soil, are capable of infecting humans; the results of these tests are also pending.

Reported by B Francis, MD, Emory University, Atlanta; JE McCroan, PhD, State Epidemiologist, RK Sikes, DVM, Georgia Dept of Human Resources; Parasitic Serology Br, Parasitology Div, Bur of Laboratories, Parasitic Diseases Div, Bur of Epidemiology, CDC.

Editorial Note: Toxoplasmosis, a systemic protozoan disease, remains incompletely understood. Caused by *Toxoplasma gondii*, it has 3 known modes of transmission: from pregnant women to their fetuses (which can cause severe neurologic and ocular abnormalities); through eating poorly cooked or raw infected meat; and presumably from infected cat feces. Cats (and all *Felidae*), the only animals capable of excreting oocysts in their feces, generally excrete the cysts only at 1 time in their lives. and then only for a period of approximately 2 weeks.

Toxoplasmosis generally causes subclinical illness. Exposure to the disease is apparently quite common: 4-30% of residents of the United States have serologic evidence of previous infection (1). Symptoms of clinical infection are protean, but among the most common ones are lymphadenopathy, myalgia, and headache. Outbreaks of toxoplasmosis are rare. A previous one occurred among 5 medical students who ate raw hamburger (2). Cases of acute toxoplasmosis, as occurred in the current outbreak, are uncommon and generally sporadic.

References
1. Remington JS: Toxoplasmosis in the adult. Bull NY Acad Med: 50:211-227, 1974
2. Kean BH, Kimball AC, Christenson WN: An epidemic of acute toxoplasmosis. JAMA 208:1002-1004, 1969

MMWR 27:343 (9/15/78)

Primary Amebic Meningoencephalitis — California, Florida, New York

Seven cases of primary amebic meningoencephalitis (PAM), a rare disease that affects the central nervous system, have recently been reported to CDC. Details of 3 of these cases follow. One, acquired in California, is the first non-fatal case described in the

United States.

California: A previously healthy 9-year-old girl was hospitalized May 27, 1978, after a 3-day history of headache, nausea, vomiting, lethargy, and stupor. Examination of cerebrospinal fluid (CSF) revealed ameboid organisms. She developed papilledema, seizures, and left focal neurologic signs and became comatose. She was treated with intravenous and intrathecal amphotericin B, miconazole—an investigational drug effective *in vitro* against *Naegleria*, the most common cause of PAM—and oral rifampin. Her condition improved after 48 hours, and within a month she had recovered completely with no significant neurologic sequellae. Culture of her initial CSF specimens yielded *N. fowleri*.

One week before onset she had bathed in a hot spring near San Bernardino. This same hot spring was implicated as the source of infection in a fatal case of PAM in 1971 (1).

Florida: On July 2, a 14-year-old boy began to complain of a progressive, severe, frontal and bitemporal headache. He had been swimming and diving in a fresh water lake for the past 3 weeks. He developed a low grade fever and malaise, and on July 4 was admitted to the hospital with mild nuchal rigidity, lethargy, and fever of 40 C. Examination of the CSF revealed a cell count of 3900/mm^3, a glucose of 13 mg/dl, and a protein of 490 mg/dl. Motile amebae (*N. fowleri*) were seen on the initial wet mounts. The patient deteriorated rapidly, becoming disoriented, agitated, and then comatose. Despite therapy with amphotericin B, neurogenic pulmonary edema ensued. Just before receiving miconazole the patient developed cerebral edema and herniation. He died 3 days later.

New York: An 11-year-old girl who had not recently traveled or gone swimming was admitted to a hospital May 27 with a 2-day history of headache, vomiting, fever, and nuchal rigidity. Spinal fluid revealed many neutrophils, and routine cultures were negative. Her condition deteriorated, and she died 8 days after onset. Autopsy revealed a vasculitis and meningoencephalitis. Amebae identified as *Acanthamoeba* species were found on fixed sections.

Reported by JS Powers, MD, Victor Valley Community Hospital; R Abbott, MD, L Boyle, M Lee, MD, R Rudas, MD, San Bernardino County Hospital; K Mackey, MPH, L Mahoney, MD, DrPH, San Bernardino County Health Dept; A Cohen, MD, J Edwards, MD, P Harmatz, MD, J Seidel, MD, PhD, J Turner, MD, Harbor General Hospital, Los Angeles; J Chin, MD, State Epidemiologist, C Powers, C Taclindo, MPH, California Dept of Health; CG Culbertson, Eli Lilly Company, Indianapolis, Indiana; S Lee, MD, RM Prudente, MD, New York City; E Galaid, MPH, C Wang, MD, MPH, New York City; JS Marr, MD, City Epidemiologist, Bur of Preventable Diseases; M Cichon, MD, Tampa, Florida; RM Yeller, MD, Acting State Epidemiologist, Florida State Dept of Health and Rehabilitative Services; Field Services Div, Parasitic Diseases Div, Bur of Epidemiology, CDC.

Editorial Note: PAM is usually caused by *N. fowleri*—a ubiquitous, free-living ameba found in fresh water ponds and lakes. Most cases occur during the summer within 8 days after swimming in warm, fresh or brackish water. The portal of entry is probably the nasal mucosa overlying the cribriform plate. Since PAM was first described in 1965 (2), over 80 cases have been reported including about 35 in the United States.

Prompt diagnosis, early treatment with miconazole, amphotericin B, and rifampin, and careful fluid management were probably responsible for the survival of the California patient. Intrathecal therapy appears critical since amphotericin and miconazole otherwise do not reach therapeutic levels in the CSF. The CDC Parasitic Disease Drug Service does not distribute miconazole but can help physicians obtain the drug for patients.

The risk of infection from water containing *Naegleria* organisms is unknown but probably small, since thousands of people swim in lakes known to contain these organisms, yet cases of PAM are rare. No U.S. case has been associated with man-made swimming pools.

Acanthamoeba, another free-living ameba, generally causes subacute or chronic infections, rather than the fulminant meningoencephalitis reported here. Its mode of transmission is unknown.

References

1. Hecht RH, Cohen AH, Stoner J, et al: Primary amebic meningoencephalitis in California. California Medicine 117:69-73, 1972

2. Fowler M, Carter RF: Acute pyogenic meningitis probably due to *Acanthamoeba* sp: A preliminary report. Br Med J 2:740-742, 1965

MMWR 28:226 (5/18/79)

Intestinal Parasites — New York City

In the fall of 1977, a pilot screening program for intestinal parasites was initiated by the New York City Department of Health's Upper West Side Tropical Disease Clinic. The object of the study was to determine the prevalence of intestinal parasites in asymptomatic immigrant children referred from the Health Department's Child Health Station.

In the 1-year period November 1, 1977—October 31, 1978, the stools of 37 asymptomatic children, 1 year or older, who had lived in the Caribbean or in Central or South America within the past 3 years and had not been tested or treated for intestinal parasites since arrival in the United States, were examined. Single stool specimens were examined by the formalin-ether concentration technique. Nineteen (51%) of the 37 specimens contained at least 1 intestinal pathogen. Seventeen of these patients were treated. (The relative frequency of each species is shown in Table 2). The overall rate of 51% for intestinal

TABLE 2. Pathogenic parasites in single, fresh stool specimen from each of 37 children, New York City, November 1, 1977—October 31, 1978

Pathogen	Positive specimens	
	Number	Percentage
Giardia lamblia	10	27.0
Dientamoeba fragilis	5	13.5
Entamoeba histolytica	3	8.1
Ascaris lumbricoides	3	8.1
Hookworm	1	2.7
Trichuris trichiura	3	8.1
Total	25	67.5

pathogens among this pilot study exceeded the rate for the general clientele of the tropical disease clinic (38.2%). Family members of the infected children in the pilot study were invited to have stools examined, and all the infected persons were appropriately treated.

Reported by SN Rosenberg, MD, MPH, CC Wang, MD, RR Pflug, RN, New York City Dept of Health; Parasitic Diseases Div, Bur of Epidemiology, CDC.

Editorial Note: Intestinal parasitic infections are frequently seen throughout the United States and in most foreign countries *(1,2).* Immigration of persons from countries where intestinal parasites are more prevalent than in the United States often raises concern about the potential for the transmission of these organisms at both the personal and community level *(3).* Although the infection rates reported here are higher than those found in most U.S. communities, infections with helminths such as *Ascaris,* hookworm, and *Trichuris* do not pose a significant public health hazard under most conditions. Eggs of these parasites require a 1- to 2-week incubation period in the soil before becoming infective. Since most immigrants in this country live and work in areas where adequate sewage disposal is available, the community is not exposed to infective eggs.

Cysts of protozoa (such as *Giardia* and *Entamoeba histolytica*) require no incubation period outside the host to develop into an infective stage. Therefore, they are directly transmissible by the fecal-oral route and do represent a potential health hazard. However, the risk of transmission is small among persons who practice good personal hygiene. Of the protozoa found in this study, *E. histolytica* has the potential for causing the greatest morbidity and should be treated promptly when detected.

References
1. Arnold K: Trends in the development of chemotherapy for parasitic diseases. Southeast Asian J Trop Med Public Health 9:177-185, 1978
2. CDC: Intestinal Parasite Surveillance Annual Summary 1977. Atlanta, CDC, 1978
3. MMWR 24:398, 1975

CHAPTER 39

Nematode Infections

MMWR 26:167 (5/20/77)

Trichinosis from Shish Kebab — California

Outbreak 1: Trichinosis was diagnosed in a 23-year-old man hospitalized in San Diego in July 1976. He and 38 other persons had attended a workshop on Santa Catalina Island. On June 10, a feral pig had been trapped, butchered, and cooked for 5 to 8 hours in an Umu (an earthen pit). The pork was described as "well cooked" and "falling from the bone" by those who ate it. However, a portion of the raw pork had been cubed and, together with commercial cubed beef, made into shish kebabs. Each participant had cooked his own shish kebab on a willow branch. Not all participants knew that 2 different meats were served and that one was feral pork.

Five (19.2%) of the 26 persons who ate feral pork became ill with trichinosis 11-26 days after the barbeque. The mean incubation period of the 2 female cases (12 days) was much shorter than that of the 3 male cases (23 days). In each case, the first symptom was periorbital edema. All patients experienced myalgia and extreme fatigue; 3 cases were hospitalized. One patient had a positive muscle biopsy. In 4 cases the bentonite flocculation test was positive, although in one case not until after 7 weeks.

Outbreak 2: A pork picnic shoulder purchased at a San Diego market in August 1976 was prepared for shish kebab and marinated with beef strips in soy sauce. The meat was then cooked approximately 3 minutes per side on a charcoal grill. Seventeen people ate the shish kebab, and 5 (29%) became ill with trichinosis 6 to 29 days later. Symptoms included facial swelling, periorbital edema, headache, nausea, fever, muscle pain, and leg swelling. Eosinophilia ranged from 28% to 44%.

Reported by M Ginsberg, MD, H Helm, RS, J Philip, MD, D Ramras, MD, and W Townsend, MD, San Diego County Health Dept; A Friedlander, MD, R Poliakoff, MD, University of California, San

Diego; K Damus, MSTH, RR Roberto, MD, California State Dept of Health; and Parasitic Diseases Div, Bur of Epidemiology, CDC.

Editorial Note: These 2 outbreaks of trichinosis illustrate the hazards of mixing pork and beef as shish kebab, and emphasize the necessity of thoroughly cooking pork products regardless of source. Consumers should be aware that commercially marketed pork is not inspected for trichinosis.

Pork products should be heated to an internal temperature of at least 137 F to kill trichinae larvae; a practical rule is to cook pork until the center is no longer pink.

MMWR 28:12 (1/12/79)

Trichinosis Associated with Bear Meat — Alaska, California

Thirteen Alaska Natives and persons of oriental descent have become ill recently with trichinosis after eating Alaskan black bear meat. The meat was eaten on multiple occasions in late October and November, sometimes after being roasted for several hours, and on some occasions after preparation in an oriental wok. Thus far, all cases have been associated with the wok-prepared meat.

The index patient, a 39-year-old man, ate the meat in early November while visiting in Anchorage, and then returned to his home in Los Angeles. On December 7, he presented to the emergency room of a hospital there with at least a 1-week history of fever, retro-orbital pain, orbital puffiness, and muscle tenderness. He was found to have 50% eosinophilia. A diagnosis of trichinosis was made, and he was admitted to the hospital. When he gave a history of eating bear meat with his relatives in Alaska, authorities notified the Alaska State Department of Health and Social Services. Investigation by the state health department uncovered the other 12 cases.

Samples of the implicated bear meat, when tested by the U.S. Department of Agriculture, were found to contain up to 1200 larvae/gram. Portions of the bear were taken to Los Angeles and Chicago by visitors returning home from Alaska. An epidemiologic investigation of potentially exposed persons in those areas and in Alaska is in progress.

Reported by J Cinqué, MD, LAC-USC General Hospital, Los Angeles; S Fannin, MD, Los Angeles County Dept of Health; R Brodsky, MD, Alaska Native Medical Center, Anchorage; J Farrell, TL Woodard, MD, Acting State Epidemiologist, Anchorage; U.S. Dept of Agriculture, Palmer, Alaska; Alaska Investigations Div, Field Services Div, Bur of Epidemiology, CDC.

MMWR 28:70 (2/16/79)

Follow-up on Trichinosis Associated with Bear Meat — Alaska, California

Twenty-seven cases of trichinosis have now been identified in the outbreak involving persons in Alaska and California who ate the meat of a single Alaskan black bear (1). Nineteen of the cases have occurred in Alaska, and 8 in California after a portion of the meat was taken to Los Angeles. Sixty-three people attended meals where the implicated meat was served, and 30 of these ate the meat. The 27 known cases indicate an attack rate of 90% in people who ate this meat.

Reported by J Cinqué, MD, LAC-USC General Hospital, Los Angeles; S Fannin, MD, Los Angeles County Dept of Health; R Brodsky, MD, Alaska Native Medical Center, Anchorage; J Farrell, TL Wood-

ard, MD, Acting State Epidemiologist, Anchorage; U.S. Dept of Agriculture, Palmer, Alaska; Alaska Investigations Div, Field Services Div, Bur of Epidemiology, CDC.
Reference
1. MMWR 28:12, 1979

MMWR 27 (A.S., 1978): 67

TRICHINOSIS — Reported Cases by Year, United States, 1950—1978

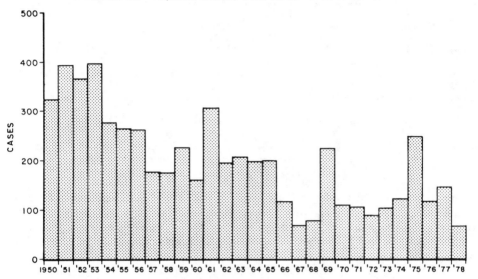

MMWR 28:346 (7/27/79)
Survey of Intestinal Parasites — Illinois

In February 1979, the Illinois Department of Public Health received several requests to screen a group of Laotian immigrants living in Kankakee and Will counties, Illinois, for intestinal parasites. Since 1977, 165 Meo Laotians have moved into these 2 counties.

In March 1979, all 165 persons submitted stool specimens to the Illinois Department of Public Health Laboratory in Chicago to be examined for ova and parasites. Stools were preserved in formalin and, in many cases, polyvinyl alcohol (PVA). All stools were examined by the formalin-ether concentration method, and, where possible, PVA smears were prepared and stained. When ova or parasites were not observed on first examination, a second stool specimen was requested and, in most instances, received.

The results of the laboratory examinations are summarized in Table 1. Hookworm was the most frequently detected parasite: its higher occurrence in females—52/72 (72%)—than in males—54/93 (58%)—accounted for the overall increased incidence of intestinal parasitism among females. Persons 4 years of age or older were significantly more likely to be infected with hookworm than children less than 4 (p<.001). Attack rates for giardiasis were significantly greater in the 4- to 9-year-olds, when compared with all other age groups (p>.01). Persons 4-14 years of age were more likely to have both ascariasis and trichiriasis when compared with all others. There were no other statistically significant differences in attack rates by age.

All infected persons have been appropriately treated.

Reported by D Safran, RN, H Wheeler, RN, Kankakee County Nurses Office; D Fazio, BS, Will County Health Dept; MK Nickels, BS, KG Hashimoto, BS, RJ Martin, DVM, BJ Francis, MD, State Epidemiologist, Illinois Dept of Public Health; Field Services Div, Parasitic Diseases Div, Bur of Epidemiology, CDC.

TABLE 1. Intestinal parasitism in Laotian immigrants, by age group, February 1979

Age group	Number tested	Helminths				Protozoans	
		Hookworm	Trichuris	Ascaris	Other	E. histolytica	G. lamblia
<1	4	0*	0	0	0	0	0 (.00)
1-3	17	0	0	1 (.9)	0	0	2 (18)
4-9	38	23 (61)	5 (13)	6 (16)	5 (13)	1 (3)	12 (32)
10-14	26	19 (73)	7 (24)	4 (15)	4 (15)	2 (8)	7 (27)
15-19	19	16 (84)	1 (5)	1 (5)	1 (5)	0	2 (11)
20-24	13	13 (100)	2 (15)	0	0	0	1 (14)
25-29	8	4 (50)	1 (12)	0	0	0	1 (20)
30-34	12	11 (92)	1 (8)	0	0	0	1 (17)
35-39	5	2 (40)	1 (20)	0	0	0	2 (40)
40-44	7	5 (71)	0	1 (14)	0	0	0 (0)
45-64	16	13 (81)	2 (12)	1 (6)	1 (6)	0	1 (6)
Total	165	106 (64)*	20 (12)	14 (9)	11 (7)	3 (2)	29 (18)

*Number of persons infected (percent infected).

Editorial Note: The high infection rates with hookworm, *Trichuris*, and *Ascaris* reported in this study do not pose a significant public health hazard because eggs of these parasites require a 2-week incubation period in the soil before becoming infective, and transmission is interrupted by adequate sewage disposal. However, early diagnosis and treatment are encouraged for the patient's benefit.

From a public health point of view, the protozoan infections pose a greater potential health risk than the other parasitic infections because the cyst stages of these parasites are infectious at the moment feces are passed. The rate of *Entamoeba histolytica* infection reported in this study is not greater than the expected U.S. level (*1*). This group of immigrants did have a high rate of *Giardia lamblia* infection, however—higher than previous groups that have been examined. Thirty percent (19/64) of children 4-14 years of age were infected with this parasite. By comparison, less than 4% of the U.S. population have a *Giardia* infection (*1*). Although the risk of *Giardia* transmission is small among persons who practice good personal hygiene, the high incidence of giardiasis among young children, especially preschoolers, may pose a public health problem where children congregate, if hygienic practices are deficient (*2*).

CDC does not consider it necessary to routinely screen all Indochinese refugees for intestinal parasites. However, testing for ova and parasites is indicated as part of a complete examination of individual refugees requiring medical care.

References

1. CDC: Intestinal Parasite Surveillance Annual Summary 1977. Issued September 1978
2. Black RE, Dykes AC, Sinclair SP, Wells IG: Giardiasis in day-care centers: Evidence of person-to-person transmission. Pediatrics 60:486-491, 1977

Part V

Data on
Infectious Diseases

CHAPTER 40

Tables on Cases and Deaths—1978

MMWR Annual Summary 1978

SOURCES OF DATA

Data on the reported incidence of notifiable diseases are routinely published in the *Morbidity and Mortality Weekly Report* (MMWR) and compiled in final form in this summary from annual reports supplied by the state and territorial departments of health. However, totals for the United States do not include data listed for Guam, Puerto Rico, the Virgin Islands, and the Trust Territory of the Pacific Islands.

CDC also maintains national surveillance programs for selected diseases, with the cooperation of state and local health departments, and publishes detailed epidemiologic analyses on a periodic basis. Data appearing in a surveillance report may not agree exactly with reports published by the MMWR because of differences in timing of reports or because of refinements in case definition.

It should be noted that the MMWR and the national surveillance program are separate systems; data from each appear in this *Annual Summary*. These data should be interpreted with caution. Some diseases such as plague and rabies that cause severe clinical illness and are associated with serious consequences are probably reported quite accurately. However, diseases such as salmonellosis and mumps that are clinically mild and infrequently associated with serious consequences are less likely to be reported. Additionally, subclinical cases are seldom detected except in the course of special studies. The degree of completeness of reporting is also influenced by the diagnostic facilities available, the control measures in effect, and the interests and priorities of state and local officials responsible for disease control and surveillance. Finally, factors such as the introduction of new diagnostic tests (e.g., hepatitis B) and the discovery of new disease entities (e.g., infant botulism and Legionnaires' disease) may cause changes in disease reporting independent of the true incidence of disease. Despite these limitations the data in this report have proven to be useful in the analysis of trends.

Mortality data, with the exception of statistics obtained from the 121 participating cities, are from the National Center for Health Statistics, Health Services Administration. Each year these data are also published in *Vital Statistics of the United States*, Vol. II.

The population data for 1978 used in computing rates are from the Bureau of the Census and are provisional estimates of the resident population as of July 1, 1978. The data are in the Bureau's *Current Population Reports* series: state estimates in Series P-25, No. 790; age estimates in P-25, No. 800 and in unpublished data; New York City data in P-26, No. 78-32. Data for U.S. Territories are provisional, unpublished estimates. Population data from those states where diseases were not notifiable or where age-specific data were not available were excluded from rate calculation. Rates were calculated using resident population with the exception of chancroid, gonorrhea, granuloma inguinale, lymphogranuloma venereum, and syphilis, for which only civilian resident population data were utilized.

In order not to delay the publication of this document, provisional data from California were included. For further modification of any of those data, contact the California Department of Health Services.

EXPLANATION OF SYMBOLS USED IN TABLES

Data not available . . . . NA

No reported cases . . . . —

Report of disease not required
by state health department
(not notifiable) . . . . NN

Case imported from outside
United States I

MMWR 27 (A.S., 1978): 3

NOTIFIABLE DISEASES – Reported Cases, United States, 1969–1978

DISEASE	1978	1977	1976	1975	1974	1973	1972	1971	1970	1969
U.S. total resident population, July 1 estimate (in thousands)	218,059	216,332	214,659	213,121	211,390	209,851	208,232	206,256	203,805	201,921
Amebiasis	3,937	3,044	2,906	2,775	2,743	2,235	2,199	2,752	2,888	2,915
Anthrax	6	2	2	—	—	2	2	5	2	4
Aseptic meningitis	6,573	4,789	3,510	4,475	3,197	4,846	4,634	5,176	6,480	3,672
Botulism, total	105	129	55	20	28	34	22	25	12	16
Foodborne	65	81	30	17	28	34	22	25	12	16
Infant	36	43	15	1	—	—	—	—	—	—
Brucellosis (undulant fever)	179	232	296	310	240	202	196	183	213	235
Chancroid	521	455	628	700	945	1,165	1,414	1,320	1,416	1,104
Chickenpox	154,089	188,396	183,990	154,248	141,495	182,927	164,114	*	—	—
Cholera	12	4	—	—	—	1	1	—	—	—
Diphtheria	76	84	128	307	272	228	152	215	435	241
Encephalitis, primary[1]	266	341	530	2,362	206	163	161	338	220	1,613
Indeterminate[1]	852	1,073	1,121	1,702	958	1,450	898	1,186	1,360	
Post childhood infections[1]	65	119	175	237	218	354	243	439	370	304
Gonorrhea	1,013,436	1,002,219	1,001,994	999,937	906,121	842,621	767,215	670,268	600,072	534,872
Granuloma inguinale	72	75	71	60	47	62	81	89	124	154
Hepatitis A	29,500	31,153	33,288	35,855	40,358	50,749	54,074	59,606	56,797	48,416
Hepatitis B	15,016	16,831	14,973	13,121	10,631	8,451	9,402	9,556	8,310	5,909
Hepatitis, unspecified	8,776	8,639	7,488	7,158	8,351	—	—	*	—	—
Legionnaires' disease	664	363	234	—	—	—	—	—	—	—
Leprosy	168	151	145	162	118	146	130	131	129	98
Leptospirosis	110	71	73	93	68	57	41	62	47	89
Lymphogranuloma venereum	284	348	365	353	394	408	756	692	612	520
Malaria	731	547	471	373	293	237	742	2,375	3,051	3,102
Measles (rubeola)	26,871	57,345	41,126	24,374	22,094	26,690	32,275	75,290	47,351	25,826
Meningococcal infections, total	2,505	1,828	1,605	1,478	1,346	1,378	1,323	2,262	2,505	2,951
Mumps	16,817	21,436	38,492	59,647	59,128	69,612	74,215	124,939	104,953	90,918
Pertussis (whooping cough)	2,063	2,177	1,010	1,738	2,402	1,759	3,287	3,036	4,249	3,285
Plague	12	18	16	20	8	2	1	2	13	5
Poliomyelitis, total	15	18	14	8	7	8	31	21	33	20
Paralytic	9	17	12	8	7	7	29	17	31	18
Psittacosis	140	94	78	49	164	33	52	32	35	57
Rabies in animals	3,280	3,130	3,073	2,627	3,151	3,640	4,369	4,310	3,224	3,490
Rabies in man	4	1	—	—	—	1	2	—	3	1
Rheumatic fever, acute	851	1,738	1,865	2,854	2,431	2,560	2,614	2,793	3,227	3,229
Rubella (German measles)	18,269	20,395	12,491	16,652	11,917	27,804	25,507	45,086	56,552	57,686
Rubella congenital syndrome	30	23	30	45	45	35	42	68	77	31
Salmonellosis, excluding typhoid fever	29,410	27,850	22,937	22,612	21,980	23,818	22,151	21,928	22,096	18,419
Shigellosis	19,511	16,052	13,140	16,584	22,600	22,642	20,207	16,143	13,845	11,946
Smallpox				Last documented case occurred in 1949						
Syphilis, primary and secondary	21,656	20,399	23,731	25,561	25,385	24,825	24,429	23,783	21,982	19,130
Total, all stages	64,875	64,621	71,761	80,356	83,771	87,469	91,149	95,997	91,382	92,162
Tetanus	86	87	75	102	101	101	128	116	148	185
Trichinosis	67	143	115	252	120	102	89	103	109	222
Tuberculosis	28,521	30,145	32,105	33,989	30,122	30,998	32,882	35,217	37,137	39,120
Tularemia	141	165	157	129	144	171	152	187	172	149
Typhoid fever (cases)	505	398	419	375	437	680	398	407	346	364
Carriers	62					NA.				
Typhus fever, flea-borne (endemic, murine)	46	75	69	44	26	32	18	23	27	36
Typhus fever, tick-borne (Rocky Mountain spotted)	1,063	1,153	937	844	754	668	523	432	380	498
Yellow fever				Last indigenous case reported 1911; last imported, 1924.						

[1] Changes in data reported for 1970-1977 reflect new diagnostic categories.

* Not previously notifiable nationally.

NOTIFIABLE DISEASES — Reported Cases per 100,000 Population, United States, 1969-1978

Disease	1978	1977	1976	1975	1974	1973	1972	1971	1970	1969
Amebiasis	1.84	1.41	1.35	1.30	1.30	1.07	1.06	1.33	1.42	1.44
Anthrax	0.00	0.00	0.00	0.00	0.00	0.00	0.00	0.00	0.00	0.00
Aseptic meningitis	3.01	2.24	1.64	2.10	1.53	2.33	2.23	2.51	3.18	1.82
Botulism, total	0.05	0.06	0.03	0.01	0.01	0.02	0.01	0.01	0.01	0.01
Foodborne	0.03	0.04	0.01	0.01	0.01	0.02	0.01	0.01	0.01	0.01
Infant	0.02	0.02	0.01	0.00	—	—	—	—	—	—
Brucellosis (undulant fever)	0.08	0.11	0.14	0.15	0.11	0.10	0.09	0.09	0.10	0.12
Chancroid	0.24	0.21	0.29	0.33	0.46	0.56	0.68	0.64	0.70	0.55
Chickenpox	80.42	97.63	96.06	78.11	72.20	97.68	87.34	*	*	*
Cholera	0.01	0.00	0.00	0.00	0.00	0.00	0.00	0.00	0.00	0.00
Diphtheria	0.03	0.04	0.06	0.14	0.13	0.11	0.07	0.10	0.21	0.12
Encephalitis, primary[1]	0.14	0.16	0.25	1.11	0.10	0.08	0.08	0.16	0.12	0.80
Indeterminate[1]	0.45	0.50	0.52	0.80	0.45	0.69	0.43	0.58	0.72	—
Post childhood infections[1]	0.03	0.06	0.08	0.11	0.10	0.17	0.12	0.21	0.20	0.15
Gonorrhea	468.25	466.83	470.47	472.91	432.12	404.92	371.62	328.11	298.52	267.86
Granuloma inguinale	0.03	0.03	0.03	0.03	0.02	0.03	0.04	0.04	0.06	0.07
Hepatitis A	13.53	14.40	15.51	16.82	19.54	24.18	25.97	28.90	27.87	23.98
Hepatitis B	6.89	7.78	7.14	6.30	5.15	4.03	4.52	4.74	4.08	3.02
Hepatitis, unspecified	4.02	3.99	3.57	3.44	3.95					
Legionnaires' disease	0.30	0.17	0.11							
Leprosy	0.08	0.07	0.07	0.08	0.06	0.07	0.06	0.06	0.06	0.05
Leptospirosis	0.05	0.03	0.03	0.04	0.03	0.03	0.02	0.03	0.02	0.04
Lymphogranuloma venereum	0.13	0.16	0.17	0.17	0.19	0.20	0.37	0.34	0.30	0.26
Malaria	0.34	0.25	0.22	0.18	0.14	0.11	0.36	1.15	1.50	1.54
Measles (rubeola)	12.32	26.51	19.16	11.44	10.45	12.72	15.50	36.50	23.23	12.79
Meningococcal infections, total	1.15	0.84	0.75	0.69	0.64	0.66	0.64	1.10	1.23	1.46
Mumps	7.81	10.02	17.93	27.99	29.00	36.23	38.42	65.33	55.55	48.65
Pertussis (whooping cough)	0.95	1.02	0.47	0.82	1.15	0.84	1.58	1.47	2.08	1.63
Plague	0.01	0.01	0.01	0.01	0.00	0.00	0.00	0.00	0.01	0.00
Poliomyelitis, total	0.01	0.01	0.01	0.00	0.00	0.00	0.01	0.01	0.02	0.01
Paralytic	0.00	0.01	0.01	0.02	0.08	0.02	0.02	0.01	0.02	0.03
Psittacosis	0.06	0.04	0.04	0.02	0.00	0.00	0.00	0.00	0.00	0.03
Rabies in man	0.00	0.00	0.00	0.00	0.00	0.00	0.00	0.00	0.00	0.00
Rheumatic fever, acute	0.60	1.23	1.32	2.01	1.79	1.92	2.01	2.16	2.45	2.48
Rubella (German measles)	8.38	9.43	5.82	7.81	5.64	13.25	12.25	21.86	27.75	28.91
Rubella congenital syndrome	0.01	0.01	0.01	0.01	0.02	0.02	0.02	0.03	0.04	0.02
Salmonellosis, excluding typhoid fever	13.49	12.87	10.74	10.61	10.40	11.35	10.64	10.63	10.84	9.12
Shigellosis	8.95	7.42	6.15	7.78	10.69	10.79	9.70	7.83	6.79	5.92
Smallpox	Last documented case occurred in 1949									
Syphilis, primary and secondary	10.00	9.50	11.14	12.09	12.11	11.93	11.83	11.64	10.94	9.58
Total, all stages	30.00	30.10	33.69	38.00	39.95	42.03	44.15	46.99	45.46	46.15
Tetanus	0.04	0.07	0.05	0.05	0.05	0.05	0.04	0.06	0.07	0.09
Trichinosis	0.03	0.07	0.05	0.12	0.06	0.05	0.04	0.05	0.05	0.11
Tuberculosis	13.08	13.93	14.96	15.95	14.25	14.77	15.79	17.07	18.22	19.37
Tularemia	0.06	0.08	0.07	0.06	0.07	0.08	0.07	0.09	0.08	0.07
Typhoid fever (cases)	0.23	0.18	0.20	0.18	0.21	0.32	0.19	0.20	0.17	0.18
Carriers	0.03	0.04	0.03	0.02	NA	0.02	0.01	0.01	0.01	0.02
Typhus fever, flea-borne (endemic, murine)	0.02	0.04	0.03	0.02	0.01	0.02	0.01	0.01	0.01	0.02
Typhus fever, tick-borne (Rocky Mountain spotted)	0.49	0.53	0.44	0.40	0.36	0.32	0.25	0.21	0.19	0.25
Yellow fever	Last indigenous case reported 1911; last imported, 1924.									

*Not previously notifiable nationally.

NOTE: Rates less than .01 after rounding are shown as 0.00.
[1] Changes in rates for 1970-1977 reflect new diagnostic categories.

NOTIFIABLE DISEASES – Deaths from Specified Notifiable Diseases, United States, 1968-1977

(Numbers after cause of death are category numbers of the Eighth Revision of the International Classification of Diseases, Adapted 1965.)

CAUSE OF DEATH	ICDA	1977	1976	1975	1974	1973	1972*	1971	1970	1969	1968
Amebiasis	006	28	36	35	25	31	52	60	59	58	51
Anthrax	022	–	–	–	–	–	–	–	–	–	–
Botulism	005.1	6	3	3	6	6	6	7	7	4	2
Brucellosis	023	–	2	–	–	1	6	3	2	3	1
Chickenpox	052	89	106	83	106	138	122	98	93	81	99
Diphtheria	032	5	7	5	5	10	10	13	30	25	30
Encephalitis, acute infectious	062-065,079.2	206	253	386	276	326	266	320	327	386	362
Gonorrhea	098	1	–	1	1	11	8	9	9	3	1
Granuloma inguinale	099.2	–	–	–	–	–	–	–	2	3	1
Hepatitis, infectious (Hepatitis A)	070	508	567	612	630	656	778	906	1,014	1,011	877
Leprosy	030	1	1	2	2	1	–	1	5	4	5
Leptospirosis	100	8	12	7	5	6	10	6	4	5	9
Lymphogranuloma venereum	099.1	–	–	2	2	2	4	2	1	4	2
Malaria	084	3	4	4	4	7	–	6	5	11	7
Measles (rubeola)	055	15	12	20	20	23	24	90	89	41	24
Meningococcal infection	036	338	330	308	305	330	350	509	550	744	741
Mumps	072	5	8	8	6	12	16	15	16	22	25
Pertussis (whooping cough)	033	10	7	8	14	5	6	18	12	13	36
Plague	020	–	2	3	–	–	–	–	–	–	1
Poliomyelitis	040-041,043	16	16	9	3	10	2	18	7	13	24
Bulbar or polioencephalitis	040	2	3	2	–	4	–	2	2	3	7
With other paralysis	041	12	1	1	–	3	–	2	2	1	3
Unspecified	043	–	12	6	3	3	2	14	4	9	14
Psittacosis	073	–	–	–	–	–	–	–	1	–	–
Rabies	071	–	1	2	–	1	2	2	2	1	1
Rheumatic fever, acute	390-392	125	149	155	175	183	180	230	256	320	363
Rubella (German measles)	056	17	12	21	15	16	14	20	31	29	24
Salmonellosis, including paratyphoid fever	002-003	73	61	67	59	76	68	81	81	82	70
Shigellosis	004	25	19	27	32	33	38	24	30	36	60
Syphilis	090-097	196	225	272	300	393	344	375	461	543	586
Tetanus	037	24	32	45	44	40	58	64	79	89	86
Trichinosis	124	–	–	1	1	1	2	4	–	–	–
Tuberculosis (all forms)	010-019	2,968	3,130	3,333	3,513	3,875	4,376	4,501	5,217	5,567	6,292
Tularemia	021	2	2	–	2	4	–	2	2	1	1
Typhoid fever	001	3	2	3	3	7	8	4	6	4	7
Typhus fever, flea-borne (endemic-murine)	081.0	–	–	–	–	1	–	–	–	–	–
Typhus fever, tick-borne (Rocky Mountain spotted)	082.0	43	41	29	49	38	50	36	29	36	21

Source: National Center for Health Statistics, Vital Statistics of the United States, Vol. II, for respective year.
*Based on 50% sample of death records.

NOTIFIABLE DISEASES — Reported Cases By Month, United States, 1978

Disease	Total	Jan.	Feb.	Mar.	Apr.	May	June	July	Aug.	Sept.	Oct.	Nov.	Dec.	Month Not Stated
Amebiasis	3,937	273	318	310	340	284	410	343	276	245	371	373	388	6
Anthrax	6	—	—	—	2	2	—	—	1	—	—	—	—	—
Aseptic meningitis	6,573	168	167	130	163	248	398	815	1,315	1,110	811	649	467	132
Botulism, total	105	2	1	2	42	8	1	4	6	6	3	14	16	—
Foodborne	65	1	—	—	38	4	1	1	1	4	1	12	5	—
Infant	36	1	2	2	3	4	—	3	5	4	2	1	10	—
Brucellosis	179	7	18	19	7	20	15	18	16	14	15	10	19	1
Chickenpox	154,089	13,075	15,106	22,081	20,616	23,994	16,157	4,893	1,624	1,163	3,010	8,455	16,271	7,644
Cholera	12	—	—	—	—	—	—	1	—	10	—	—	1	—
Diphtheria	76	5	7	8	8	7	9	4	11	10	2	8	5	—
Hepatitis A	29,500	1,933	2,142	2,517	2,438	2,522	2,430	2,157	2,654	2,489	2,622	2,459	2,771	366
Hepatitis B	15,016	1,124	1,150	1,428	1,224	1,302	1,230	1,156	1,316	1,204	1,187	1,198	1,289	208
Hepatitis, unspecified	8,776	545	658	711	679	676	742	611	852	780	761	765	966	30
Legionnaires' disease	664	29	19	22	28	38	52	65	163	139	61	28	18	2
Leprosy	168	4	4	14	16	14	15	24	21	13	10	12	20	1
Leptospirosis	110	4	2	1	8	8	8	19	15	11	9	1	28	—
Malaria	731	42	39	46	39	74	75	93	95	64	59	46	49	10
Measles (rubeola)	26,871	960	1,800	3,977	4,531	5,486	3,996	1,471	923	899	554	1,064	1,180	30
Meningococcal infections, total	2,505	188	277	275	266	252	182	162	144	118	157	190	258	36
Military	34	—	3	6	6	2	3	2	1	1	3	1	1	7
Civilian	2,471	186	270	260	258	242	178	155	143	115	148	182	250	84
Mumps	16,817	1,388	1,723	2,320	2,080	2,205	1,532	677	418	374	479	802	1,411	1,408
Pertussis (whooping cough)	2,063	196	205	144	127	121	133	204	201	207	142	164	133	86
Plague	12	—	—	1	1	—	1	2	3	1	1	2	3	—
Poliomyelitis, total	15	—	—	—	1	—	1	—	2	2	4	2	3	—
Paralytic	9	—	—	—	1	—	1	—	2	1	2	1	2	—
Psittacosis	140	5	3	19	19	7	14	10	10	13	6	9	22	3
Rabies in man	4	—	—	1	—	—	1	—	1	—	1	—	1	—
Rheumatic fever, acute	851	86	80	82	92	82	44	47	35	30	44	67	40	122
Rubella (German measles)	18,269	573	708	1,943	3,303	4,606	2,908	810	466	316	260	454	531	1,391
Rubella congenital syndrome	30	1	9	—	1	1	4	4	3	—	2	—	5	—
Salmonellosis, excl. typhoid fever	29,410	1,642	1,594	1,710	1,595	1,976	2,364	2,750	3,439	3,275	3,128	2,699	2,737	501
Shigellosis	19,511	1,193	987	1,178	1,182	1,386	1,457	1,669	2,130	2,037	1,902	1,922	2,168	300
Syphilis, primary & secondary	21,656	1,539	1,705	1,745	1,758	1,742	1,721	1,675	1,880	2,012	1,974	1,994	1,911	—
Tetanus	86	3	3	6	9	8	7	12	10	5	7	6	10	—
Trichinosis	67	3	1	15	2	3	9	5	12	3	3	—	9	—
Tularemia	141	5	4	6	7	8	13	22	13	17	12	16	16	2
Typhoid fever	505	17	54	62	37	42	33	42	48	42	39	48	37	4
Typhus fever														
Flea-borne (endemic, murine)	46	2	2	6	2	2	2	10	3	7	3	1	6	—
Tick-borne (Rocky Mountain spotted)	1,063	—	3	5	23	136	232	239	178	147	58	22	17	3

NOTIFIABLE DISEASES — Reported Cases By Age, United States, 1978

Disease	Total	<1	1-4	5-9	10-14	15-19	20-24	25-29	30-39	40-49	50-59	60+	Age Not Stated
Cholera	12	—	—	—	1	2	—	—	1	3	3	2	—
Diphtheria	76	—	4	2	1	1	6	7	16	13	17	8	1
Gonorrhea	1,013,436	(......11,958......)				254,928	387,984	202,374	119,360	26,413	(....10,419....)		—
Hepatitis A[1]	28,835	59	847	2,476	2,002	3,637	5,890	4,445	4,067	1,813	1,357	1,069	1,173
Hepatitis B[1]	14,723	13	41	84	126	2,220	4,197	2,633	2,220	1,036	839	795	519
Hepatitis, unspecified[1]	9,734	18	297	730	583	1,241	2,122	1,420	1,180	529	510	544	560
Measles (rubeola)	26,871	718	2,054	3,601	4,723	3,273	392	129	106	27	4	10	11,834
Meningococcal infections, total	2,505	489	640	191	175	270	129	85	83	96	83	119	145
Military	34	1	1	—	3	5	11	3	—	—	—	—	10
Civilian	2,471	488	639	191	172	265	118	82	83	96	83	119	135
Mumps	16,817	36	738	3,092	1,526	400	117	82	88	53	25	16	10,644
Pertussis (whooping cough)	2,063	677	431	163	95	37	26	23	21	12	1	4	573
Plague	12	—	1	—	2	3	1	—	1	1	2	1	—
Poliomyelitis, total	15	4	1	—	1	3	2	1	3	1	—	—	—
Paralytic	9	4	1	—	1	3	—	—	3	—	—	—	—
Rubella (German measles)	18,269	342	444	619	1,051	4,543	2,540	363	259	91	36	8	7,973
Salmonellosis (excl. typhoid fever)	29,410	4,885	4,365	1,938	1,160	1,504	1,696[2]	1,267[2]	1,535	1,056	1,152	2,223	6,601
Shigellosis	19,511	853	5,895	2,671	872	623	1,026	1,094	1,052	409	321	358	4,337
Syphilis, primary & secondary	21,656	(......154......)				3,032	6,044	5,125	4,879	1,746	(....676....)		—
Tetanus	86	4	3	3	3	3	2	2	5	4	17	42	1
Tuberculosis	28,521	(....836....)		(....651....)		(....2,098....)		(.........24,870.........)					66
Typhoid fever	505	3	42	58	44	39	64	54	61	41	31	49	19

[1] Age distribution of Hepatitis A cases (665) and Hepatitis B cases (293) reported by the state of Georgia included in Hepatitis, unspecified.

[2] Does not include cases reported by state of Arizona.

NOTIFIABLE DISEASES — Reported Cases by Geographic Division and by State, United States, 1978

Area	Tot. Resident Population (in thousands)	Amebiasis	Anthrax	Aseptic Meningitis	Botulism Foodborne	Botulism Infant	Botulism Unspecified	Brucellosis	Chancroid
United States	218,059	3,937	6	6,573	65	36	4	179	521[1]
New England	12,256	17	2	224	–	–	–	15	1
Maine	1,091	1	–	26	–	–	–	1	–
N. H.	871	3	2	23	–	–	–	–	–
Vt.	487	–	–	6	–	–	–	8	–
Mass.	5,774	2	–	73	–	–	–	3	1
R. I.	935	1	–	15	–	–	–	1	–
Conn.	3,099	10	–	81	–	–	–	2	–
Mid. Atlantic	36,825	2,033	–	1,183	4	6	–	12	51
Upstate N. Y.	10,599	45	–	277	–	–	–	11	2
N. Y. City	7,149	1,931	–	192	2	–	–	–	47
N. J.	7,327	42	–	379	–	2	–	–	2
Pa.	11,750	15	–	335	2	4	–	1	–
E. N. Central	41,233	181	–	1,237	1	–	–	6	84
Ohio	10,749	71	–	329	–	–	–	1	1
Ind.	5,374	24	–	196	–	–	–	–	1
Ill.	11,243	77	–	238	–	–	–	1	33
Mich.	9,189	9	–	377	–	–	–	2	49
Wis.	4,679	–	–	97	1	–	–	2	–
W. N. Central	17,018	226	1	303	–	–	1	32	1
Minn.	4,008	37	–	–	–	–	–	1	–
Iowa	2,896	161	–	38	–	–	–	18	–
Mo.	4,860	20	–	145	–	–	–	3	1
N. Dak.	652	–	1	6	–	–	–	1	–
S. Dak.	690	–	–	4	–	–	–	2	–
Nebr.	1,565	–	–	43	–	–	–	5	–
Kans.	2,348	8	–	67	–	–	1	2	–
S. Atlantic	34,579	157	2	1,029	3	3	–	24	314
Del.	583	–	–	13	–	1	–	–	–
Md.	4,143	17	–	258	–	1	–	–	2
D. C.	674	12	–	2	–	–	–	–	20
Va.	5,148	35	–	193	1	–	–	6	3
W. Va.	1,860	–	–	24	–	–	–	1	1
N. C.	5,577	9	2	195	–	–	–	3	49
S. C.	2,918	60	–	33	–	–	–	1	2
Ga.	5,084	2	–	–	1	1	–	3	226
Fla.	8,594	22	–	311	1	–	–	10	11
E. S. Central	14,001	8	–	441	–	–	–	24	11
Ky.	3,498	1	–	104	–	–	–	5	–
Tenn.	4,357	NN	–	145	–	–	–	6	3
Ala.	3,742	5	–	148	–	–	–	4	–
Miss.	2,404	2	–	44	–	–	–	9	8
W. S. Central	22,046	259	–	631	4	–	–	41	29
Ark.	2,186	13	–	54	–	–	–	7	3
La.	3,966	6	–	97	–	–	–	3	15
Okla.	2,880	30	–	75	–	–	–	8	–
Texas	13,014	210	–	405	4	–	–	23	11
Mountain	10,289	94	1	219	42	15	–	13	9
Mont.	785	–	–	31	–	–	–	–	1
Idaho	878	2	1	19	–	–	–	9	7
Wyo.	424	–	–	3	–	–	–	–	–
Colo.	2,670	29	–	69	8	–	–	2	–
N. M.	1,212	7	–	44	34	2	–	1	1
Ariz.	2,354	37	–	12	–	3	–	1	–
Utah	1,307	14	–	37	–	10	–	–	–
Nev.	660	5	–	4	–	–	–	–	–
Pacific	29,811	962	–	1,306	11	12	3	12	21
Wash.	3,774	28	–	129	2	–	–	–	1
Oreg.	2,444	12	–	205	–	–	1	–	1
Calif.	22,294	909	–	860	9	12	2	11	19
Alaska	403	–	–	34	–	–	–	1	–
Hawaii	897	13	–	78	–	–	–	–	–
Guam	99	4	–	1	–	–	–	–	–
P. R.	3,378	1	–	10	3	–	–	4	15
V. I.	105	–	–	–	–	–	–	–	–
Pac. Trust Terr.	116	2,294	–	26	–	–	–	–	NA

[1] Civilian cases only.

NOTIFIABLE DISEASES — Reported Cases by Geographic Division and by State, United States, 1978 — Continued

Area	Chicken-pox	Cholera	Diphtheria	Encephalitis Primary	Encephalitis Indeterminate	Encephalitis Post Childhood Inf.	Gonorrhea	Granuloma Inguinale
United States	154,089	12	76	266	852	65	1,013,436[1]	72[1]
New England	16,173	–	–	4	19	7	25,708	–
Maine	3,262	–	–	–	–	–	2,109	–
N. H.	515	–	–	1	1	–	1,171	–
Vt.	200	–	–	–	–	–	618	–
Mass.	5,895	–	–	–	9	1	11,189	–
R. I.	2,827	–	–	–	–	–	1,966	–
Conn.	3,474	–	–	3	9	6	8,655	–
Mid. Atlantic	13,865	–	1	19	111	6	110,009	9
Upstate N. Y.	8,447	–	–	6	46	4	19,491	1
N. Y. City	2,733	–	1	7	24	2	40,571	7
N. J.	NN	–	–	3	13	–	20,222	1
Pa.	2,685	–	–	3	28	–	29,725	–
E. N. Central	64,725	1	–	104	266	23	162,046	4
Ohio	7,593	–	–	27	120	12	41,366	–
Ind.	8,304	–	–	NA	NA	NA	15,691	–
Ill.	14,471	–	–	13	74	3	54,190	4
Mich.	20,078	1	–	12	59	5	36,647	–
Wis.	14,279	–	–	52	13	3	14,152	–
W. N. Central	19,035	–	2	68	78	3	51,309	–
Minn.	30	–	–	49	8	–	8,517	–
Iowa	6,978	–	–	15	32	–	5,432	–
Mo.	4,048	–	1	–	28	1	22,840	–
N. Dak.	417	–	–	–	–	–	876	–
S. Dak.	441	–	–	–	–	–	1,726	–
Nebr.	1,118	–	1	2	1	–	3,653	–
Kans.	6,003	–	–	2	9	2	8,265	–
S. Atlantic	13,580	–	–	36	154	15	242,635	56
Del.	223	–	–	–	1	–	3,522	–
Md.	1,432	–	–	–	38	1	30,480	1
D. C.	35	–	–	–	–	–	16,286	–
Va.	1,076	–	–	3	31	5	24,034	–
W. Va.	5,597	–	–	–	22	–	3,313	–
N. C.	NN	–	–	4	28	6	34,479	2
S. C.	380	–	–	–	7	–	23,914	–
Ga.	80	–	–	4	4	1	46,219	52
Fla.	4,757	–	–	25	23	2	60,388	1
E. S. Central	3,862	–	–	13	69	3	85,108	–
Ky.	2,637	–	–	–	16	2	11,445	–
Tenn.	NN	–	–	3	30	–	31,072	–
Ala.	915	–	–	8	10	1	24,436	–
Miss.	310	–	–	2	13	–	18,155	–
W. S. Central	6,486	11	–	8	87	6	133,940	–
Ark.	323	–	–	4	11	2	9,926	–
La.	NN	11	–	–	15	–	22,367	–
Okla.	NN	–	–	–	20	2	12,704	–
Texas	6,163	–	–	4	41	2	88,943	–
Mountain	6,040	–	4	9	23	1	38,909	1
Mont.	870	–	–	1	15	–	2,127	–
Idaho	916	–	–	–	–	–	1,600	1
Wyo.	19	–	–	–	–	–	983	–
Colo.	3,339	–	2	2	3	1	10,835	–
N. M.	54	–	–	3	–	–	5,525	–
Ariz.	NN	–	1	3	4	–	10,064	–
Utah	711	–	–	–	1	–	2,118	–
Nev.	131	–	1	–	–	–	5,657	–
Pacific	10,323	–	69	5	45	1	163,772	2
Wash.	7,689	–	64	3	24	–	13,487	–
Oreg.	55	–	–	2	14	1	11,243	–
Calif.	1,273	–	2	NA	NA	NA	131,136	2
Alaska	621	–	3	–	7	–	5,132	–
Hawaii	685	–	–	–	–	–	2,774	–
Guam	289	–	–	–	–	–	16	–
P. R.	467	–	–	–	10	2	2,170	1
V. I.	15	–	–	–	–	–	289	–
Pac. Trust Terr.	449	–	–	NA	NA	NA	NA	NA

[1] Civilian cases only.
[2] Notifiable only for 16 years of age and over.

NOTIFIABLE DISEASES — Reported Cases by Geographic Division and by State, United States, 1978 — Continued

Area	Hepatitis A	Hepatitis B	Hepatitis Unsp.	Legionnaires' Disease	Leprosy	Leptospirosis	Lympho-granuloma Venereum	Malaria
United States	29,500	15,016	8,776	664	168	110	284[1]	731[2]
New England	817	598	189	87	–	4	4	34
Maine	94	23	14	4	–	–	–	2
N. H.	67	27	6	4	–	–	–	4
Vt.	60	19	9	5	–	–	–	–
Mass.	313	250	132	10	–	2	4	11
R. I.	104	72	–	–	–	–	–	5
Conn.	179	207	28	64	–	2	–	12
Mid. Atlantic	2,576	2,499	928	118	12	–	38	142
Upstate N. Y.	685	455	280	22	2	–	1	22*
N. Y. City	499[3]	493[3]	268[3]	37	6	–	27	65*
N. J.	653	750	216	26	2	–	3	30
Pa.	739	801	164	33	2	–	7	25
E. N. Central	4,171	2,236	665	95	2	5	11	69
Ohio	1,147	474	–	3	–	1	2	11
Ind.	245	201	190	43	–	–	3	6
Ill.	1,304	705	179	21	2	2	3	29**
Mich.	1,206	705	263	22	–	2	3	21
Wis.	269	151	33	6	–	–	–	2
W. N. Central	2,371	777	361	46	4	2	14	26
Minn.	942	253	12	2	1	1	–	4
Iowa	140	100	60	24	1	–	–	–
Mo.	552	231	192	5	–	1	12	10
N. Dak.	100	10	–	11	–	–	–	–
S. Dak.	242	14	24	–	–	–	–	1
Nebr.	126	53	18	3	2	–	–	5
Kans.	269	116	55	1	–	–	2	6
S. Atlantic	3,776	2,628	1,175	94	7	29	138	124
Del.	35	51	11	–	–	1	1	2
Md.	411	477	172	9	1	3	–	26
D. C.	34	72	5	2	–	–	71	6
Va.	272	331	166	12	4	2	4	23
W. Va.	171	56	17	5	–	–	–	1
N. C.	331	230	128	7	–	1	7	12
S. C.	102	152	93	2	–	–	–	4
Ga.	665	293	–	19	–	–	47	10
Fla.	1,755	966	583	38	2	22	8	40
E. S. Central	1,627	896	164	83	–	2	6	14
Ky.	268	164	35	14	–	–	–	2
Tenn.	687	490	72	63	–	–	5	8
Ala.	224	168	57	4	–	1	1	2
Miss.	448	74	–	2	–	1	–	2
W. S. Central	4,006	1,080	1,670	53	31	22	41	40
Ark.	427	125	73	5	–	2	1	2
La.	550	212	193	8	3	6	6	4
Okla.	333	157	206	2	–	–	–	1*
Texas	2,696	586	1,198	38	28	14	34	33*
Mountain	3,027	652	1,406	11	4	5	7	10
Mont.	196	27	28	–	–	–	3	–
Idaho	229	12	16	2	–	–	3	–
Wyo.	29	9	8	–	–	–	–	–
Colo.	477	243	236	2	1	–	–	5
N. M.	454	94	115	1	–	1	–	2
Ariz.	1,227	172	813	1	2	NN	1	2
Utah	326	39	150	4	1	1	–	–
Nev.	89	56	40	1	–	3	–	1
Pacific	7,129	3,650	2,218	77	108	41	25	272
Wash.	932	223	277	7	2	1	2	12
Oreg.	1,105	393	165	2	–	11	3	9
Calif.	4,803	2,923	1,733	68	75	12	20	225
Alaska	130	46	14	–	–	–	–	4
Hawaii	159	65	29	–	31	17	–	22
Guam	46	14	45	–	–	–	–	–
P. R.	186	53	211	–	15	–	2	4
V. I.	9	–	7	–	–	–	–	2
Pac. Trust Terr.	–	–	125	–	10	–	NA	–

[1] Civilian cases only.
[2] All cases imported except 4 induced (*) and 1 congenital (**).
[3] Classifications based on HBsAg test results.

NOTIFIABLE DISEASES — Reported Cases by Geographic Division and by State, United States, 1978 — Continued

Area	Measles	Meningo-coccal Infections	Mumps	Pertussis	Plague	Poliomyelitis		Psittacosis
						Total	Paralytic	
United States	26,871	2,505	16,817	2,063	12	15	9	140
New England	2,046	143	905	61	–	–	–	10
Maine	1,320	9	588	9	–	–	–	1
N. H.	82	11	18	7	–	–	–	2
Vt.	55	3	6	–	–	–	–	–
Mass.	253	53	97	23	–	–	–	5
R. I.	8	20	56	11	–	–	–	–
Conn.	328	47	140	11	–	–	–	2
Mid. Atlantic	2,288	391	807	201	–	–	–	13
Upstate N. Y.	1,439	137	256	115	–	–	–	3
N. Y. City	405	88	165	54	–	–	–	3
N. J.	72	77	200	2	–	–	–	1
Pa.	372	89	186	30	–	–	–	6
E. N. Central	11,599	370	6,843	599	–	6	2	8
Ohio	492	98	1,410	140	–	1	1	–
Ind.	227	57	373	105	–	1	–	1
Ill.	1,381	110	2,100	260	–	3	–	5
Mich.	8,006	87	1,628	47	–	1	1	1
Wis.	1,493	18	1,332	47	–	–	–	1
W. N. Central	583	108	2,149	106	–	–	–	5
Minn.	46	26	24	23	–	–	–	1
Iowa	73	21	192	3	–	–	–	3
Mo.	154	41	1,211	45	–	–	–	1
N. Dak.	211	3	15	8	–	–	–	–
S. Dak.	–	4	11	11	–	–	–	–
Nebr.	5	–	26	2	–	–	–	–
Kans.	94	13	670	14	–	–	–	–
S. Atlantic	5,572	585	1,035	257	–	3	3	16
Del.	7	2	62	3	–	–	–	1
Md.	51	41	86	13	–	–	–	6
D. C.	48	2	2	–	–	–	–	–
Va.	2,837	73	196	18	–	1	1	3
W. Va.	1,066	17	200	22	–	–	–	1
N. C.	125	110	82	45	–	1	1	–
S. C.	199	43	18	12	–	–	–	–
Ga.	36	65	71	82	–	1	1	2
Fla.	1,203	232	318	62	–	–	–	3
E. S. Central	1,409	196	1,313	118	–	–	–	–
Ky.	122	31	311	46	–	–	–	–
Tenn.	952	58	471	60	–	–	–	–
Ala.	102	52	437	3	–	–	–	–
Miss.	233	55	94	9	–	–	–	–
W. S. Central	1,454	339	2,254	184	–	–	–	14
Ark.	17	26	659	35	–	–	–	3
La.	385	149	68	4	–	–	–	3
Okla.	19	20	NN	13	–	–	–	3
Texas	1,033	144	1,527	132	–	–	–	5
Mountain	257	55	502	109	11	3	1	20
Mont.	88	7	140	9	–	–	–	–
Idaho	1	4	28	4	–	–	–	– –
Wyo.	–	–	2	–	1	–	–	–
Colo.	50	3	115	21	2	1	–	10
N. M.	–	12	20	42	5	1(1)	1(1)	–
Ariz.	57	16	26	24	2	1	–	2
Utah	44	7	162	8	–	–	–	8
Nev.	17	6	9	1	1	–	–	–
Pacific	1,663	318	1,009	428	1	3	3	54
Wash.	442	56	223	59	–	1	1	5
Oreg.	562	39	138	103	–	–	–	20
Calif.	649	209	595	247	1	1	1	29
Alaska	1	11	15	18	–	–	–	–
Hawaii	9	3	38	1	–	1	1	–
Guam	28	1	40	–	–	–	–	–
P. R.	326	13	1,718	21	–	–	–	–
V. I.	9	5	4	1	–	–	–	–
Pac. Trust Terr.	649	2	120	–	–	–	–	–

NOTIFIABLE DISEASES — Reported Cases by Geographic Division and by State, United States, 1978 — Continued

Area	Rabies In Animals	Rabies In Man	Rheumatic Fever, Acute	Rubella	Cong. Syndrome	Salmonellosis	Shigellosis	Syphilis Primary & Secondary	Syphilis All Stages
United States	3,280	4	851	18,269	30	29,410	19,511	21,656[1]	64,875[1]
New England	96	–	9	826	1	2,495	666	563	1,716
Maine	79	–	2	158	–	121	17	11	80
N. H.	2	–	–	108	1	130	33	7	14
Vt.	1	–	4	51	–	66	156	3	6
Mass.	7	–	NN	261	–	1,464	303	342	1,003
R. I.	–	–	–	42	–	162	19	29	146
Conn.	7	–	3	206	–	552	138	171	467
Mid. Atlantic	86	–	–	3,108	7	4,922	2,318	2,965	10,185
Upstate N. Y.	62[2]	–	NN	580	5	969	551	223	772
N. Y. City	–	–	NN	152	–	1,283	764	2,058	5,648
N. J.	13	–	NN	1,625	2	1,331	472	357	1,813
Pa.	11	–	NN	751	–	1,339	531	327	1,952
E. N. Central	215	–	441	8,995	5	4,826	2,504	2,494	9,719
Ohio	21	–	224	1,390	–	490	177	463	1,600
Ind.	12	–	26	649	1	498	220	166	934
Ill.	75	–	177	1,972	–	1,748	1,578	1,535	5,684
Mich.	10	–	NN	3,373	3	1,155	263	257	1,133
Wis.	97	–	14	1,611	1	935	266	73	368
W. N. Central	694	–	156	716	–	1,832	1,216	434	3,048
Minn.	209	–	–	128	–	513	155	146	353
Iowa	147	–	26	72	–	210	85	36	235
Mo.	90	–	88	118	–	487	443	144	1,583
N. Dak.	104	–	21	83	–	48	76	4	18
S. Dak.	103	–	–	112	–	102	185	3	19
Nebr.	7	–	NN	34	–	103	22	15	89
Kans.	34	–	21	169	–	369	250	86	751
S. Atlantic	521	1	7	1,411	5	6,075	2,553	5,647	15,179
Del.	3	–	1	37	–	98	12	12	63
Md.	19	–	4	305	–	793	269	441	1,859
D. C.	–	–	–	1	–	90	85	407	1,276
Va.	13	–	NN	247	1	990	142	474	1,653
W. Va.	14	1	–	342	–	47	39	29	590
N. C.	16	–	–	204	3	865	171	611	1,672
S. C.	119	–	2	32	–	400	265	288	662
Ga.	290	–	–	29	–	1,168	713	1,402	2,751
Fla.	47	–	NN	214	1	1,624	857	1,983	4,653
E. S. Central	172	–	74	555	2	1,868	897	1,127	2,711
Ky.	78	–	61	155	1	261	221	150	548
Tenn.	35	–	NN	215	–	513	225	385	815
Ala.	53	–	11	25	–	486	246	199	415
Miss.	6	–	2	160	1	608	205	393	933
W. S. Central	927	1	36	977	2	2,151	2,650	3,538	8,138
Ark.	160	–	3	58	–	419	247	77	357
La.	17	–	8	494	–	178	122	727	1,631
Okla.	194	–	NN	18	–	355	416	94	366
Texas	556	1 (1)	25	407	2	1,199	1,865	2,640	5,784
Mountain	129	1	105	237	–	1,308	1,968	418	1,396
Mont.	26	–	3	22	–	40	118	8	19
Idaho	–	1	12	3	–	79	54	9	13
Wyo.	11	–	16	–	–	11	2	6	26
Colo.	29	–	9	53	–	475	496	124	398
N. M.	25	–	25	4	–	265	551	87	275
Ariz.	23	–	–	103	–	263	553	113	509
Utah	8	–	40	40	–	110	159	14	49
Nev.	7	–	–	12	–	65	35	57	107
Pacific	440	1	23	1,444	8	3,933	4,739	4,470	12,783
Wash.	5	–	–	149	–	420	233	265	544
Oreg.	11	1	4	174	–	257	263	170	415
Calif.	411	–	12	1,100	8	2,719	4,084	3,979	11,686
Alaska	13	–	7	8	–	63	28	12	56
Hawaii	–	–	NN	13	–	474	131	44	82
Guam	–	–	3	5	–	70	35	–	–
P. R.	31	–	6	17	2	288	81	535	1,659
V. I.	–	–	–	1	–	6	6	18	90
Pac. Trust Terr.	–	–	5	3	–	–	244	NA	NA

[1] Civilian cases only.
[2] Includes N. Y. City.

NOTIFIABLE DISEASES — Reported Cases by Geographic Division and by State, United States, 1978 — Continued

Area	Tetanus	Trichinosis	Tuberculosis	Tularemia	Typhoid Fever Cases Endemic	Typhoid Fever Cases Imported	Typhoid Fever Carriers	Typhus Fever Murine	Typhus Fever Rocky Mt. Spotted
United States	86	67	28,521	141	242	263	62	46	1,063
New England	3	8	970	3	8	72	1	—	14
Maine	—	—	70	—	—	—	—	—	—
N. H.	—	1	21	1	—	5	—	—	—
Vt.	2	—	41	—	1	—	—	—	—
Mass.	—	1	580	—	—	63	—	—	6
R. I.	—	—	72	—	—	4	—	—	1
Conn.	1	6	186	2	7	—	1	—	7
Mid. Atlantic	6	36	4,341	8	50	23	5	—	60
Upstate N. Y.	3	2	753	5	10	—	—	—	29
N. Y. City	—	7	1,307	1	32	15	5	—	4
N. J.	—	2	1,003	—	—	8	—	—	13
Pa.	3	25	1,278	2	8	—	—	—	14
E. N. Central	5	5	4,599	2	27	35	5	—	76
Ohio	1	2	890	1	5	1	—	—	30
Ind.	1	—	544	—	2	—	—	—	6
III.	2	2	1,645	1	13	25	5	—	40
Mich.	1	1	1,260	—	7	8	—	—	—
Wis.	—	—	260	—	—	1	—	—	—
W. N. Central	8	2	989	27	16	5	—	—	56
Minn.	2	—	175	—	6	1	—	—	—
Iowa	—	—	103	1	—	2	—	—	1
Mo.	2	2	456	21	7	—	—	—	29
N. Dak.	—	—	33	—	—	—	—	—	—
S. Dak.	1	—	76	—	—	—	—	—	7
Nebr.	—	—	30	1	—	1	—	—	12
Kans.	3	—	116	4	3	1	—	—	7
S. Atlantic	23	2	6,171	14	49	13	7	6	569
Del.	—	—	58	—	2	1	—	—	5
Md.	2	1	755	5	5	8	3	3	119
D. C.	—	—	314	2	1	—	—	—	1
Va.	1	—	722	5	1	3	2	1	111
W. Va.	—	—	216	—	7	—	—	—	11
N. C.	6	—	943	—	3	—	—	1	204
S. C.	4	—	563	—	8	—	2	—	56
Ga.	—	—	876	—	3	1	—	—	50
Fla.	10	1	1,724	2	19	—	—	1	12
E. S. Central	5	1	2,712	8	7	2	3	3	177
Ky.	2	—	649	3	1	1	1	—	42
Tenn.	—	—	842	4	4	—	—	2	108
Ala.	—	—	672	1	2	1	—	1	13
Miss.	3	1	549	—	—	—	2	—	14
W. S. Central	17	2	3,571	62	33	20	11	33	97
Ark.	1	—	417	34	4	—	—	—	13
La.	2	—	648	7	4	—	—	—	2
Okla.	3	—	346	15	5	—	2	—	54
Texas	11	2	2,160	6	20	20	9	33	28
Mountain	4	3	924	10	15	5	1	—	11
Mont.	—	—	58	—	3	—	—	—	2
Idaho	1	—	38	3	4	1	—	—	3
Wyo.	—	—	15	2	—	—	—	—	1
Colo.	1	1	143	1	2	3	1	—	2
N. M.	—	—	149	—	2	—	—	—	—
Ariz.	—	2	406	1	4	—	—	NN	1
Utah	2	—	42	3	—	1	—	—	—
Nev.	—	—	73	—	—	—	—	—	2
Pacific	15	8	4,244	7	37	88	29	4	3
Wash.	1	—	305	—	7	—	3	—	1
Oreg.	—	—	204	4	—	1	—	1	2
Calif.	13	8	3,351	3	24	86	22	1	—
Alaska	1	—	94	—	—	—	—	—	—
Hawaii	—	—	290	—	6	1	4	2	—
Guam	1	—	67	—	—	—	—	—	—
P. R.	11	—	375	—	3	—	—	1	—
V. I.	—	—	NA	—	2	—	—	—	—
Pac. Trust Terr.	—	—	59	—	—	—	—	—	—

MMWR 27 (A.S., 1978): 77

NON-NOTIFIABLE CONDITIONS — Cases of Acute Conditions *Optionally* Reported by Certain States, 1978

Area	Giardiasis[1]	Histo-plasmosis	Infectious Mono-nucleosis	Meningitis (Bacterial & Unspecified)	Reye Syndrome[2]	Streptococcal Sore Throat & Scarlet Fever	Toxo-plasmosis
No. Cases Reported	12,947	771	16,027	4,331	236	397,039	579
No. States Reporting	—	(18)	(27)	(43)	—	(40)	(17)
New England	483	—	904	191	12	32,314	74
Maine	7			10	1	2,676	5
N. H.	38			19	—		1
Vt.	56		27	11	—	3,979	
Mass.	—				2	8,719	
R. I.	115		39	39	4	7,129	
Conn.	267		838	112	5	9,811	68
Mid. Atlantic	577	2	8,545	896	38	9,969	14
Upstate N.Y.	27		7,468	356	27[3]	5	
N. Y. City	400			328		831	
N. J.	132				3		
Pa.	18	2	1,077	212	8	9,133	14
E. N. Central	545	324	1,439	900	76	70,728	125
Ohio	64	3	813	76	23	2,277	41
Ind.	118	307	101	135	12	15,076	84
Ill.	32	12		485	18	12,714	
Mich.	203			130	22	29,759	
Wis.	128	2	525	74	1	10,902	
W. N. Central	939	386	1,374	320	27	48,947	223
Minn.	620	68		42	—		44
Iowa	66	4	1,157	74	14		1
Mo.	83	310	169	93	3	20,555	168
N. Dak.	27				1	4,792	
S. Dak.	8	2	46	26	2	3,509	10
Nebr.	18			36	5	11,168	
Kans.	117	2	2	49	2	8,923	
S. Atlantic	4,158	8	1,090	765	32	51,099	132
Del.	5			39	—	1,386	
Md.	167			139	1	12,512	
D. C.	—				—	1,907	
Va.	231	7	805	201	10	482	9
W. Va.	97		273	27	1	14,299	
N. C.	186			288	—		
S. C.	676		12	71	1	1,976	
Ga.	591				15	2,957	121
Fla.	2,205	1			4	15,580	2
E. S. Central	1,796	15	472	314	17	16,966	3
Ky.	181	13	246	140	2	3,051	
Tenn.	236				8		
Ala.	894		104	105	4	4,702	
Miss.	485	2	122	69	3	9,213	3
W. S. Central	1,359	22	42	210	7	29,487	—
Ark.	224	20	37	59	1	54	
La.	724	2	5		5		
Okla.	104			151	—		
Texas	307				1	29,433	
Mountain	369	2	181	273	22	97,085	3
Mont.	47		2	30	2	3,989	1
Idaho	29		45	19	—		
Wyo.	1			2	3	22,855	
Colo.	69			78	10	60,002	
N. M.	22			50	1		
Ariz.	26	2		26	4		
Utah	172		133	65	2	10,171	2
Nev.	3		1	3	—	68	
Pacific	2,721	12	1,980	462	5	40,444	5
Wash.	320			181	3	9,393	
Oreg.	35		1,917	79	—	6,369	
Calif.	2,246	12	17	151	2	19,723	5
Alaska	—			38	—		
Hawaii	120		46	13	—	4,959	
Guam	—		11	12		812	
P. R.	107		10	165		38	
V. I.	32					3	
Pac. Trust Terr.				26		336	

[1] Source: Parasitic Diseases Division, Bureau of Epidemiology. Refers to stool specimens containing *Giardia lamblia.*
[2] Source: Viral Diseases Division, Bureau of Epidemiology.
[3] Includes New York City.

NON-NOTIFIABLE CONDITIONS — Cases of Acute Conditions *Optionally* **Reported by Certain States, 1978 — Continued**

Fungal Diseases

Actinomycosis	Mass. 2; Minn. 2; Okla. 1; Va. 1
Blastomycosis	Ariz. 1; Ark. 14; Fla. 7; Ill. 1; Ky. 3; Minn. 3; Mo. 14; Nev. 1; N.C. 1; Va. 7; Wis. 1
Coccidioidomycosis	Ariz. 85; Ark. 2; Calif. 1096; Fla. 1; Idaho 1; Minn. 4; Mo. 6; Nev. 2; Oreg. 11; S. Dak. 2; Utah 1; Va. 1
Cryptococcosis	Ark. 5; Calif. 1; Fla. 2; Ind. 1; Ky. 4; La. 1; Md. 4; Minn. 4; Miss. 1; Mo. 15; Ohio 1; Pa. 8; S.C. 2; S. Dak. 1; Va. 5
Nocardiosis	Ind. 7; Minn. 1; Mo. 12; Va. 2

Rickettsial Diseases

Q Fever	Ariz. 7; Calif. 10; Colo. 1; Iowa 2; Maine 5; Oreg. 4; Wash. 3; Wis. 1

Viral Diseases

Colorado Tick Fever	Calif. 6; Colo. 104; Idaho 7; Mont. 18; N. Mex. 1; Oreg. 1; S. Dak. 9; Utah 21; Wash. 1; Wyo. 2
Trachoma	Calif. 5; N. Mex. 6; Oreg. 1; Utah 1

Conditions included in this table are not officially notifiable to the Center for Disease Control but are reported *optionally* by some states. These data should be used with great caution and should in no way be considered a representative national sample. We have not included a summary of every optionally reported condition because of the limitations of space and infrequency of reports. Unpublished data will be made available to individuals on specific request.

NON-NOTIFIABLE CONDITIONS — Deaths from Selected Acute Conditions, United States, 1968–1977

(Numbers after cause of death are category numbers of the Eighth Revision of the International Classification of Disease, Adapted 1965)

CAUSE OF DEATH	ICDA	1977	1976	1975	1974	1973	1972*	1971	1970	1969	1968
Abortion											
Septic	640.0,641.0,642.0,643.0,644.0,645.0, 640.2,641.2,642.2,643.2,644.2,645.2	4	10	15	14	24	46	64	94	94	84
Non-septic	640.1,640.9,641.1,641.9, 642.1,642.3,642.9, 643.1,643.9,644.1,644.9, 645.1,645.9	16	6	12	13	12	24	35	42	38	49
Diabetes mellitus	250	32,989	34,508	35,230	37,329	38,208	38,674	38,256	38,324	38,541	38,352
Fungal infections											
Actinomycosis	113	12	11	9	9	8	10	12	18	15	16
Aspergillosis	117.3	112	66	63	50	55	42	32	38	36	28
Blastomycosis	116.1-116.2		2	2	1	—	—	3	3	2	—
Coccidioidomycosis	114	58	66	60	61	37	30	37	42	60	58
Cryptococcosis	116.0	134	123	131	122	125	136	119	112	117	96
Histoplasmosis	115	55	49	59	58	53	62	55	56	61	58
Moniliasis	112	237	244	215	190	173	138	159	153	114	112
Nocardiosis	117.8	18	36	24	37	20	22	13	27	24	26
Unspecified	117.9	60	63	37	61	54	42	43	35	45	36
Giardiasis	007.1	—	1	—	1	—	—	1	—	—	—
Herpes zoster	053	136	113	132	112	95	86	75	79	82	69
Hydatid disease	122	2	4	3	5	4	4	7	3	9	6
Meningitis, excluding meningococcal and tuberculous	320	1,526	1,589	1,630	1,539	1,523	1,482	1,553	1,701	1,719	1,707
Mononucleosis, infectious	075	13	18	11	24	25	18	22	19	21	14
Renal disease	400.3,403,581-584,590-595	22,140	22,584	22,304	23,536	24,651	25,856	26,019	27,197	28,199	28,921
Reye syndrome	347.9	2,650	2,317	2,266	2,388	2,071	1,872	1,741	1,654	1,484	1,423
Respiratory infections											
Bronchitis, acute	466	697	854	737	750	905	1,146	1,154	1,310	1,286	1,432
Influenza	470-474	1,304	7,877	4,277	2,201	5,131	4,986	1,504	3,707	5,971	7,062
Pneumonia (primary cause of death)	480-486	49,889	53,989	51,387	52,576	57,428	57,594	55,690	59,032	62,394	66,430
Upper respiratory infections, acute	460-465	368	384	342	377	453	504	522	574	621	784
Rheumatoid arthritis	712,718	1,396	1,343	1,311	1,356	1,402	1,292	1,304	1,291	1,302	1,418
Sepsis of childbirth	635,670	13	16	11	17	9	38	30	18	27	32
Streptococcal sore throat and scarlet fever	034	14	14	15	22	20	16	23	29	41	28
Toxoplasmosis	130.0,130.1,130.2,130.9	19	13	11	13	13	14	21	21	14	20

Source: National Center for Health Statistics, Vital Statistics of the United States, Vol. II, for respective year.

*Based on 50% sample of death records.

Index